THE MINDFULNESS MATTERS PROGRAM
FOR CHILDREN AND ADOLESCENTS

Also Available

Teaching Mindfulness Skills to Kids and Teens
Edited by Christopher Willard and Amy Saltzman

The Mindfulness Matters Program for Children and Adolescents

Strategies, Activities, and Techniques for Therapists and Teachers

Randye J. Semple
Christopher Willard

Foreword by Lisa Miller

THE GUILFORD PRESS
New York   London

Copyright © 2019 The Guilford Press
A Division of Guilford Publications, Inc.
370 Seventh Avenue, Suite 1200, New York, NY 10001
www.guilford.com

Printed in the United States of America

This book is printed on acid-free paper.

Last digit is print number: 9   8   7   6   5   4   3   2   1

The authors have checked with sources believed to be reliable in their efforts to provide
information that is complete and generally in accord with the standards of practice that are
accepted at the time of publication. However, in view of the possibility of human error or
changes in behavioral, mental health, or medical sciences, neither the authors, nor the editor and
publisher, nor any other party who has been involved in the preparation or publication of this
work warrants that the information contained herein is in every respect accurate or complete,
and they are not responsible for any errors or omissions or the results obtained from the use of
such information. Readers are encouraged to confirm the information contained in this book with
other sources.

Library of Congress Cataloging-in-Publication Data

Names: Semple, Randye J., author. | Willard, Christopher (Psychologist), author.
Title: The mindfulness matters program for children and adolescents : strategies, activities, and
    techniques for therapists and teachers / Randye J. Semple, Christopher Willard.
Description: New York : Guilford Press, [2019] | Includes bibliographical references and index.
Identifiers: LCCN 2019019325| ISBN 9781462539307 (pbk. : alk. paper) |
    ISBN 9781462539369 (hardcover : alk. paper)
Subjects: LCSH: Mindfulness (Psychology) | Meditation for children. | Meditation—
    Therapeutic use.
Classification: LCC BF637.M56 S46 2019 | DDC 158.1/2—dc23
LC record available at *https://lccn.loc.gov/2019019325*

Illustrations by Laila A. Madni.

About the Authors

Randye J. Semple, PhD, is a clinical psychologist and Associate Professor in the Department of Psychiatry and Behavioral Sciences at the University of Southern California (USC). She has authored over 40 scientific journal articles, book chapters, and other professional publications. Dr. Semple is Consulting Editor for *Spirituality in Clinical Practice* and serves on the steering committees for Mindful USC and the Center for Mindfulness Science, USC's mindfulness initiatives, and on the research committee of the American Mindfulness Research Association. She is the lead developer of mindfulness-based cognitive therapy for children (MBCT-C), an evidence-based group psychotherapy that is being researched and implemented worldwide. Dr. Semple presents and publishes widely and provides workshops, consulting, invited lectures, and other training opportunities. Her website is *https://sites.google.com/site/randyesemplephd*.

Christopher Willard, PsyD, is a clinical psychologist and educational consultant with a specialty in mindfulness. Based in Boston, he speaks on the topic of mindfulness and meditation with young people nationally and internationally, and teaches at Harvard Medical School. Dr. Willard is on the board of directors of the Institute for Meditation and Psychotherapy and is past president of the Mindfulness in Education Network. He has been practicing sitting meditation since 1999. Dr. Willard is coeditor of *Teaching Mindfulness Skills to Kids and Teens*, among other books. His website is *www.drchristopherwillard.com*.

Foreword

This book provides readers looking for ways to teach mindfulness to kids with an outstanding opportunity. It takes decades of direct experience to cultivate a deep understanding of how to deliver an intervention, how the process takes hold and transforms a young person's life, and how to harness state-of-the-art clinical science to tailor and focus an intervention. In 2002, Randye Semple launched the first systematic clinical trial on mindfulness with youth, and together with her colleagues showed that anxiety and depression could be ameliorated in children through group mindfulness interventions. Until the publication of her research, there were only studies showing how mindfulness could alleviate symptoms of psychopathology in adults. Dr. Semple opened a new field of clinical science by establishing that the benefits of mindfulness held equally true, sometimes even more robustly, for youth. Meanwhile, Christopher Willard was sharing mindfulness with hundreds of young people in schools, treatment centers, and community settings. Together, Semple and Willard have amassed over 30 years of experience introducing mindfulness to children and adolescents, through both clinical work and clinical science, both of which inform their approach to delivering mindfulness interventions. Their work addresses the unique needs of a range of different youths, across a broad set of disorders, environments, and developmental challenges.

How does all this condensed experience of the authors benefit the reader, a seeker of mindfulness work?

The exercises in this book clearly have been used over and over, tweaked and revised to stand as extensive, workable, and practical strategies for providers and teachers in youth settings. These practices are engaging and helpful to youth; they feel real and have a proven track record.

For a solo provider or teacher, particularly one who is "flying blind," there is plenty of clear, detailed, and practical help in these pages, where the positive end results of mindfulness, as well as the challenges to implementation, are clearly spelled out. Semple and Willard anticipate almost all of the questions and confrontations you may face from the youths themselves, as well as parents and professional colleagues, and they supply you with well-founded answers. The authors equally know what obstacles to expect in delivering these interventions to youth, who might resist, laugh at, and likely be unfamiliar with mindfulness. They have seen nearly all of this before and provide text to inform your responses. You never are alone in the room; the two authors are always by your side throughout the pages of this book.

Equally valuable, when you set up your mindfulness work, you may find enthusiasm, interest, and skepticism in equal measure from the community. Semple and Willard have engaged many youth systems, school districts, mental health centers, community organizations, and treatment facilities, so they have realistic advice to provide here too.

At the crossroads of clinical science and practice, the authors have identified pathways for working with youth populations facing specific developmental challenges, stresses or losses, or mental disorders, organizing the interventions around profiles of need. Programmatic options are derived from clinical science.

The text offers versatility to address the needs of specific groups, whether around low emotional quotient, impulsivity, or inoculation to socioecological stress. Nimble architecture here allows the clinical trials and meta-analyses that inform "best practices" to meet with the "nitty-gritty" delivery of mindfulness. In addition, the reader quickly discovers that mindfulness can be delivered in many ways through awareness exercises that focus on the body, emotion, thought, outward setting, or relationship.

Semple and Willard rightly empower teachers and providers to be themselves and to use their own judgment and acumen as they guide and share mindfulness techniques. These experienced authors know that most teachers and providers come to the work with lived wisdom, a sense of calling to the work, and inspiration to deliver it. A tightly prescriptive manual, by contrast, can effectively remove the teacher or provider from the work and expunge the wisdom and knowledge that could benefit youth. Herein mindfulness exercises are not delivered through a lockstep manual but are presented as a multifaceted resource from which you can select appropriate options, adapt the practices, and learn how to caringly share these with children and adolescents. The creative, at times almost playful, tone and nature of these exercises will speak to the heart of teachers, therapists, and counselors. In short, the text reads less like a DMV manual of instruction and is more akin to an NFL playbook of proven options to be used wisely by a coach. And just as a football coach ultimately relies on the players, this book implicitly views youth as curious knowers able to draw connections and serve as co-contributors.

Semple and Willard know how to establish new ground with institutions. Even if a school has never before used mindfulness, these exercises have a familiar, school-friendly quality. Often the exercises draw on materials that are customarily used in a classroom: found objects, classical art, and musical sounds. The authors often use catchy acronyms (such as CALM and HALT) to hold processes and sometimes engage students in paired listening exercises and the use of small toys as "breathing buddies." These closely resemble normative school lessons, but the lesson here is mindful awareness and attention. An added bonus for providers and teachers is that most of the practices cost nothing or need only a low level of funding.

If you are considering a foray into the implementation of mindfulness with youth, Semple and Willard can support you in a way that can be applied to the setting in which you work, is attuned to the needs of the kids with whom you work, and offers you the reassurance of having a constant colleague by your side.

Mindfulness interventions have burgeoned since the pioneering work of Semple and Willard. Ultimately the book makes mindfulness fun, credible, and well within reach of nearly any youth organization. Enjoy; you have a treat in store!

LISA MILLER, PhD
Department of Counseling and Clinical Psychology
Teachers College, Columbia University

Contents

PART I   **Introduction to the Mindfulness Matters Program**   1
for Children and Adolescents

PART II   **Mindfulness Activities**   15

GROUP 1 Introductory and Core Activities   17

GROUP 2 Mindfulness of the Breath Activities   29

GROUP 3 Mindfulness of the Body Activities   42

GROUP 4 Mindful Awareness Activities   65

GROUP 5 Sensory-Based Mindfulness Activities   84

GROUP 6 Mindfulness of Thoughts   115

GROUP 7 Mindfulness of Emotions   123

GROUP 8 Concluding Activities   185

PART III   **Pathways to Mindfulness**   193

Pathway through Stress and Anxiety   195

Pathway through Depression   201

Pathway through Attention Problems   211

Pathway through Problems of Emotion Regulation   221
and Impulse Control

Pathway through Trauma, Abuse, and Neglect   231

PART IV **Research Support for Mindfulness with Kids**   241

References   249

Index   256

Purchasers of this book can download and print the handouts
at *www.guilford.com/semple-forms* for personal use or use with clients
or students (see copyright page for details).

PART I

Introduction to the Mindfulness Matters Program for Children and Adolescents

Welcome to the *Mindfulness Matters* program, an adaptable, modular approach to teaching mindfulness to children and teens. This program is designed to be implemented in a variety of settings and schools, and for kids and teens ages 8–18 with a broad range of backgrounds and concerns, including mental health, learning, emotional, or behavioral issues with which they may be struggling.

Who Are We?

Randye and Chris are both licensed clinical psychologists. We are clinicians, educators, and researchers who are experienced at working with the youth populations for whom this book is intended. We both have our own long-standing mindfulness practices, which support our basic approach to teaching mindfulness. We have studied most of the popular or effective mindfulness programs in our search to build a user-friendly, practical, and versatile mindfulness resource for you and the unique kids with whom you work. And we have implemented all the activities we describe with kids of varying ages, from different backgrounds, with different needs, and in different settings. One thing we have discovered in our work as researcher-practitioners is that although dozens of excellent programs abound, a "one-size-fits-all" manual might well be impossible, especially when we work in so many diverse settings. So, the *Mindfulness Matters* program was developed with a clear focus on adaptability and flexibility of implementation.

What Is the Purpose of This Book?

Most of us live in worlds that are full of competing demands, never-ending challenges, and stress. These circumstances inevitably affect not only ourselves, but also the children and teens with whom we interact. One key purpose of the *Mindfulness Matters* activities is to teach, experientially, how paying attention in a particular way (i.e., intentionally, in the present moment, and without judgment), can change how we relate to ourselves and to our own experiences. Developing mindfulness helps kids (and ourselves) become more aware of both pleasant and unpleasant experiences that often slip by unnoticed or unappreciated. Bringing greater awareness to pleasant experiences often increases the wonderful richness of those experiences. Bringing greater awareness to unpleasant experiences can help us respond to our kids, and help our kids to respond to themselves and each other, with greater understanding and skill.

For both children and adolescents, learning to practice mindfulness is a powerful tool with which to develop essential social–emotional competencies. These competencies include the qualities of self-awareness, responsibility, personal initiative, planning and implementation of goal-directed behaviors, inhibition of inappropriate behaviors, conscious decision making, empathic communications, compassion for others, and interpersonal skills in conflict resolution. Children and adolescents who are socially and emotionally competent are more likely to be successful in a wide range of areas, including family and peer relationships, academics, sports, and other extracurricular activities (Mak, Whittingham, Cunnington, & Boyd, 2017). Furthermore, these skills lay the foundation for mindful self-management of emotions and behaviors throughout life.

Embedded in the practice of mindfulness are opportunities to observe feelings as they arise and tolerate them just as they are. As kids improve their ability to stay present with distressing and uncomfortable feelings, they are less inclined to react impulsively or hastily to emotional triggers. Tolerance and acceptance of distressing thoughts and emotions are cornerstones of our mindfulness and social–emotional literacy approach. Staying present with distress is a skill that lets us see where we are right now, and lets us see our choices—before we even begin to choose adaptive and constructive ways to respond. As the psychologist Carl Rogers (1961) once noted, "The curious paradox is that when I accept myself just as I am, then I can change" (p. 17). So we teach staying present long enough to see choices and recognize our freedoms. Trying vainly to control what happens to us is not freedom. Freedom is making conscious choices in how we respond to the events in our lives.

For Whom Was This Book Written?

This book was written for a few audiences: clinically trained mental health providers working in outpatient clinics, residential facilities, inpatient settings, and for those in the welfare and juvenile justice systems. It is also for those who are not clinically trained and who work with kids and teens in nonclinical environments such as schools, community recreation centers, or libraries. Parents who would like to bring mindfulness into the home and to work with their own children may also find this book helpful.

Because you are each working in different settings with different children who have different issues, we decided to base the structure of this book less on a traditional treatment manual or class curriculum format, and make it more like the "choose your own adventure" books that many of us may remember from childhood. Why? Because the developmental paths of childhood and certainly child- or adolescent-focused treatments are rarely as linear and predictable as the developmental theories that some of us learned in graduate school might suggest. The paths are unpredictable, take surprising twists and turns along the way, and often get stuck or end up in a different place than we might have expected. Developmental trajectories are often based not only on the genes and environment that were given to us, but also on the adventures that we choose, or that are chosen for us as, we grow and develop. As far as we know, there aren't any other mindfulness programs out there like this one, which made the writing and makes the reading of this book both challenging and somewhat unconventional.

How to Use This Book

The *Mindfulness Matters* program offers instruction and practice in the essential skill of being present with each moment of our lives. Over the course of the program, children and teens learn to bring intentional awareness to their thoughts, feelings, body sensations, speech, and behaviors as they move through their daily lives. We do encourage you to read this entire book cover to cover, soaking in all of the practices, theory, research, and rationales as you go. However, in the 21st-century lives of extremely busy teachers and clinicians, we understand that many folks might just read the introductory sections and then flip to the activities or the pathway that has the most relevance for their immediate needs. The book will work just fine if you choose to use it that way. It really is okay if you don't read the whole book! But by reading all of the material, you may develop a greater depth of understanding and be more comfortable with this approach, particularly if you are not already experienced with integrating mindfulness and positive psychology practices into your work with young people.

One benefit that we built into the *Mindfulness Matters* program is "guided and informed customization." Some lucky educators, clinicians, parents, and other professionals have unlimited time and no financial restraints; others have kids for a handful of 30-minute sessions every other week; still others are restricted to working in large classrooms with a wide variety of kids and what feels like too many educational demands on their time already. This variability makes a "one-size-fits-all" approach effectively impossible. For that reason, in Part II we offer detailed descriptions of conducting broadly applicable activities, along with suggested uses and adaptations to make depending on the age of the kids; your setting and time constraints, the unique stressors, and the developmental and diagnostic presentations in your group. We have included nearly 60 activities, presented in a similar format and structure, which generally follow the outline shown in Table I.1.

The first activities we describe teach basic settling and attending skills, which include mindful breathing, mindful body, and mindful movement activities. The next section provides kids with opportunities to become more observant and mindful of perceptual–sensory experiences that are often performed with little awareness such as mindful eating, seeing, and hearing. Through these activities, children learn to notice the differences between mindfully observing their moment-by-moment experiences and letting them pass by unnoticed. They experience what happens when they react emotionally or judgmentally versus responding with attention, thoughtfulness, and compassion. Later activities are designed to guide kids in applying these mindfulness skills to relate more adeptly to their own thoughts and emotions, while also cultivating and expanding their social–emotional awareness.

TABLE I.1. General Structure of Each Mindfulness Activity

Time Requirement
- Explains time required or recommended for the activity and the follow-up inquiry.
- Most activities aim to take from less than 5 minutes up to 30 minutes.

Themes

Themes include the focus and underlying goals of each activity.

Background

This narrative section goes into greater depth about the rationale and offers a brief description of the activity.

Materials Needed

This section describes any materials needed to conduct the activity.

Vocabulary for Grades K–3 and for Grades 4–8

Developmentally appropriate vocabulary helps children understand the practices and offers a way to reinforce the experience of mindfulness and related practices through shared language related to mindfulness, mental health, and social–emotional concepts, between and among kids and adults.

Mindfulness Activity
- This section includes instructions for conducting the activity.
- Many activities include sample scripts, sample dialogues, and examples of charts.

Challenges and Tips
- This section offers tips for overcoming challenges that may arise with a particular activity, both for the kids practicing and for the facilitator leading the activity.
- Some sections include sample responses from kids and how to work with them.

Suggested Practice Activities

Practice activities are recommendations for activities that kids can practice (in class and/or at home), and additional "homework" activities they can do related to the aim of that activity.

Additional Discussion Questions for Children/Teens
- This section includes a few general inquiry questions.
- Note that each pathway includes more specific, pathway-relevant discussion questions to promote insight for that particular group of children or teens.

Variations
- Variations of the activities are provided that can further deepen the children's practices and facilitate their engagement by using creative alternatives on the same theme.
- Some activities include age-appropriate adaptations.

In Part III, you can choose to work within one of five suggested "pathways" through the activities that we described in Part II. We begin with a brief introduction to the five pathways to mindfulness. Each pathway is focused on a specific problem area.

- Pathway through Stress and Anxiety
- Pathway through Depression
- Pathway through Attention Problems

- Pathway through Problems of Emotion Regulation and Impulsive Behaviors
- Pathway through Trauma, Abuse, and Neglect

Within each pathway, we emphasize certain aspects of mindfulness that might yield more clinical or educational benefits for addressing commonly seen problems. We offer tips for avoiding clinical complications and identify specific contraindications along the way. We describe adaptations for different settings and age groups. Nevertheless, you may wish to, or need to, do more customization with your treatment or with a specific group that is beyond our recommendations. This is perfectly okay. Ultimately, you will know your kids, classrooms, and each group's dynamics far better than we do, and we believe that you should trust your own experiences of mindfulness, using compassion and good judgment as your guide. Of course, knowing when you need to seek consultation is also an important component of good judgment.

Creating these pathways was one of the most enjoyable and yet most challenging aspects of writing this book. The *Mindfulness Matters* approach consists of core practices and parent-, teacher-, and clinician-friendly resources for adults to implement with children at home, in classrooms, and in clinics. Whereas there is abundant and growing research on the use of mindfulness practices with adults from a variety of clinical and nonclinical populations, high-quality research on children and teens is less advanced. Research with juveniles is harder to conduct than research with adults. In part, this is due to the unique challenges of obtaining institutional review board approval to conduct research with minors, particularly in the context of entire classrooms or schools. There are also design and logistic challenges of matching sample populations, recruiting, screening, and consenting participants, selecting control interventions and randomizing participants, and perhaps most challenging with kids and their parents, consistent scheduling. The assessment of mindfulness in children also has special challenges, which are beyond the scope of this book. For those who may be interested in this topic, we suggest several reviews that discuss issues associated with assessment of mindfulness in adults (Baer, Walsh, Lykins, & Didonna, 2009; Grossman, 2008) and in youth (Goodman, Madni, & Semple, 2017, 2019).

The research community has not yet begun to investigate the effectiveness of individual mindfulness activities for particular disorders, albeit programmatic research is progressing (Part IV offers an overview of current research on mindfulness with kids and teens). For that reason, the choice of specific activities for each pathway was informed by the small amount of available research in combination with our own experience, clinical training and judgment, review of the existing clinical literature, and consultation with other experienced clinicians, mindfulness researchers, and child development experts. For each of the five pathways, we consulted with experts who specialize in that problem area. We also consulted with clinicians who are knowledgeable about cultural translations of mindfulness.

Each pathway explanation follows a similar structure. We begin with an overview of the problem area or syndrome and indications that might suggest whether or not your group will be appropriate for that pathway. We examine the ways symptoms manifest uniquely in children at different developmental stages, and how the symptoms "look" behaviorally in school, at home, and in other contexts, as well as how a child might describe them. We explain the theoretical and research rationale underlying each pathway; discuss the particular challenges of working with each population, gaining buy-in and engagement, and dealing with common forms of resistance in sessions and out; and we provide tips for teaching and working with each population. Suggested inquiry and discussion questions along with a specific emphasis for each group are also covered. We highlight possible contraindications or significant adaptations that may need to be made with certain populations. We then lay out each pathway with a recommended sequence of activities:

- Introductory Activities
- Core Activities
- Intermediate Development Activities
- Advanced Deepening Activities
- Maintenance, Generalization, and Concluding Activities

Getting Started

Composing Your Group

If you are a classroom teacher, you likely have little or no flexibility regarding the size or composition of your group. We do suggest, however that you consider the specific issues or dynamics that may be present in your classroom. These may include the overall number of kids in your classroom, their ages, the gender ratio, the school environment (e.g., inner city, urban, or rural), and a wide variety of intellectual, emotional, or behavioral issues that may be present. The more individual attention a child or teen requires, the more important it will be to have a support person or co-facilitator in the room. If you are a clinician, you may have more flexibility in constructing your groups. In clinic settings, groups are generally smaller than in classrooms because the kids often need more individual attention. You may consider creating groups of similar ages (no more than 1–2 years apart), similar stages of development, or similar clinical diagnoses or problem areas. This selective grouping lets you provide more focused guidance than can occur in more heterogeneous groups. When the group is composed entirely of kids who require a high degree of individual attention (e.g., those with attention-deficit/hyperactivity disorder [ADHD] or conduct problems), we recommend keeping the group size small (no more than seven or eight kids) and, when possible, including another clinician as co-facilitator. Another factor to consider is if the kids already know each other or if they meeting for the first time. If the latter, you will probably need to spend more time on icebreaker activities to create a sense of safety and to cultivate cohesion in the group.

Group Logistics

We recognize that scheduling groups with children, especially in a school setting, always presents challenges. We have included an estimated amount of time needed for each activity, but not for each "session." A teacher may have only 10– 15 minutes to do one or two activities at a time, whereas a clinician or after-school program facilitator may have 45 or 50 minutes, and can complete four or five activities in one "sitting." Instead of thinking of the *Mindfulness Matters* program as a structured curriculum, we encourage you to be creative, while broadly following the basic structure of introduction, core activities, intermediate development activities, advanced deepening activities, and then the final maintenance, generalization, and concluding activities. How much time you spend in each area should fit into the logistics of the time and space you have available and the needs of the group with whom you are working. We encourage you to modify any of the activities or pathways necessary to meet the needs of your group members. When each level of practice has been suitably mastered, then move on to the next level. Many of the activities described in Part II include a number of variations for repeated practice, adaptations for different age groups, and suggested home practices that help the kids integrate mindfulness into their daily lives, outside of your group time with them.

Where to Conduct Your Group

A busy and loud school may not seem like the ideal environment in which to cultivate mindfulness, but we all have to work with what we've been given. If you can keep your environment relatively quiet and free of distractions, so much the better for learning anything, not just mindfulness. Elementary-age students do well sitting in a circle, either on chairs or on the floor using cushions or mats. Middle school kids might be better off seated in rows to reduce social distraction. When creating a seating arrangement for teens in high school, we recommend that you base seating decisions on the personalities and dynamics of the group. School desks or chairs are fine for sitting; you don't need any special mats or cushions, unless you would like to use them.

Basic Supplies

There are actually very few "essential" supplies needed to conduct the *Mindfulness Matters* program. When a particular activity requires additional materials, they are listed at the beginning of the activity. None of these are expensive—most are common household or classroom items that are free or readily accessible. A few activities will require some advance preparation. For example, the mindful drawing activities require drawing supplies and paper, and the activities involving mindfulness of smell require a few small jars and an assortment of scents. If you would like to seat your group on the floor rather than in chairs, providing small cushions or pillows is helpful. Yoga mats or bath towels can be used for activities such as the body scan, which can be done sitting up or lying down.

    The only item that we do recommend you purchase is a bell or chime of some sort. We use mindfulness bells to start and end each activity. Very quickly, the sound of the bell becomes an invitation to let go of whatever the mind might be occupied with and bring attention to whatever is happening in that moment. At the beginning of each group, we invite anyone who feels the desire to become more present in that moment to ring the bell for him- or herself. We also encourage participation by inviting individual group members to ring the bells to begin and end an activity. This can be a useful technique for engaging an unruly or disruptive child. Bells come in many different forms. Some readily accessible choices include chimes, rain sticks, a classic handheld or hanging bell, or a small percussion musical instrument, such as a triangle or xylophone. If you are working in a school, we recommend bells or chimes that do not denote any spiritual or religious significance.

Suggestions for Creating a Safer Space

We suggest that guidelines and "rules" be kept to a minimum to allow enthusiastic and creative mindfulness practices to flourish. The most important benefit to using guidelines is that they create a sense of physical and emotional safety for all and a positive environment conducive to learning. To that end, teaching a mindfulness class will probably have similar rules and expectations as other classes: students are to speak quietly and respectfully to you and their peers, to participate, and not to disrupt the group. However, even when in a mandatory classroom or therapy group, children should be still free to participate or not. We sometimes joke that as long as kids are not disruptive, they are welcome to daydream or plan their summer vacation while we practice—although they are less likely to get much out of the class if they do!

The main difference in a mindfulness class in contrast to a regular academic class is that the inquiries and discussions can get quite personal, which sometimes may feel strange or even unsafe, especially for vulnerable kids. Adult facilitators may feel out of their element if children begin to disclose deeply personal or disturbing information. Guidelines about not sharing what group members have talked about outside of the group might be in order, even when working in classroom settings. Occasional reminders that practices are "invitational," not mandatory, can also help. As kids get older, invite them to create guidelines for their group themselves—thereby increasing their sense of empowerment and ownership of the group and its norms. Of course, the exception to confidentiality involves our role as mandated reporters. Anything a child discloses to you that concerns his or her safety or well-being, or that of others, should always be followed up on with the appropriate staff at your school, or with child protective services as mandated in your state.

Safety and Risk Management

We know that not everyone reading and using this manual will be a mental health clinician. You may be a teacher, recreation worker, parent, or even a librarian who runs children's groups. If you do work with groups of clinically diagnosed kids (e.g., in a therapeutic school or in the juvenile justice system), we strongly recommend that you co-facilitate or work in close consultation with a mental health professional. Have a safety plan and contact information handy, particularly if you have concerns about any child or teen in your group. About one in five children have a diagnosable mental disorder (Merikangas et al., 2010). So, even as a mainstream classroom teacher, you are almost certain to have some kids who are struggling with depression, anxiety, or other emotional or behavioral problems.

You may find students opening up emotionally during the inquiry process. This probably means that you are doing a great job of creating a wholesome space in which kids feel emotionally safe enough to share. At the same time, particular settings or aspects of certain group dynamics may make the group a relatively unsafe space to share deep-rooted thoughts or fears, intense emotions, or past traumatic experiences. Kids may not always be the best judge of whether their secrets are safe in their peers' hands. We suggest talking about the importance of confidentiality at the initial session. Everyone in the group should agree that "what happens and is said in mindfulness class, stays in mindfulness class." Of course, as an adult professional who works with children, you most likely also have a duty to protect, and you probably are mandated to report abuse, neglect, or other safety issues. If you haven't worked with children in a while, we highly recommend you refresh your knowledge of your jurisdiction's requirements as they relate to minor children.

You may encounter children who are at risk of bullying or victimization from other kids, or alternatively those who may be bullying, aggressive, or threatening violence to others. You may learn about illicit alcohol or substance use (particularly with the older kids). You may also encounter kids who are at risk to themselves in terms of self-injurious behaviors or suicidal behaviors. These too should be dealt with according to your professional ethical standards, the protocols of your jurisdiction, the policies at your place of work, and the needs of the child. We have included a section on suicide risk management in the Pathway through Depression, and we strongly recommend you read this section even if the kids you work with don't appear to be depressed or suicidal.

Facilitating the Postactivity Inquiries and Discussions

To be an effective mindfulness facilitator, you need to embody mindfulness in the way that you present each activity and in how you guide the inquiries and respond to children during the discussions that follow. Just imagine trying to learn mindfulness from a tense, indifferent, frustrated, or burned-out teacher—it would be a less-than-ideal experience. Conveying an attitude of open curiosity and acceptance about child experiences will be more helpful than trying to provide explanations about their experiences. One way to facilitate curiosity and acceptance is to ask open-ended questions. It is also helpful to *invite* participation rather than calling on a specific child to respond and catching him or her off guard or unwilling to share. We model freedom to choose by inviting children to respond to our questions. This can sometimes be challenging for classroom teachers who are used to calling on children to elicit a single correct answer. We encourage you to practice taking off your "teacher hat" during the mindfulness activities, and also to share your own observations about the practice. Kids with language delays or English language learners can be given the freedom to write or brainstorm their ideas before having to share verbally. Moreover, not every response needs to be verbal or written. Communications can be powerful when conveyed through pictures, songs, or dance and other movements. The main purpose of the postactivity inquiries is to help kids connect their experiential wisdom to intellectual and practical understandings. The general structure of each inquiry follows three lines:

1. *"What was this experience like for you?"* Invite the kids to describe (without judging) the thoughts, emotions, and body sensations that they experienced during the activity. A feelings chart or vocabulary prompts might be helpful here too. We practice looking closely in order to better see what is actually happening inside us in each moment.
2. *"How was this experience different from what you normally do?"* We invite exploration of what might change when we bring mindful awareness to our activities. Often, the kids discover that the experience is richer, more interesting, more pleasant, or even less unpleasant than other, similar experiences.
3. *"How might you practice what you've just learned in everyday life?"* Throughout the program, we emphasize the "everydayness" of mindfulness practices. Learning and

practicing in the group will not be helpful unless the knowledge and skills are integrated into their daily lives.

After many of the activities described in Part II, we offer suggested questions and guidance for conducting the inquiry. Some general questions to consider after a practice include:

- "What did you notice? In your mind? In your emotions? In your body?"
- "What felt familiar or unfamiliar?"
- "What surprised you?"
- "What parts of the experience were pleasant, unpleasant, or neutral?"
- "How did you decide if you liked or didn't like something?"
- "What were you curious about?"
- "What did you learn?"
- "When might it be helpful to you to use that practice?"
- "What urges or impulses did you notice?"
- "What changed . . . before, during, and after the activity?"

You might also ask kids to describe or reflect on their experiences using Daniel Siegel and Tina Bryson's (2012) acronym SIFT: "What did you notice in Sensations, Images, Feelings and Thoughts?" (p. 105). You can also use the mindful SEAT acronym to elicit responses by asking, "What Sensations, Emotions, Awareness, and Thoughts were present during that activity?" Speak slowly and clearly, with warmth and confidence, as you guide the practices. If you are truly present, calm, and centered, and express nonjudgmental curiosity and interest, the kids will be right with you.

Home Practice

Social norms can help facilitate compliance with home practice, as it does for school homework. Asking at the start of each class for examples of when or how kids used or didn't use their skills encourages them to learn from peers who are practicing and experiencing benefits. You might seed your inquiry with guiding questions such as "Who used mindfulness skills to help with homework, with stress, or with managing emotions with your family or friends or during sports or other activities?" Initially, you might choose to ask kids to write down their experiences if they are feeling shy, and perhaps share a few anonymous responses with the rest of the class. As group members become more comfortable with each other, you can encourage them to share their favorite mindfulness practices with family members or friends, and then ask about their experiences of sharing mindfulness with others in their lives.

Gaining Buy-In from Kids and Teens

Teaching mindfulness may feel unfamiliar, and new facilitators often think "Where do I begin?" or "How will I get my students to engage and focus?" Remember, though, that this is the question of teachers from time immemorial, and we usually manage to get kids to sit still and learn subjects like history or math that may not be so exciting to them. Mindfulness is no different; it's just another new topic—new to both teachers and students, and one with which kids may not have any familiarity or understanding. For that reason, we suggest building on their current experiences and understandings by asking questions such as "When have you ever felt peaceful?" "What are the times when you feel the most present?" Conversely, you might ask about moments of "absent-mindedness" when they weren't present and missed out on something, forgot what they were reading or watching, or when something unexpected occurred. Questions like this help kids identify familiar experiences that, in turn, help them relate to concepts of mindfulness. With younger kids, mindfulness might be considered a superpower, and truly, staying calm in the face of frustrating, sad, triggering, or other emotional situations *is* a superpower. You might connect mindfulness with a child's existing passion for sports, music, arts, or socializing, exploring how mindfulness can make these activities more enjoyable, help the child to be more present with the experience, and even improve his or her skillfulness with that activity.

There are dozens of mindfulness role models in sports, pop culture, the arts, and even the business and political worlds. Movies such as *Kung Fu Panda* and *Avatar* feature characters that gain power and peace of mind through meditation. The Jedi Knights of *Star Wars* consistently preach mindfulness to each other, specifically as a way to foster compassion and restraint. Mindfulness is also totally Gucci (which, for those of us who aren't Gucci, means very cool, at least at the time of the writing of this book!). Celebrity meditators include Emma Watson, Kendrick Lamar, Jerry Seinfeld, Goldie Hawn, Miley Cyrus, Angelina Jolie, Richard Gere, Arnold Schwarzenegger, RZA and other members of the Wu-Tang Clan, and even Kourtney Kardashian. Mindfulness is seriously macho—it's being used to train police officers, first responders, and U.S. Army and Marine Corps personnel. Famous athletes such as Kobe Bryant, LeBron James, and Derek Jeter practice mindfulness. Entire sports teams are now incorporating mindfulness into their trainings. Examples include the Los Angeles Lakers, Chicago Bulls, and Seattle Seahawks. A simple Internet search, often accompanied by quotes about mindfulness or short videos featuring celebrities and potential role models, can offer motivation to engage in mindfulness practices.

Mindfulness can be presented as at least a partial solution to a particular problem or challenge, to improve attention or sleep, or to reduce stress and anxiety. Many kids of all ages are excited by the research and brain science of mindfulness. Still others can engage using a (half-serious) competitive approach. "Last year's class could do 15 whole minutes of silent breathing by the end of the year. There's no way you guys could do that . . . or could you?" Group projects can also engage kids in learning and sharing mindfulness with each other, not just sit and listen to us adults prattle on at them. These can include preparing an assembly for parents, doing a presentation to a class on the brain science of mindfulness, a group of senior students offering to lead mindfulness groups for the younger students, or the AV club creating videos to teach mindfulness.

You will almost inevitably face resistance from some proportion of your students when you teach mindfulness, but remember that this is true when teaching any topic. There are some basic tips for handling resistance that we are happy to share. First, we might examine our own role as we face resistance, in terms of the conditions we may be creating that lead to resistance. How much time have we spent building trust with these kids? Are we an insider or outsider? How can we gain their trust through other staff or through their peers? Next, are we pushing the kids too hard, or not hard enough? Resistance may come in the form of acting out, giggling, or being disruptive during the practice activities. Passive resistance may be present as well—like simply ignoring the practice instructions, or not showing up at all. As clinicians, we believe all behaviors mean something. Behaviors can even be diagnostic. What might the "resistant" behavior tell you about what the child really needs or is trying to get via that behavior? The acceptance of peers? To avoid something uncomfortable or challenging physically or emotionally? As the well-known psychologist Robert Leahy (2001) has suggested, there is no such thing as a resistant patient—only a therapist who doesn't get it. How can we help kids get their needs met in other ways, or maybe set those needs aside during the group? Can the "resistant" kid be engaged on some other level, perhaps as a timekeeper, bell ringer, or even as co-facilitator, if doing the practice feels too difficult at that moment?

Gaining Buy-In from Administrators and Organizations

Between the two of us, we've consulted in well over 100 schools, hospitals, clinics, and other institutions, with varying degrees of success and buy-in from the administrators and organizations. Based on our experiences and conversations with others, we've collected a few basic tips to help you gain organizational buy-in. Some degree of buy-in from parents, educators, administrators, and other stakeholders is necessary to work effectively and also to avoid feeling undermined by certain systems and organizational cultures. The first question many organizational representatives will ask (just like when engaging kids) is "What's in it for us?" We have learned that taking time to learn the issues and needs of that particular agency, school, or district is never wasted. Presenting generic or "canned" information that doesn't address the needs of that organization is rarely a good strategy.

People are influenced by facts. For that reason, we suggest including research on the effectiveness of mindfulness in improving classroom behaviors, academic performance, or mental health issues in your initial presentations. Up-to-date research (much of which is presented in Part IV of this book), particularly neuroscience research, certainly helps bolster your credibility. The American Mindfulness Research Association (AMRA) maintains an online library of research information on their website at *http://goamra.org*. People are also influenced by their own personal experiences, and so we always include at least one short mindfulness practice in all of our presentations. We often discuss the impact of stress and burnout on teachers and clinicians, as well as the effects it has on the academic performance and behaviors of the kids with whom they're working. You might ask your audience to imagine being with "un-stressed-out" kids—and the ways in which the absence of stress might positively influence their achievements and behaviors.

Common objections are generally related to the costs—in time and money—associated with bringing mindfulness training into a school or clinic. These costs can include the fees required to hire trained facilitators; the time and expense of training teachers or clinical staff; the cost of the necessary space and supplies; and what may be most important to address, the amount of time that the program takes when multiple other demands may already feel overwhelming for a time- and cash-strapped organization. There is no one "right" way to address these concerns, but we often suggest starting with something very short and simple—like inviting teachers to practice 3 minutes of mindful breathing with their kids at the beginning of each class for just 1 week and observing what might change.

We generally don't push a "hard sell" when offering an overview of mindfulness to schools; instead, we simply suggest that mindfulness could be one more tool for educators to use if it resonates with them. As an outsider to the organization, this is particularly important in winning over skeptical staff who may have already had dozens of "miracle programs" thrown at them over the years. Another challenge may arise when outside facilitators begin mindfulness work within a school or clinic, and there are already staff members doing this work. Your mere presence may trigger them to feel challenged or undermined. We strongly encourage you to seek out and partner with those staff members—to establish yourself as a supporter and collaborator, rather than as a competitor.

The Importance of Cultivating Your Own Practice

As a mindfulness facilitator, it is essential to remain mindfully aware of what's going on with the kids throughout the class—checking in with them and observing their body language, tone of voice, breath rate, and nonverbal cues to monitor their engagement and involvement. Our own authenticity is key as well; not promising what mindfulness may deliver to the kids, only suggesting possibilities; embodying mindfulness ourselves through our choice of words, our attitudes, and our presence; and showing the kids we have no hidden motives.

Our own practice is key to all of this; when we practice cultivating presence, nonreactivity, and nonjudgment, we model the qualities that mindfulness fosters. We also model mindfulness as a means of embodying and expressing our authentic selves. Mindfulness is not about raising expectations; on the contrary, it's about removing expectations altogether and learning to accept ourselves and our lives just as they are. It's about freeing ourselves from the tyranny of our own thoughts and emotions, which in turn frees us to live a more fulfilling life.

What's more, mindfulness and compassion, as is the case for other mood states, appear to be contagious. This supports our belief that the best way to teach mindfulness is to *practice* mindfulness. As noted earlier, imagine trying to teach mindfulness to kids when you are tense and stressed out, or trying to learn mindfulness from a tense and anxious teacher. It's not a pretty sight! When we cultivate our own practice, we also teach from our personal experiences. We can speak to the challenges and successes that we ourselves have discovered. Depending on your relationship with the kids and your own personal level of comfort, you may wish to be more or less explicit about your personal experiences of mindfulness. In any case, it is our own practice that helps us maintain emotional equanimity, to be nonreactive in response to kids who are expressing their own distress, to be compassionate in the face of resistance, to be flexible and adaptable when the unexpected inevitably arises, and to be as fully present as we can be—for the benefit of the kids we serve.

PART II
Mindfulness Activities

In Part II, you will find comprehensive instructions for conducting a wide variety of mindfulness activities. These generally follow the same structure. An approximate time required to conduct each activity is noted, followed by background information for the facilitator and themes to guide the group discussions. When relevant, we describe the materials needed and provide vocabulary definitions. Many of the activities include sample scripts or charts that support the discussions, additional discussion questions, potential challenges and tips for addressing them, and suggested variations and other practice activities. Some of these additional practice activities are intended for in-session or classroom practice, and others can be assigned as home practices.

We have grouped the activities in Part II into eight groups. These groups are helpful when selecting specific activities within a chosen pathway (see Part III). The groups are:

- Introductory and Core Activities
- Mindfulness of the Breath Activities
- Mindfulness of the Body Activities
- Mindful Awareness Activities
- Sensory-Based Mindfulness Activities
- Mindfulness of Thoughts
- Mindfulness of Emotions
- Concluding Activities

Introductory and Core Activities

Introductory practices are written to be simple enough for children to enjoy successful experiences and engaging enough for children and teens to want more. The intention for this group of activities is to engage and interest kids enough that they have a positive (or, at least, not a negative) experience. We hope this initial exposure will leave them wanting to learn the basic principles of mindfulness and to engage in more practices. Your group can move on to the next set of activities once the kids have demonstrated mastery of these basics.

Activity 1. Introduction to Mindfulness

Background

The whole idea of cultivating mindfulness and living with mindfulness may be new to many children. For that reason, throughout the program, but especially during the initial sessions, it can be helpful to reinforce a few important points.

- Mindfulness is simply attention—unbiased, nonjudgmental attention to present-moment experiences. Kids with mental health or learning issues might respond better to the word *awareness* than to *attention,* but most would probably like to learn how to pay better attention.
- Mindfulness can be cultivated with practice and patience, just like any other skill, such as sports or academic proficiencies.
- When the mind wanders into the past or to the future, the emotional response is often one of unhappiness.
- When the mind is judging or criticizing the present moment, the emotional response is often one of unhappiness.
- When the mind wants the present moment to be different from what it actually is, the emotional response is often one of unhappiness.
- Mindfulness can help manage all this unhappiness. We do this by bringing our awareness to what is actually happening in our Sensations, Emotions, Actions, and Thoughts

17

(getting in our "SEAT"), and to the events going on around us—right here, right now. Simply noticing the wanderings of the mind. Noticing the judgments. Noticing the wanting. Then refocusing our attention to describe what *is* happening, rather than what we think *should be* happening, with openness, acceptance, curiosity, and delight.

- We cannot control our thoughts, and we frequently can't control what goes on around us, but we always have choices in how to respond—rather than react—to those thoughts and events.

- Choices live only in the present moment. We can think about choices we have made in the past. We can think about and plan to make a choice in the future. But the only time that we can actually make a choice is in the present moment. When we are paying attention to the present moment, we can better see just how our past- and future-oriented thoughts affect our emotions, and how our emotions affect our choices. We often discover that our own thoughts, judgments, beliefs, desires, and expectations influence many of the choices we make.

- We don't need to be pushed around by our thoughts and emotions. Even when strong thoughts and emotions trick us into believing that we have no choices at all, we can still remember that we *do* have choices. Seeing clearly, we may see more choices than we thought we had. And when we do, we tend to make better choices—and better choices usually mean better outcomes and less unhappiness.

Vocabulary for Grades 4–8

Mindfulness means giving our attention to whatever is happening in the present moment, with curiosity, openness, and acceptance, whether or not we happen to like it.

Vocabulary for Grades K–3

Mindfulness means paying attention to what is going on right now.

Introduction to Mindfulness

Mindfulness must be introduced to children in developmentally appropriate language, and illustrated with concrete examples. The following is a sample script for introducing mindfulness. We encourage you not to read it aloud verbatim. Rather, read this script first to yourself (and other sample scripts that we provide) a few times, then communicate the concepts in your own voice—using your own words. You may not address all these points in the first sessions, but it is helpful to use creative repetition and reaffirm these ideas on a regular basis.

"Sometimes, our minds wander into the past—thinking about things that have already happened. Wondering why we (or someone else) said '_____' or acted in a certain way. Sometimes we spend time feeling sad and regretting our own behaviors. Sometimes we are angry about something someone else said. At other times, our minds might wander into the future, worrying about what might happen if _____, or maybe planning how to respond if someone says '_____' to us.

"Our minds are often in a completely different place than our bodies, remembering the movie we saw last Saturday at our friend's house, or thinking about the class field trip that is coming up. We might be reliving the exam we took this morning, reviewing every question over and over again in our heads. We might be planning exactly how to ask our parents for a bigger allowance, or figuring out what to say to a friend that you forgot to invite to your party. In fact, most of the time, our minds are wandering all over the place.

"Sometimes, we can be on complete on *automatic pilot* or *autopilot* for short. On an airplane, the pilots can turn on the autopilot feature to let the plane fly itself, and they hardly pay attention any more. Our brains and bodies can go on autopilot too, often without us noticing. So, *autopilot* is when we do things without our minds being present at all. Have you ever walked down the hall at school and right past your classroom door because your mind was a million miles away? Or gone to school 'absent-mindedly' with your shirt buttoned wrong—and never even noticed until your best friend laughed? How many times are we so 'lost in thought' that we don't even hear someone talking to us? What about reading a book or watching a show and then realizing a few minutes had gone by— and we have no memory of what we just saw or read? The mind loves to wander, which is actually a bit odd, because all this wandering doesn't seem to make us any happier. When the mind is in the past, we can sometimes feel sad, or upset, angry, remorseful, guilty, or even ashamed. When the mind is in the future, we might feel worried or anxious, fearful, frustrated, or scared. Where the mind seems to spend the least amount of time is in the present moment—right here and right now. When the mind does come back and hang out in the same time and the same place as the body, we may discover that the present is actually a pretty interesting place—and there is lots more going on than we ever imagined.

"Mindfulness is a way of learning to bring our minds back to what is happening right here, right now, in the present moment. When we do that, we might discover new and exciting things that we would never have seen . . . or heard . . . or tasted . . . smelled . . . or touched. We might discover that in the present moment, there isn't a lot of sadness about things that have already happened (that we can't do anything about), and there aren't as many worries about things that haven't yet happened (and may never happen). In fact, the present can be a pretty nice place for the mind and the body to hang out together.

"A big part of mindfulness practice is being kind to ourselves. We practice each of the mindfulness activities in class [or in session] and at home as best we can. With awareness, we see that training the mind is a little like training a bouncy puppy who is always running around. When our puppy minds wander off, we don't need to get mad or down on ourselves. Instead, we just notice that the mind has wandered, and then with kindness for ourselves, we bring our attention back to where we choose to place it. If you train a puppy by being mean to it, you probably end up with a mean puppy. If you train it by being kind, well, just like your mind, you end up with a kind puppy.

"Another key part of mindfulness practice is patience. In order to learn to ride a bicycle, we must first learn how to get on the bicycle. We need to learn how to pedal and brake, how to steer the bicycle, and how to balance. When we begin, all this can seem very complicated with many things to remember at once. We might even fall off a few times. But then we learn to ride . . . slowly and carefully at first, but with practice and patience, we begin to see changes. In the same way, we ask you to practice the mindfulness activities in class [or in session] and at home with patience—even if you do not see changes right away."

Activity 2. What Does Mindfulness Mean to Me? (Part I)*

Time Requirement

15–20 minutes.

Themes

- What is mindfulness?
- What does *mindfulness* mean to each of us?
- How is practicing mindfulness different from what we do every day?

Background

Growing mindfulness is like growing a plant. We plant the seeds, provide food, water, and sunlight, and then we wait. Given the right conditions, the seeds will gradually emerge and grow. As we wait, we practice growing our mindfulness by bringing awareness to ordinary, everyday activities. We form the intention to bring more mindful awareness into our lives, and we practice giving mindful attention to what we think, feel, say, and do. Then our mindfulness grows and blossoms like a garden.

When we practice mindfulness, we practice being more aware and awake. Mindfulness is a different kind of awareness than we might be used to. It is focused on what is happening right here and right now. We practice simply looking at, rather than judging, our experiences. We can practice bringing mindful awareness to everything we do, and doing so can get interesting and fun. We might learn some new things about our world and ourselves that we thought we knew so well. We can be adventurous explorers making wonderful new discoveries—right here, in the rich and diverse "nowscape" of our lives.

Materials Needed

- Drawing paper.
- Colored pencils, markers, or crayons.

Vocabulary for Grades 4–8

- *Mindfulness* means paying attention, with openness and curiosity, to whatever is happening right now (even if we don't like it).
- *Judging* means deciding if something is good or bad; often it means being critical about what is happening.
- *Observing* means watching carefully and noticing what is happening, without being critical or making judgments about it.

---

*Part II of this activity is in Group 8, Activity 55 (pp. 185–187).

Vocabulary for Grades K–3

- *Mindfulness* means paying attention to what is going on.
- *Judging* means deciding that you like or don't like something.
- *Observing* means watching what's going on.

Mindfulness Activity

During this activity, each child is invited to create a drawing—using any shapes, colors, images, or words he or she wishes—to express what mindfulness means to him or her. Instructions for this activity are simple: "Draw whatever mindfulness means to you." Allow 10–15 minutes, encouraging children to stop every few minutes to check in with their own thoughts and feelings about mindfulness, and then give their mindful attention to creating the drawing. The aim of this drawing activity is to give each child an opportunity to express a personal meaning about mindfulness in a way that doesn't require verbal fluency. Some children might feel a bit self-conscious about their drawing skills, so it can be helpful to emphasize that there is no "right" or "wrong" way to draw mindfulness, and the quality of the drawing is not important.

Additional Discussion Questions for Children/Teens

Afterward, children can be invited (not instructed) to show the others in the group their new drawing and describe what mindfulness means to them. Focus on descriptions of the drawings and on the children's experiences of drawing with mindful awareness. We suggest that you avoid calling on a specific child *and* avoid judging the quality of the drawings, either with praise or with criticism. Rather, express interest using encouraging, objective comments, while praising the child's intent and effort. For example, "Wow, that's quite a detailed picture of what's happening in your brain. Can you tell me more about what [some element of the drawing] means to you?" We model nonjudgmental acceptance with our own choice of words, tone of voice, and empathic attunement with each child. Convey openness and interest by eliciting descriptive adjectives of the drawing. Asking about specific elements in a drawing may help shy children express themselves, but no one should ever be required to speak. The child's awareness and mindful engagement in the activity are the focus, not the product of his or her efforts. If the child seems comfortable with this, you might include questions that elicit thoughts and feelings along with the nonjudgmental description of the drawing.

Challenges and Tips

Some children may disparage their own drawings or compare them negatively to others' drawings. Critical self-judgments have become habitual for some children. The challenge of avoiding self-judgments can be normalized—perhaps with a gentle observation that the drawing and the child's thoughts about the drawing are not the same. Without minimizing the doubts expressed by the child, the self-criticisms can be framed as being more thoughts about which he or she can practice being aware. Likewise, kids criticizing the drawings of others should be gently, but firmly, discouraged.

Suggested Practice Activities

For example, you might say something like the following:

- "Take your drawing home. Describe the drawing and explain to your parents, brother, or sister what mindfulness means to you."
- "Invite a friend or a sibling to practice mindfulness with you by creating another drawing together. You might each draw one element, going back and forth, or alternately, draw for 30 seconds each, or create your shared image using different colors. Work together without talking at all, creating a shared image of what mindfulness means to two of you."

Activity 3. A Cup of Mindfulness

Time Requirement

10–15 minutes.

Themes

- We live much of our lives on autopilot.
- Mindfulness can be cultivated.

Background

This activity provides an excellent introduction to the concept that mindfulness can be cultivated like a plant, and with practice, it can improve and increase. Some children come to a mindfulness group believing that they are already as mindful as they can possibly be. We feel it's important to discuss this point at the beginning, not from an intellectual perspective, but rather from an experiential one. You might start by sharing one of your own personal experiences of *not* being mindful, and then invite each child to offer one of his or her own personal experiences. This approach conveys that no one is expected to always be mindful and validates "absent-minded" experiences as being normal and expected. Some examples might include:

- Walking right past a door you intended to enter because your mind was a thousand miles away.
- Going to another room to get something and then forgetting what you went to get.
- Eating an entire bag of chips while watching television and only becoming aware of it when the whole bag is empty.
- Not noticing that you put on two different shoes because your mind was occupied elsewhere.
- Reading a few pages of a book and then realizing you have no idea what you just read.
- Watching a show and realizing your mind had wandered for the past few minutes.
- Spacing out during a sports game.
- Playing a video game on autopilot.

- Absent-mindedly putting the box of cereal in the refrigerator instead of in the cabinet.
- Being lost in thought while walking to school, and when you get there, realizing that you can't remember the walk at all.
- Not noticing something that you see every day (e.g., the colors on the flowers of the bush outside your door, or how many windows there are in your classroom).

Materials Needed

- Three small plastic or Styrofoam cups; glass and paper cups are not recommended.
- Water.

Mindfulness Activity

Mindfulness in a Cup is an introductory activity that lets children experience shifts in mindful attention as we place increasing demands on their attentional skills. Children and the facilitator sit close together in a circle, so that each person can easily reach the hand of the person on either side. Group members generally sit cross-legged on the floor or on small cushions.

Fill three small cups about half full with water. Explain that this activity is to provide an experience of what it's like to gradually increase mindful attention, and that it is helpful to learn through contrasting experiences. Encourage children to give their full attention to each task. This is a mindfulness activity that is done in silence, so children should be reminded not to talk until all the tasks are completed.

The activity involves three tasks. The first is for each child to simply pass each half-full cup of water to the next child, while being careful not to spill any water. Not spilling water when the cup is only half full is not difficult and does not demand a high level of attention. All three cups are passed all the way around the circle. Using three cups provides sufficient engagement that the children won't be bored waiting for a cup to come around the circle.

After the cups have been passed once around the circle, stop them, and then fill each one almost to the brim with water. The second task is to pass these three completely filled cups of water around the circle again. Handing the cup to the next child without spilling any water now demands more mindful attention. We must pay greater attention to our own movements and the movements of the person sitting next to us. We also need to communicate and coordinate our movements using our eyes, ears, and sense of touch, but without speaking to the other person.

The final task is to pass the completely full cups of water around the circle for the second time. The difference this time is that the window shades should first be closed and the room lights turned off. Darken the room as much as possible. Alternatively, if you and the kids would be comfortable doing this, ask the children to close their eyes and keep them closed for the rest of this activity, or put a scarf or mask over their eyes. In the absence of vision, attention to our other senses increases. As the task demand increases, so does mindful awareness of the small nuances and fine details of the task. It rarely happens, but if a little water happens to get spilled? Well, a little water never actually hurt anyone.

After all three parts of this activity are complete, guide a discussion by eliciting descriptions of the thoughts, feelings, and body sensations experienced, and exploring how these

might have changed with each task. Children can discuss their felt experiences as the growing challenges of each round demanded an increase in mindful attention. Explore ways in
which cultivating greater mindfulness might be helpful to them in everyday life.

Variation for Older Kids and Teens

The difficulty of the third (eyes closed) task can be increased by using three cups of different
colors and asking them to also remember what color cup they are holding. Several times as
the cups travel the circle, pause, and then ask each person holding a cup to name the color
of that cup.

Challenges and Tips

When working with children who have a high level of anxiety about spilling the water, it can
be helpful during the postactivity discussion to first validate and normalize the experience of
anxiety, and then nonjudgmentally explore the child's anxious thoughts and how they relate
to his or her emotions and body sensations. You might also ask the children who endorse feeling anxious how they knew that they were anxious; that is, where and how in their bodies did
they experience that emotion, and what words would they like to use to describe that anxiety
(e.g., *worried, nervous, scared*)?

Suggested Practice Activities

- Open by generating a list of brief, everyday activities that are often done with little mindful
  awareness. The list of "autopilot activities" may include things like brushing teeth, combing
  hair, showering, getting dressed, or walking to school. Daily chores might include setting
  the table, washing dishes, or taking out the trash.
- Tell the children to select one activity that they do every day and commit to doing it, as
  best they can, with mindful awareness for 5 days. Explain: "Each day, briefly describe in
  your mindfulness journal the thoughts, feelings, and body sensations that you experienced
  during the activity." To enhance the intentional quality of awareness, kids might play with
  doing these tasks with their nondominant hand. In either case, the children are asked to
  observe ways in which the experience might have changed over the course of the week.

Activity 4. Listening to Silence

Time Requirement

1 minute.

Background

Children often enjoy ringing the bells of mindfulness themselves. The sound of the bells
creates a lovely reminder to stop, check in with ourselves, and take a few mindful breaths.

We encourage children to ring the bells whenever they themselves feel the need for this reminder. In addition to listening to the sounds, we invite them to listen to the silence in between the sounds.

Materials Needed

Bells of mindfulness: These may be chimes, a clapper bell, a singing bowl, a small gong, or small *tingsha* cymbals.

Mindfulness Activity

This activity takes only a moment and can be repeated several times. This simple activity unfailingly engages the interest of children. You can experience an almost palpable awareness of the concentrated listening energy in the room. Brief moments like this may have a larger impact than we might expect, as they add up. And we have many opportunities each day to practice mindful awareness of whatever is present—whether sounds or silence. We don't need much sensory stimulation to practice mindful listening. Small moments are all that's necessary.

Open by inviting the children to form an intention to be mindful, as best they can, of the sounds of the bells and the silence between the sounds. Ring the bells of mindfulness one time, listening carefully until the sound fades away. Then listen to silence for a few moments. Now ring the bell twice more, each time with a long space of silence in between.

Variations

You can explore using different bells, ringing them at different volumes, and moving them in different ways to bring more attention to them. You might even ring two bells at once, inviting the children to notice the sounds of both bells, as well each individual bell, as they shift their attention.

Additional Discussion Questions for Children/Teens

You might invite children to describe the experience of listening to silence. Alternatively, you may choose to return to the previous activity without further discussion.

Challenges and Tips

Whether in the classroom or a clinic setting, we prefer that you do not use the bells as a way to "quiet down" or discipline children if they become noisy or unruly. Mindfulness is about choice and self-empowerment, not coercing children into silence. We do let them know that the bells are available as a reminder to bring mindfulness to what is happening in that moment. We offer children many opportunities to ring the bells. In particular, if any child personally feels the need for a reminder to practice mindfulness, he or she is permitted to ring the bells at any time. In our experience, children do not abuse this privilege.

Activity 5. Taking a Mindful Posture

In the formal practice of mindfulness, we first form an intention (as best we can) to bring our awareness to the present moment. We can express this intention by taking a mindful posture. Help the children settle into a comfortable sitting position, either on a straight-backed chair or on a mat or a cushion on the floor. If a child uses a chair, it can be helpful to instruct him or her to sit without leaning into the back of the chair, so that the spine is self-supporting and both feet are firmly on the floor, with the body balanced stably like a tripod or three-legged stool. With the legs uncrossed, invite the children to place both of their feet flat on the floor about hip-width apart. If children sit on the floor cross-legged, they may be more comfortable if both knees touch the ground. Adjust the height of the cushion until the child feels comfortable and firmly supported. Invite each child to sit in an upright and comfortable position, not rigid or stiff, with the spine straight. Whether sitting in a chair or on a cushion, the hands should be resting loosely, separately, and comfortably in the lap. To help straighten the spine, the chin can be tucked slightly inward. You might suggest that the children imagine that their heads are like balloons that are gently floating up toward the sky, or that they are sitting tall like or a king or queen on their throne, or sitting tall and still like a mountain, or imagining a string holding them upright from the crown of their heads. This is "taking a mindful posture."

Invite the children to gently close their eyes, but only if they wish to do so. It is important to let them know that this is optional, because some children may not be comfortable closing their eyes. This point can be particularly relevant when working with children who have experienced trauma or those who have significant anxiety. You may offer them the alternative of softly gazing (unfocused attention) upon a space about 3 feet in front of them on the floor or at the desk in front of them.

As breathing and mindfulness practices become more prolonged, some children may find themselves getting sleepy. This is perfectly okay! Getting drowsy or spacing out is completely normal and nothing to worry about. At times, the mind may feel like it's trapped in a thick fog. When this happens, it is difficult to maintain awareness, alertness, and the ability to focus. You may see this fogginess often with teens, who are frequently short on sleep. One way to spot when a child or teen might be falling asleep is to observe if his or her head begins making small, downward bobbing motions. At these times, it can be helpful to invite the child or teen to open his or her eyes halfway and let in some light. This is perfectly okay too. In some contemplative traditions, all the practices are done with eyes half or fully open for the entire duration of the practice. Correcting a slumping posture by suggesting that the child or teen sit up a little straighter can help maintain alertness too. Invite the children to experiment to see what works for them, while continuing to focus attention on the breath or body, or whatever the focus of that mindful awareness activity might be.

To counter extreme sleepiness, taking a few minutes to quietly practice mindful walking or another gentle movement activity can be helpful. Getting more sleep certainly wouldn't hurt either. Ironically, one of the first benefits of mindfulness practices that many people report is sleeping better. Mindfulness may allow intrusive, disturbing, or stressful thoughts or physical tension in the body to be released more easily, which facilitates the relaxation needed for sleep to arise more naturally. And better sleep, of course, helps with stress, anxiety, depression, cognitive functioning, and impulse control.

Activity 6. Taking a Mindful SEAT

Time Requirement

5 minutes.

Themes

- Sitting in a mindful posture.
- Checking in with our experience in the present moment.

Background

The mindful SEAT: Sensations, Emotions, Actions, and Thoughts.

Materials Needed

None.

Vocabulary

For kids of all ages: We are introducing the notion of making contact with what is happening in the present moment.

Mindfulness Activity

We often may find our thoughts racing back to the past and forward to the future, feel overwhelmed by our emotions, or be distracted by perceptions and sensations. What's more, it is often our sense perceptions and body sensations that lead to emotions and thoughts. We can learn to find these first in the body and then to respond to them in different ways. So, we begin by taking a SEAT in a mindful, upright posture.

S Is for Sensations

"Start by checking in with your body. What sensations are you noticing right now? Now set aside awareness of those sensations and turn your attention to. . . . "

E Is for Emotions

"What emotions are present in this very moment? Now set aside awareness of those emotions and turn your attention to. . . . "

A Is for Actions

"What do you feel like doing in this moment? Do you feel any urges or impulses to take action? Now set aside awareness of those actions and impulses and turn your attention to. . . . "

T Is for Thoughts

"What thoughts are present in this moment? Now set aside awareness of those thoughts and turn your attention to whatever is happening in this moment."

Challenges and Tips

Children might want to write down for themselves or share aloud what happens when they take their mindful SEAT. The mindful SEAT can also be an inquiry process, to ask kids how they feel about each letter of the acronym after this mindfulness activity.

Suggested Practice Activities

Encourage kids to take a mindful SEAT during transition times or at potentially triggering moments during the day—really, at any time in their lives. It can be as simple as identifying a mundane if uncomfortable moment:

> **Sensation:** *I feel itchy.*
> **Emotion:** *I hate mosquito bites!*
> **Action:** *I want to scratch it!*
> **Thought:** *Why do mosquitos bite me more than everyone else?*

This check-in would be more nuanced and complex, of course, with more challenging emotions and actions such as aggression, avoidance, self-harm, and other unhelpful emotions or behaviors.

Mindfulness of the Breath Activities

Group 2 activities include a number of simple and introductory practices focused on mindfulness of breath. The goal of these activities is for children to become aware of the breath and to learn how to comfortably focus on the breath in engaging and useful ways. A strong emphasis is placed on not having to breathe "perfectly" and on stepping away from self-judgment in the process. Children and teens might also become increasingly aware of their moods and emotions before, during, and after each mindful breathing practice.

Activity 7. Mindfulness of the Breath

Time Requirement

For initial introduction to mindfulness, 10–15 minutes; with repeated practice, 3–5 minutes.

Themes

- Introduce mindfulness of the breath.
- Explain how practicing mindfulness is different from what we do every day.

Background

We believe that mindfulness is cultivated primarily by *practicing* it. Each activity is taught in such a way that kids first experience the activity and then describe their experience. The goal is to cultivate experiential knowledge first and develop an intellectual understanding afterward. Keeping this approach in mind, explanations of each activity should be kept very brief. It is better to say too little than too much, especially when talking to kids!

Breathing is a particularly valuable activity with which to develop mindfulness because it is rarely done with mindful awareness. Our breath is always with us—we need only consciously direct our attention to it. This seemingly simple activity also helps children understand how challenging it can be to be fully mindful and aware. Children gain first-hand, experiential knowledge of how frequently thoughts and emotions can distract them from bringing present-focused awareness to this moment. This experience is an essential first step in helping children understand the concept of mindfulness. Mindful breathing practice offers children direct exposure to a new way of relating to their experiences, and provides an opportunity to contrast it with their usual autopilot way of doing things. The first lesson learned by most of us is that the mind is like a monkey, or even feeling like the mind seems to have a mind of its own. With the best intention in the world, we sit down to watch our breath and the next thing we know, we are off daydreaming somewhere in a different time or miles away. But each wandering of the mind is less a problem than it is an opportunity to train our attention and practice being kind to ourselves as we guide our attention back to the breath, rather like gently training a pet. Cultivating mindfulness of the breath is a core skill, which, like all skills, develops with patience and practice.

Materials Needed

- One firm cushion or chair per child.
- Activity handout: *Mindfulness of the Breath.**

Vocabulary for Grades 4–8

- *Mindfulness* means paying attention to things as they occur in any given moment, however they are, rather than as we want them to be (Williams, Teasdale, Segal, & Kabat-Zinn, 2007).
- *Autopilot* means being in a state of mind in which we act without awareness of what we're doing.

Vocabulary for Grades K–3

- *Mindfulness* means paying attention as best you can.
- *Autopilot* means acting, feeling, or thinking without paying attention to what's really going on.

Mindfulness Activity

Invite the children to take a mindful posture and gently close their eyes, but only if they wish to do so. It is important to let them know that this is optional, because some children may be not be comfortable sitting in a group with their eyes closed. You may invite them to take "a soft [unfocused] gaze," looking about 3 feet in front of them on the floor or at the desk in front of them.

> "Let's begin by bringing your awareness to the sensations of touch in your body where it meets the floor, cushion, or whatever you are sitting on. Taking a moment to feel where

---

*All activity handouts are at the ends of groups.

your legs or feet touch the floor. Feeling yourself connected with the ground, sitting like a mountain, strong and still. Then, when you're ready, shifting your attention to your breath. Bringing your awareness to each of the sensations in the belly as you breathe in and out. It may be helpful to place your hand on your lower belly to become aware of the changing sensations where the hand touches the belly. Afterward, you may remove your hand and continue to focus on the sensations of breathing. Focus your awareness on the sensations in your body as the belly rises with each inbreath, and as the belly falls with each outbreath. As best you can, following the changing sensations down into the belly, as the breath enters on the inbreath, and as the breath leaves on the outbreath. Noticing the slight pauses between the inbreath and the outbreath.

"There is no need to try to control the breathing in any way—allow the breath to breathe itself. A good way to think of it is taking the kind of breath you would if you were sleeping. Not really big breaths and not really short breaths, but just the kind of breath you would take if you weren't paying attention to it. Except that now, we are practicing paying attention. If one breath is long and another short, that's totally okay. With mindfulness, we practice just noticing what is already there. The breath may be long or short, rough or smooth, loud or soft, cool or warm, just noticing all of these.

"Sooner or later, the mind will wander away from the focus on the breath in the lower belly to thoughts or daydreams. This is perfectly okay. This is simply what minds do. It is not a mistake. It doesn't mean you are doing it wrong. When you notice that your awareness is no longer on the breath, congratulate yourself—you have come back and are again aware of your experience! You may wish to briefly note where the mind has been. Then, gently bring your awareness back to the changing sensations in the belly. Pay attention to the movement of the inbreath and the movement of the outbreath.

"Each time you notice that the mind has wandered (and this will happen over and over again), just gently bring your attention back to your breath. Your only job is to follow the changing sensations that come with each inbreath and with each outbreath. As best you can, be kind to yourself. You don't need to worry about doing it right. There is no wrong way to be mindfully aware of the breath. It's okay if your mind wanders. That's just what minds do. No big deal, just practice bringing your attention back to the breath."

Remind the children from time to time that the goal is simply to be aware of their experience in each moment. Each time they notice that the mind has wandered, gently bring attention back to the breath to reconnect with the here and now.

Challenges and Tips

Mind Wandering

Remember to emphasize that a wandering mind is not a problem but is a natural part of these practices. The intent of all mindfulness practices is not to control the mind, but rather to bring nonjudgmental awareness to whatever arises in each moment.

Being Kind to Yourself

Explain to kids that thoughts of "I'm not doing this right" or "I'm no good at this" aren't helpful; they're just negative self-judging thoughts. As we cultivate mindfulness, we may begin to notice how often these negative self-judging thoughts come into our heads. Believing that thoughts are true often creates unhappiness. All thoughts are just thoughts . . . even the ones that tell you they're not. Suggest to the kids that they try some more encouraging wording, such as "This is hard, but I'm still learning."

Suggested Practice Activities

- Brainstorm with the kids the several times every day that they might practice mindful breathing. For example, right when they wake up, before meals, when they leave their house for school, before each class, etc.
- Suggest that they practice mindful breathing with a classmate, friend, or family member. Better yet, teach that classmate, friend, or family member!
- Keeping a mindfulness journal is also a good idea. Suggest: "Record your thoughts about how mindfulness might be helpful to you in your own life." Examples:
  - "Mindfulness could help me to be less afraid when I have to take a test."
  - "Mindfulness could help me not lose my temper at my little brother."
  - "Mindfulness could help me to pay attention in class, so that multiplication might be easier to learn."
  - "Mindfulness could help me make better choices, so maybe I won't get into trouble at school so often."

Activity 8. Taking Three Mindful Breaths

Time Requirement

1 minute.

Theme

We can always choose to practice being mindful of our next breath.

Background

The breath is always with us—every moment of every day. Even when we have been on auto-pilot for a while, we can always choose to bring mindful awareness to the very next breath we take. Taking three mindful breaths can be done at many different moments throughout the day.

Materials Needed

None.

Mindfulness Activity

Invite the kids to take a mindful posture and gently close their eyes, if they wish to do so.

"We can practice bringing mindful awareness to every breath we take. We will start by being mindfully aware of just three breaths. For this practice, you may wish to focus on the breath in your nostrils. Bringing attention to the first long inbreath and the first slow outbreath, perhaps noticing that the air feels cool as it enters your body and feels slightly warmer as it leaves. Noticing the space between the outbreath and the next inbreath. Attending to the sensations as the second slow inbreath begins. Bringing awareness to that moment between the end of the inbreath and the beginning of the outbreath. Breathing out . . . then resting in the quiet space between the outbreath and the next inbreath. Now taking one more long breath in. You may notice that this inbreath has a beginning, a middle, and an end. Pausing. Breathing out, letting go. Resting for a moment in the place of stillness at the end of the outbreath."

Challenges and Tips

Remembering

You can take the mindful breathing further for the kids by pointing out that it is easy to forget to use it. For example:

"Taking three mindful breaths is not difficult, but it can sometimes be difficult to remember to do. It might be easier to remember if you practice taking three mindful breaths before an activity that you already do every day. You might choose brushing your teeth in the morning, for example, or before getting into your pajamas at night. You could post a brightly colored note in your bathroom or bedroom that can also help you remember, or even in your notebook, or ask your parents and teachers to help you remember."

For Younger Children

You may wish to include imagery with your guidance to help younger children focus on their breathing. Examples include, "Breathe in like you are smelling soup; blow out like you are cooling it off" or "Breathe in and pretend that you are a big balloon filling up with air; breathe out slowly as you let all the air out of the balloon."

Suggested Practice Activities

- Suggest to the kids that for 1 week, they practice taking three mindful breaths before one activity that they do every day—for example, before eating a meal, before starting their schoolwork, or before doing chores.
- In addition: "Notice how you feel before, during and after, and if taking three mindful breaths beforehand changes how you experience doing these things."
- Going further: "You might try using your imagination or counting to help focus—for example, breathing in while imagining you are smelling your favorite meal, and blowing out imagining cooling it off."
- And to complete the mindful experience: "Record in your mindfulness journal what might have changed in your experience. For example, was it easier to pay attention? Did the food taste any different? Were you calmer? If you practiced before a chore that you don't much like to do, were you less bothered about it? What changed?"

Activity 9. Mindful Smiling While Waking Up

> Mindfulness is about setting an intention to pay attention in the present moment, with kindness and curiosity, so we can then choose our next action or behavior.
>
> —CARLA NAUMBURG

Time Requirement

1–2 minutes.

Themes

- We practice starting the day with few mindful breaths, a smile, and an intention to meet our day with presence, kindness, and care.
- We commit to facing our experiences with openness, curiosity, and acceptance of whatever arises.

Background

Forming an intention to be present (as best we can) is the essential first step in cultivating mindfulness. That's why making a conscious choice to pay attention to something is so important. Intentions are not the same as goals. Goals are something that we strive to achieve. Goals can and do provide us with direction and purpose. There is absolutely nothing wrong with having goals. Nonetheless, by definition, goals live in the future.

Intentions, however, live in the present moment and aim our self-awareness toward that moment. Intentions are something to which we can always return—with each new moment—with each new breath. Clear intentions are the foundation of our mindfulness practice.

Materials Needed

Activity handout: Mindful Smiling While Waking Up

Mindfulness Activity

Explain the process of mindful smiling while waking up to the kids:

"Place a photograph of your own favorite 'happy place' on the ceiling or on the wall by your bed where you can see it as soon as you wake up. Alternatively, you may wish to color one or more of the smiley faces or emojis included here and place them where you can see them while lying in bed. This photo or smiley face is your reminder to practice mindful smiling while waking up every morning for the next week. Before you get out of bed each morning, take a few moments to practice mindful breathing. Breathe in slowly three times and breathe out slowly three times while keeping a gentle half-smile on your lips and in your eyes. You are practicing being aware of each inbreath and each outbreath. Then form an intention to remember (as best you can) to be fully present with your experiences and to be kind to yourself and others today. Now putting a slightly bigger smile on your face, breathe three more times—slowly—in and out, while bringing awareness to the movements of each breath in your body."

Challenges and Tips

Mindfulness may be simple, but it isn't easy. Many people say that the hardest part of mindfulness is just remembering to practice. Starting each day by forming an intention to practice, aiming to practice, and forming an intention or aiming to be kind to ourselves and others, can make remembering easier. Suggest to the kids that they think of a moment in the morning when they can set their intention—perhaps while heading to school, while brushing their teeth, or when they're at the breakfast table.

Activity 10. Belly Breathing

Time Requirement

5 minutes.

Theme

Mindful body awareness begins with mindfulness of the breath in the belly.

Background

Mindful awareness can be practiced at any time and any place. Physical sensations are experienced only in the present moment, and our bodies are always with us every moment of every day. So, we can use body sensations to ground ourselves in the present—especially when our minds are a million miles away, or racing back to the past or toward the future. We start cultivating mindfulness of body sensations by bringing awareness to what the body feels when we breathe. Belly breathing is not about lying on the couch or sleeping in bed; rather, it is a mentally engaged activity that leaves the mind focused and alert, while the body feels relaxed and calm.

Materials Needed

Clean carpeted floor or one yoga mat per child.

Vocabulary for Grades 4–8

- *Body sensations* are present-moment experiences of seeing, hearing, tasting, smelling, and touching. Body sensations play an important role in how we relate to the world around us.
- *Belly breathing* is deep breathing in a way that makes the abdomen rise on the inbreath and fall on the outbreath.

Vocabulary for Grades K–3

- *Body sensations* are what we see, hear, taste, smell, and feel.
- *Belly breathing* means breathing slowly and deeply.

Mindfulness Activity

Invite the children to lay flat on their backs and, if they wish to do so, gently close their eyes. Ask them to place the left hand on the belly and the right hand over the heart.

> "Start by bringing your attention to the sensations of touch and pressure on your body where it touches the floor. Taking a few moments to notice how your body connects with the ground. Feeling the sensations of the palms of your hands connecting with your body. Then shifting your attention to the rise and fall of your belly as you breathe in and breathe out. As best you can, bring awareness to all the different sensations in your body as the belly rises with each inbreath, and as the belly falls with each outbreath. It's perfectly okay if your mind wanders—that's what minds do. Each time you notice that the mind has wandered, gently nudge your attention back to the sensations as your belly rises on the inbreath and falls on the outbreath. For 3 minutes, we are just following the changing sensations that come with every inbreath and with every outbreath."

Challenges and Tips

Difficulty Feeling the Movements of the Body

It can sometimes be difficult initially for a child to feel sensations in his or her body. With older children, you might prop up their heads with pillows, and then lay a book on each child's belly. Invite them to keep their eyes open—watching as the book rises and falls with each breath. The additional visual and sensory input can help focus attention on the sensations in the body. For younger children, proceed in the same way with the pillows, and then place a small stuffed toy, bean bag, or heavy stuffed animal—a "breathing buddy"—on each child's abdomen. Invite each child to watch carefully as his or her breathing buddy moves up with each inbreath and down with each outbreath.

Suggested Practice Activities

Here are some variations on belly breathing that you can suggest to your kids:

- "Practice belly breathing for 3–5 minutes right after you wake up and before you go to sleep. But don't practice this lying in bed, as you just might fall asleep! Instead, lie on your back on the floor or a mat."
- "Practice belly breathing with a classmate, friend, or family member. You can even look at each other and smile as you practice!"
- "Watch your breathing buddy rise and fall like you are rocking it to sleep."
- "Record in your mindfulness journal how your mind and body feel right after you practice belly breathing."

Activity 11. Mindful Breath Counting

Time Requirement

10 minutes.

Themes

- Focusing on counting with the breath can reduce distractions from intrusive thoughts or strong emotions.
- Bringing attention to counting with the breath during times of stress can be calming and relaxing.

Background

When children, or even adults, are stressed out or experiencing anger, anxiety, or other strong emotions, they tend to either breathe more shallowly or hyperventilate. In some cases, they may temporarily stop breathing altogether. Learning "how to breathe" during difficult moments sustains a normal rate of breathing, which provides the appropriate amount of oxygen to the brain and body, and opens up and "massages" the organs in the torso. As children learn to breathe in ways that are more efficient and more aligned with normal, nonstressed breathing, the parasympathetic nervous system response produces a calming effect on their bodies and minds. This ability to down-regulate intense emotions through the breath and body is an important and powerful skill that can help manage uncomfortable emotional states.

Materials Needed

None.

Vocabulary for Grades 4–8

Diaphragmatic breathing. As we breathe in, we should see the stomach rise slightly. As we breathe out, both the chest and the stomach fall and come to rest.

Vocabulary for Grades K–3

Belly breathing means breathing through the belly like filling a balloon.

Mindfulness Activity

You might introduce this activity by explaining that learning to pay attention to the breath—learning to breathe deeply and more slowly—can be very relaxing. Deep breathing can also help in managing anxiety, anger, and other strong emotions. Invite the children to notice that, when we become anxious or scared, one thing that happens is that our breathing gets faster and shallower. When we slow down the anxious, scared breathing, the anxiety and fear may decrease as well.

Breath counting can also help strengthen children's ability to focus on the breath with fewer distractions. It is always important, however, to normalize the inevitable wanderings of the mind when thoughts or other distractions arise, while also encouraging them to continue to focus on counting along with the breath. Using brief phrases such as "*when* the mind wanders" (rather than "*if* the mind wanders") or brief statements such as "wandering is just what the mind does" can be helpful in validating the universal nature of the experience.

This mindful breath counting activity can be done sitting up in a mindful posture or lying on the back with arms and legs away from the body a little and comfortably straight. Invite the children to close their eyes if they wish, without insisting that they do so. Some children will be more comfortable with their eyes open and taking a "soft gaze." The following activity was adapted from an intervention developed for acutely burned, traumatized adults (Briere & Semple, 2013). We offer gentle verbal guidance through the three stages of the activity.

1. Begin by inviting the children to breathe through their noses, paying careful attention to the feeling of the breath as it flows in and flows out. Ask them to note how long each inhale and each exhale lasts, without trying to speed up or slow down the breath. Do this for three breath cycles (three inhalations and three exhalations).

2. Next, invite the children to shift their attention to the breath in the belly—feeling the belly rise with each inbreath and fall with each outbreath. You may suggest they place one hand on their belly to feel more easily the rising and falling of the diaphragm with each breath. This type of breathing can feel different from normal breathing. Some children may say that it "feels funny" or observe that breathing in this way makes each breath feel deeper than normal. Some might find it helpful to imagine the breath coming in and out like an ocean wave. Continue this diaphragmatic breathing for another three breath cycles.

3. Once the children are breathing more deeply and fully into the belly, the next step is to slow the breath down even further. Ask the group to slowly (silently) count to three with each inbreath, pause, and then slowly count to four for each outbreath: inbreath for the count of three, long pause for a count of four, then outbreath for the count of five. Then rest in another long pause before beginning the next inbreath. You can remind them that each outbreath should take a little longer than each inbreath. The speed of the counting is left up to each child. Although it should be slower than usual, the pace should not be so slow as to feel uncomfortable. Children may need to experiment a little bit to find a comfortable rate of breathing. Once they have found a comfortable pace, they can continue at that pace for another 3 or 4 minutes. It can be helpful periodically to remind the kids to focus on counting with each inbreath and each outbreath, and to redirect their attention back to counting whenever they become aware that they have been distracted by a thought, an emotion, a sensation, a sound, or other distraction. Validate that losing track of the counting is completely okay, and that they can always just start again at "one" with the next inbreath. Mindful awareness is noticing that the attention has wandered, and then with gentle kindness, choosing to return to counting with each breath.

Additional Discussion Questions for Children/Teens

- Elicit descriptions of the kids' experiences by inquiring about the thoughts and feelings that came up during the activity.
- Explore how practicing mindful breath counting might be useful when intrusive thoughts or memories become distressing, or when strong emotions like anxiety or anger emerge. This practice can sometimes also help in managing physical discomfort or pain. Invite the children to explore "breathing into" discomfort.
- Invite exploration of other times when self-relaxation might be helpful (e.g., before taking a test, when meeting new people, before an arts or sports performance).

Challenges and Tips

Some children and adolescents can be so habitually self-critical that they interpret the perfectly normal challenge of keeping their attention on counting as further "evidence" to support their negative self-image. This not uncommon self-criticalness is why emphasizing two points is important. First, the wandering of the mind is a perfectly normal and expected experience. Second, the need for self-kindness when noticing that the mind has wandered, and then in making the choice to return attention to the breath, is essential. A metaphor of training a puppy to heel can be useful here. Over and over, the bouncy puppy-mind tries to run off, and over and over, with gentle kindness, we bring it back, perhaps also noticing where it had gone.

Suggested Practice Activities

- Invite the children to practice the breath-counting activity at home for 5–10 minutes each day for 1 week. It can be helpful to choose a specific time of day to make it easier to remember to do this as a regular part of their daily routine.
- Children can more readily notice sensations by placing a hand on their bellies, or if lying down, by placing a heavier beanbag, doll, or stuffed animal on their bellies, to rise gently as they feel the breath fill their bellies. If group members are comfortable with the idea, perhaps they could pair up and one child could lie down and place his or her head or hand on the partner's belly.

Encourage children to notice times when mindful breathing practices have been helpful (or when mindful breathing might have been helpful). Suggest that the children use a separate page in their journals to create a list of these opportunities. If this feel challenging, they can consider when mindful breathing might help a friend, family member, or a teacher!

Mindfulness of the Breath

Take a mindful posture by sitting upright in a comfortable position. Rest your hands on your thighs. Gently close your eyes or take a "soft gaze," looking at the floor about three feet in front of you. If you're sitting in a chair, it is helpful to sit upright—without slouching—keeping your back away from the back of the chair. Place your feet flat on the floor with your legs uncrossed. If you're sitting on the floor, you may want to sit with your legs crossed and your bottom supported by a cushion.

- Start by paying attention to the sensations of touch and pressure in the parts of your body that are touching the floor or the chair you are sitting on. Spend a minute or two exploring these body sensations.

- Now shift your attention to the sensations in the belly as you breathe in and out. You may want to place your hand on the lower belly for a moment to focus your awareness on the sensations of breathing. Feel the belly rise with each inbreath, and the belly fall with each outbreath. As best you can, follow the sensations down into the belly as the breath enters on the inbreath and out of the body as the breath leaves on the outbreath. Notice the slight pauses between the inbreath and the outbreath.

- There's no need to control your breathing in any way—just let the breath breathe itself. As best you can, simply allow your breath to be what it is—without wanting it to be anything else.

- Then, the mind will wander away from the breath to other thoughts, memories, or daydreams. This is perfectly okay. It is simply what minds do. It is not a mistake or a failure. When you notice that the mind has wandered (this will happen many times), you are once again being mindful of your experience.

- Congratulate yourself on reconnecting with your experience. You may wish to note to yourself, "thoughts" or "thinking." Then, gently bring attention back to the breath, and continue to follow the sensations of each inbreath and each outbreath.

- As best you can, be kind to yourself. Remember that each wandering of the mind is just one more opportunity to cultivate mindfulness.

- Continue practicing mindfulness of the breath for 3 to 5 minutes, or more.

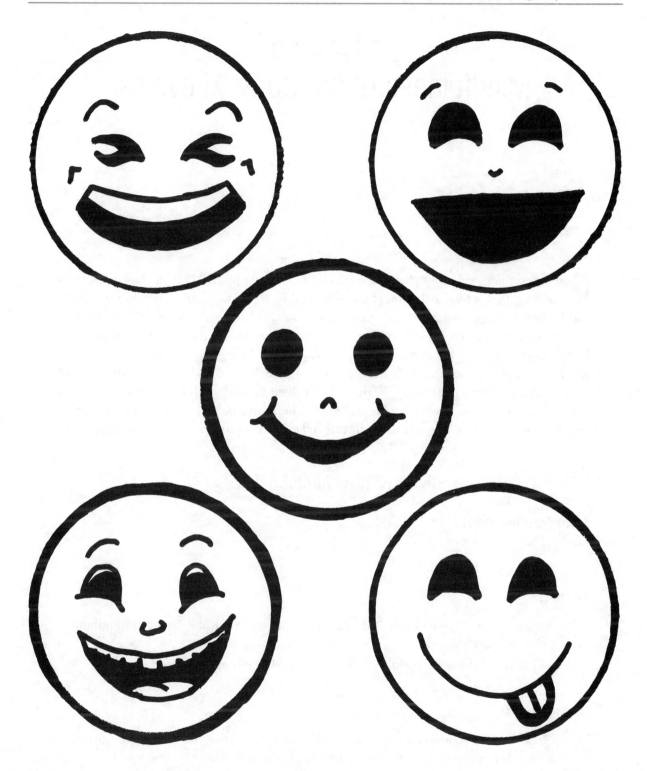

Mindfulness of the Body Activities

Group 3 includes activities that foster mindfulness of the body. Many of these are movement oriented, which makes them more fun and engaging for young, often fidgety minds and bodies. These movement-based body activities may also serve as easy anchors for kids with trauma, anxiety, depression, and/or attentional issues that make sitting in stillness and silence more challenging. For this reason, movement may be a great place to start with kids who are struggling to settle. Further, body awareness can help kids identify the physiological manifestations of emotions, which in turn allows them to work with those strong emotions before they morph into uncomfortable thoughts or impulsive behaviors. Movement also may help improve children's general mental health and cognitive function (Fedewa & Ahn, 2011).

Activity 12. Mindful Silliness

Time Requirement

5 minutes.

Themes

- To engage children, we feel that it is both necessary and desirable to teach mindfulness with playfulness and laughter.
- Practicing mindfulness is possible every day and in everything we do and say.

Background

This activity can be done as an initial icebreaker for a new group. It serves two purposes. First, it provides an opportunity for the children to learn each other's names, which is essential in cultivating a cohesive group. The interactive nature of this activity creates connections between children as they coordinate with each other. Second, it introduces mindfulness of the body *in motion*—requiring mindful attention to both one's own body movements and the movements of others, in a fun way.

Materials Needed

None.

Mindfulness Activity

In this activity we play catch with an invisible ball. The children stand in a circle facing each other (you, as the facilitator, are part of the circle). Hold both of your hands out in front of you, as if you are holding a ball that is about 12–14 inches in diameter. Explain that you are holding an invisible ball. Describe its size, color, weight, texture, and other qualities, and then invite the children to play catch with the invisible ball. Before they toss the ball, they must say their own name, and then point to another person and mime throwing the ball to that person, who mimes catching the ball. Then, that person says his or her own name and throws the ball to someone else. After the ball has been tossed around the circle for a few minutes and everyone has said their own names at least once, stop for a moment to announce a change in the rules. Now, instead of saying their own names, children must say the name of the person to whom they are throwing the ball. When everyone knows each others' names, you might increase the mindfulness component of this activity by introducing a second invisible ball of a different size and weight into the circle.

Challenges and Tips

Some children can become quite anxious when being required to engage in sports or athletics. The way this activity is structured, however, does not seem to arouse anxiety in even highly anxious children. Although you'll want to have the simulated throwing and catching be as realistic as you can, it's actually not possible to be either "good" or "bad" at this activity.

Activity 13. Mindful Flower Stretch

Time Requirement

5–10 minutes.

Theme

The idea here is to help children bring themselves into their bodies in a mindful way, while also practicing breath awareness and building feelings of self-confidence and self-efficacy.

Background

When we are down or feeling sad, worried, ashamed, or scared, our bodies and brains might shut down and go into "freeze-and-give-up" mode. Our bodies might shrink or slump down, and we may feel lifeless inside. Constricted postures can make us feel less self-confident, and may even affect neurotransmitters such as serotonin and gamma-aminobutyric acid (GABA), or hormones such as oxytocin, which play important roles in the regulation of our moods. By mindfully reconnecting with our breath and mindfully adopting a posture of confidence, we may be able to actually change our body chemistry to overcome negative emotions such as shame, depression, and fear (Briñol, Petty, & Wagner, 2009).

Materials Needed

None.

Mindfulness Activity

The group can be seated in chairs, sitting with both feet on the floor, or preferably standing up, especially if the kids could use a break from sitting. Invite them to close their eyes if they wish, or to gaze softly at the floor in front of them. Begin by asking them to slump over in a posture of defeat, shame, depression, or fear, like a wilted flower. The kids might even imagine a situation in which they, or someone in their lives, or even someone from popular culture has felt that way. Invite the children or teens to notice what it feels like in their brains and bodies to be all slumped over.

> "Take a few breaths like this [demonstrate]. What do things look and feel like? What are your emotions? Now take another deep breath in, and as you breathe in, stand or sit up just a little bit taller and more upright. On the outbreath just hold yourself in this slightly more upright posture. Breath by breath, slowly lift and stretch your body and back upward until you are standing or sitting completely upright. Now lift your hands until they are stretching up, palms outward, blossoming like a flower. If there's not enough space in which to stretch all the way out, just hold your hands upright, or rest them akimbo, arms on your hips. From this pose of fully blossoming, begin to notice how your breath, body, and mind feel a bit different than when you were slumped over."

Challenges and Tips

This practice is particularly helpful for kids who are feeling down, ashamed, depressed, or afraid. There is even some evidence that our moods (Peper, Lin, Harvey, & Perez, 2017) and body chemistry (Carney, Cuddy, & Yap, 2010) change in different poses in ways that can make us feel better and more confident.

Suggested Practice Activities

Tell the kids that they can practice the mindful flower stretch "throughout your day when you are feeling good and want to feel even better, or if you are feeling down, or scared and need some confidence." They can also try it before taking on a big challenge—a test, or class presentation, or a big game or performance.

Activity 14. Three Minutes in My Body

Time Requirement

5 minutes.

Theme

Becoming more aware of our bodies in this moment.

Materials Needed

None.

Mindfulness Activity

Lead the group through a few minutes of mindfulness practice that is focused on body sensations. This activity can be done sitting in a chair, sitting on the floor, or while standing.

"Take a moment and bring your attention to your breath while slowly counting down from 10 to 1. Bring your attention to the bottoms of your feet where they touch the floor. Notice any sensations where your feet touch your socks or your shoes. Now slowly bring your focus up to your legs. In your mind's eye, find the exact spot on one of your legs where it first meets the chair. Slowly observe all of the places on the back of your leg that are touching the chair. Now move your attention to your back. If your back is against the chair, observe how that feels. What physical sensations do you notice where your back and the chair meet? If your back is not touching the chair, observe how your shirt feels against your back. Finally, bring your attention to your arms and hands, and with all of your attention, notice whether they are resting on your lap, your desk, or by your sides. Bring your full attention to any sensations on your arms wherever they are touching something. Maybe you feel your clothing, or the air, or another part of your body. Then pat yourself on the back for growing your mindful attention."

Activity 15. Mindful Walking

Time Requirement

5–15 minutes. One rule of thumb is to walk for the duration of the child's age minus 3 minutes; for example, 8-year-old children walk for 5 minutes, 15-year-old teens walk for 12 minutes. Being attentive to when children become distracted or restless, continue the walking for 1 more minute, and then end the activity.

Theme

Mindfulness isn't just about *what* we do, it's about *how* we do it.

Materials Needed

None.

Vocabulary for Grades 4–8

- *Parallel*
- *Intention*

Vocabulary for Grades K–3

- *Muscles*
- *Experiment*

Mindfulness Activity

Lead the children to a space that is large enough in which to walk around comfortably. It can be inside a building (e.g., in a classroom, gym, stage, hallway), or outside (e.g., in a courtyard, in a quiet space in a park or playground). It can be helpful if there is some privacy so that the children do not need to be concerned about being watched by others, as older kids often feel self-conscious when practicing mindful walking. Demonstrate what you are inviting them to do as you offer the following guidance:

"Start by standing with your feet parallel to each other, about 4–6 inches apart, with your knees 'unlocked' or relaxed so that they can gently bend. Allow your arms to hang comfortably by your sides or hold your hands loosely together in front of your body. Lower your eyes and take a soft gaze on a spot about 3–4 feet in front of you on the ground.

"Bringing your awareness to the sensations in the bottom of your feet. Noticing each sensation and each spot on your foot where the foot touches the ground. Noticing the weight of your body pressing onto your legs, onto your feet, and onto the ground. You may find it helpful to bend your knees slightly a few times, like you're bobbing gently up and down, to feel the weight of your body on your legs and feet. Is your body balanced evenly on both legs or are you shifting your weight from one leg to another?

"When you are ready, first notice your decision to move, and then slowly begin shifting the weight of your body onto one leg. It doesn't matter which one you choose. As you're shifting your weight onto the leg, pay attention to all of the movements and other sensations that emerge in the body. How does the leg holding your weight feel different from your other leg?

"Now focusing on your 'empty' leg, the leg that is not supporting your weight. When you are ready, slowly lifting the heel of the empty leg while noticing any sensations in your calf muscles. Noticing how this movement feels in your foot and toes. Keep lifting the empty foot until only the toes are touching the ground. Raising the empty leg until it comes off the floor completely. Carefully and slowly moving this leg forward. Feeling the foot and leg as they move through the air. Next, carefully placing the heel of the empty leg on the floor. After the heel touches the ground, slowly let the rest of the foot make contact with the floor.

"Once this foot is on the floor, slowly start to shift your weight onto it. Now this will become the 'full leg.' Once all your weight is on the full leg, begin to lift the heel of the empty leg up. What sensations do you notice in the calf of this empty leg? Where do you feel pressure? Keep lifting this foot until only the toes are on the floor. Then lifting the empty leg completely off the ground. Slowly moving the empty foot forward and placing the heel on the ground. What sensations do you notice as the heel makes contact with the floor? Becoming aware of all the sensations as the rest of the foot begins to press against the floor.

"Continue walking in this way for a few more minutes. As best you can, bringing attention to all the different body sensations as you slowly walk. Which muscles do you notice as your legs swing forward? How many different parts of your body are involved in taking a single step? Paying close attention to the bottoms of your feet as they make contact with the ground.

"It's okay if your mind starts to wander away from the movements of your body and its sensations. That's just what the mind does. Congratulate yourself for being aware of this and bring your attention back to walking with mindfulness.

"By slowing down an activity that we do every day, we have more opportunities to become aware of the amazing variety of sensations that happen in our body with every simple movement. Once you feel comfortable walking slowly with awareness, you can experiment with walking at other speeds."

Inquiry: Describing Experiences

After the walking activity is complete, ask children to sit in a circle to discuss their experiences. It is common for children to express appreciation for how complex a seemingly ordinary task is when one attends to what is actually involved. For example:

> FACILITATOR: What were some of the things you noticed while doing this activity?
>
> CHILD: I never realized how much walking makes your legs feel so many different things. I guess I never really paid attention to what it feels like to walk.
>
> FACILITATOR: Thank you, Casey. Would you mind telling us what body sensations you noticed while you were walking mindfully. (*Pauses for response.*) Did anyone else have the same experience as Casey?

It is also common for children to express how strange or odd it felt to experience a routine event, such as walking, in such a novel way when they pay greater attention. It is particularly helpful if the facilitator points out that this is the power of bringing mindfulness to our everyday life: It changes how we experience the world! For instance, an exchange might go like this:

> CHILD: When I did the walking, it made me feel weird, like I was walking, but I really wasn't walking. It was like I was doing something totally different.
>
> FACILITATOR: In what ways did mindful walking feel different to you from autopilot walking?

Variations

Different prompts can elicit different responses and observations. For example:

- Invite the children to focus on different places in their bodies (e.g., the soles of their feet, the movement of muscles in their legs, the level of their belly buttons as they walk).
- Invite the children to notice the surface beneath them: bumps, small hills, rough or smooth textures, even warmer or cooler areas through which they might be walking.
- With older kids who might feel self-conscious, invite them to become curious about this feeling. When did they feel self-conscious? Where in their bodies did they notice this self-conscious feeling? What happened when they approached someone else's space, or someone entered their personal space?
- You can also make this activity playful by walking silently like a ninja, for example, or carefully as if walking on ice, or walking while pretending to feel different emotions or to be different people.
- Experiment with different speeds between walking slowly and walking more quickly.

Challenges and Tips

Remembering

Doing a simple activity like walking with mindful awareness is not difficult, but it can sometimes be very hard to remember to be mindful. Visible or audible reminders can make it easier to remember. For example, kids can be encouraged to set a reminder on their smartphones, leave a note about mindful walking in their shoes, or post a brightly colored note in their sock drawer as a helpful means of remembering.

Suggested Practice Activities

Additional practice activities may be introduced in the following general way:

"Think about all the simple physical activities that you normally do on autopilot—like buttoning your jacket, combing your hair, or opening your bedroom door. Pick an activity that you do every day and practice doing it with mindful awareness for 7 days. As with the mindful walking activity, *slow down* so that you have time to observe all the various aspects of the activity.

- "What do you observe about the sensations in your body as you perform the activity? Anything surprising or new?
- "Does bringing your full attention to an activity change how you experience it? If so, in what ways?
- "How might practicing mindful awareness be helpful in other areas of your life?"

Activity 16. Mindful Movements

Time Requirement

10–20 minutes.

Themes

- Body sensations are always experienced in the present moment.
- Paying attention to body sensations gets us out of our heads and into our bodies.
- Grounding awareness in the body can help calm down turbulent thoughts and strong emotions.

Background

Some teachers and clinicians are already familiar with basic stretching or yoga postures, but for those who are not, we offer brief instructions to guide a few simple postures. Some of the many kid-friendly yoga poses include downward facing dog, cat and cow, butterfly, cobra, and the tree pose. Remember that the aim of any mindful movement activity is simply to cultivate mindful awareness of body sensations. Discourage competition between children or struggles to achieve a "perfect" posture—or work with it mindfully and compassionately when it arises. Verbal guidance should focus on using body movements to creatively cultivate mindful awareness of body sensations.

Materials Needed

- One yoga or gym mat for each child and facilitator.
- If mats are not available or floor space is limited, you may prefer to guide only standing movements and poses.

Mindfulness Activity

Yoga Postures for Children*

Downward Facing Dog

- Stand at one end of the mat with both feet flat, about hip-width apart.
- Slowly bend at the waist until both hands reach the ground. Knees may be bent if needed to place the hands on the mat. Palms are facing down and about shoulder width apart.
- Walk the hands forward—out to nearly the height of the child.
- Raise buttocks in the air, arms and legs straight, with the back straight and the head hanging down. This posture resembles an upside-down V.
- Bark like a dog.

---

* From Semple and Lee (2011, pp. 154–155). Reprinted with permission from New Harbinger Publications.

Cat and Cow

- Start by getting down on all fours—on hands and knees on the mat.
- Arch the back up high, like a cat. At the same time, point the head down and meow or hiss like that cat.
- Gently let the back fall into a sway downward, belly toward the floor, while lifting the chin and tailbone. Then moo loudly.
- Repeat, slowly swaying the spine upward and downward, accompanied by the appropriate sound effects. Meowing, hissing, and mooing are encouraged.

Butterfly

- Start by sitting on the floor with the back pressed against a wall and the soles of the feet together.
- Take a moment to relax and let the knees sink closer to the floor.
- Sit up tall, pulling the feet as close to the torso as is comfortable. With both hands, hold the soles of the feet together.
- Begin to gently "flap" both legs (wings) up and down—like a butterfly flying. Perhaps the butterfly is gathering nectar or flying up high just for the fun of it.

Cobra

- Lie flat, with stomach prone on the mat and legs together and straight behind the torso.
- Place hands on either side of the chest with elbows pointed upward, fingers point forward.
- Push the upper body upward as far as is comfortable with the head and eyes lifting toward the ceiling in a gentle curve.
- Hiss like the cobra.

Tree Pose

- Start by standing with both legs together and arms straight down at the sides of the body.
- Slowly slide the bottom of one foot up the inside of the other leg to the calf or thigh. Be careful not to press the sole of the foot against the kneecap.
- As best possible, keep the knee on the lifted leg pointed out to the side.
- Gaze at a single, stable point (something that is motionless).
- When the balance feels stable, slowly lift both arms out to either side, and then stretch them overhead, fingers toward the ceiling, palms together.
- Let the arms sway back and forth like a tree in the wind while making soft wind sounds.

Challenges and Tips

Although mindful movement activities are often helpful in managing stress and anxiety, bringing awareness to body sensations can also trigger traumatic memories or trauma responses. If any mindfulness activity triggers overwhelming anxiety or fear, then it is counterproductive to continue. If traumatic memories are sufficiently intense, a child may start crying or even dissociate. Be tuned into any expressions of distress. You might want to shift to a grounding activity, such as mindfulness of the soles of the feet. Because attention is focused on the connections between the outside of the body and the environment around us, focusing on touch points (described below) can also create a sense of safety and stability in the body. Alternatively, you can quietly go over to that child and start him or her on a silent breath-counting activity.

Suggested Practice Activities

- Any of these activities or variations on them can be practiced at home. Invite each child to pick three mindful movement poses and teach them to his or her parents or siblings.
- Suggest that the children practice mindfulness movements by bringing attention to the "touch points" of their bodies as they practice each pose. Touch points are places where the body touches itself or the world. For example, while practicing the butterfly pose, the soles of the feet touch each other, the back touches the wall, the sit bones touch the floor, the palms of the hands touch the feet, the lips may touch the tongue, and the eyelids touch each other.

Activity 17. Matching Movement Moments

Time Requirement

5 minutes.

Themes

- Bringing mindful attention to our own movements is one way to increase awareness of our own bodies.
- Bringing mindful attention to another person's movements is a way of increasing our emotional attunement, recognition, and connection to others.

Background

Children benefit from engaging in frequent physical activity, both to revitalize themselves and to help maintain their focus throughout the day. Teachers and parents may also notice fewer behavior problems when children are given regular opportunities to move around. Matching Movement Moments is a brief activity that can be done in limited space, and can be repeated in a variety of different ways during a therapy session or throughout the school day.

Materials Needed

None.

Mindfulness Activity

Invite the children to think about all the different ways that they might move their heads, faces, hands, feet, arms, legs, and bodies. They might slide, stamp, or tap their feet; stand on their toes or heels, clap their hands; bob their heads back and forth; move their fingers or arms up, down, forward and back, or around in circles; or move their whole bodies by bending, stretching, jumping, or squatting down. The body is capable of making thousands of different movements. What's more, each movement can be done fast or slowly or be repeated rhythmically or randomly, or in any combination of these. The variety is infinite.

Divide the children into pairs to stand or sit facing each other about 2–3 feet apart. One child will assume the role of leader and the other will be the follower. It does not matter which child takes which role, because the roles will be reversed in the second part. You may like to use a mindfulness bell to start and end each half of the activity. When you ring the bell, the leader begins making his or her movements, while the follower tries to match those movements as precisely as he or she can, until the bell rings to end that segment. Then the children switch roles, and the new leader determines the matching movements for the dyad.

Each segment generally lasts for only 30–60 seconds. The Matching Movement Moments activity should be done with no touching of the other child and in complete silence. Initially, you may want to conduct a group discussion after the activity to elicit descriptions of the experiences, in what ways mindful movements differ from ordinary movements, and how this knowledge could be useful in their daily lives. After this (or any) activity is repeated several times, you may subsequently prefer to move on to the next activity without further discussion.

Variations

Variations are limited only by your time and creativity. Following are a few of the variations we have offered:

- "Pretend to swim like a fish, move as slowly as a turtle, walk as heavily as an elephant, stretch as tall as a giraffe, slither like a snake, flap your wings like a bird, trot like a horse, or hop like a bunny rabbit."
- "Make up a brief pattern of movements to do over and over again. One pattern, for example, might be three handclaps, then cross the arms and pat your opposite shoulder twice with each hand. Repeat the same pattern slowly for 1 minute until the bell rings. What does it feel like to match your movements in rhythm with another person?"
- "Do the matching movements activity sitting down. This might include leg or foot movements such as tapping the heels together; rocking the toes and heels back and forth; or turning the palms of the hands up and down, back and forth. The leader selects a repeating pattern and performs it for the follower. Then the follower joins in and matches the leader's movements."
- "Limit the allowable movement to facial expressions only. Be mindful that this variation can be hard to do without bringing lots of giggles into the room."

Additional Questions for Children/Teens

- "What did you observe about your own body movements while you were the leader?"
- "What did you observe about the body movements of the person following your movements? For example, did that person mirror your actions [reversing left and right] or match exactly what you did?"

- "What thoughts did you notice during the activity?"
- "Did different movements affect your mind or mood differently? If so, in what ways?"
- "Did anything you did just now feel different from the usual way that you move?"
- "As the follower, were your thoughts trying to anticipate the movements of the leader?"
- "Did your thoughts and feelings change when your role changed?"

Challenges and Tips

- Monitor the activity level carefully, as some children can quickly become wilder in their movements and start jumping or running around. At that point, they may have forgotten that the aim of this activity is to practice mindfulness of their own body movements and attunement to the movements of others. A gentle reminder of this point is typically all that is needed. Also, be aware that children may try to make the activity a competition with the other child, or deliberately make movements that are hard to follow. You might remind them that there are no "good" or "bad" ways to move, and there are no winners or losers. Instead, they ought to make moves their partner can follow.
- To increase energy in the room, invite the leaders of each pair to start by making their movements very slow, and then gradually increase the speed. Explore what it feels like to speed up and slow down and "shift gears," regulating themselves from fast to slow, silly to serious, large to small.
- To decrease energy in the room, invite the leaders of each pair to start by making their movements very fast, and then, like a battery wearing down, gradually decrease the speed until the battery goes completely "dead," and the children come to a complete stop.
- Another way to reduce the energy in the room is to invite the children to make their movements very small and as slow as molasses throughout, focusing on making the smallest movements possible. One example of this would be to make a very slow tapping pattern with one finger while keeping the rest of the hand motionless on a table or lap.

Activity 18. Mindfulness While Lying Down

Time Requirement

3 minutes.

Themes

- Particularly when caught up in the grip of strong emotions, practicing mindfulness for just a few minutes while lying down can help us to calm down and remember that we have choices.
- Even just changing our posture can change how we are feeling emotionally.

Materials Needed

Yoga mats (optional).

Mindfulness Activity

"Lie on your back on a firm, flat surface. Keep your arms loosely at your sides and your legs slightly apart, stretched out straight. Closing your eyes if you wish or allowing your eyes to take a soft, fuzzy gaze, bring a gentle half smile to your face. Breathing in and out smoothly, keeping your attention focused on each of the sensations in your body as your breath moves in and moves out. Bringing your awareness to all the points where your body touches the surface underneath you, the outline of the points of contact. Feeling as each muscle in your body relaxes. Letting go of whatever uncomfortable emotions and sensations you might be experiencing. Letting all those feelings flow out of your body and quietly disappear as they sink into the floor. Letting every muscle in your body go limp. Relaxing each muscle—just as if you are a soft and flowing piece of silk hanging in the breeze to dry. Letting go completely, keeping your attention only on your breath and your half smile. You might choose to pretend that you are a cozy cat or pet—completely relaxed as you lay in front of a warm fireplace. Then slowly count 15 inbreaths and 15 outbreaths."

Additional Questions for Children/Teens

- "How did your body feel when you began the activity?"
- "How does your body feel now? Is there a difference? If so, describe what changed."
- "Try holding your breath for 10 or 15 seconds. How did it feel while you were holding your breath? How did it feel when you released the breath?"

Tip for Working with Younger Children

To encourage stillness of the body and to help keep the focus on the breath, younger children may enjoy placing a small stuffed animal on their bellies and then watching their "breathing buddy" move up and move down as they slowly breathe in and breathe out. If a child still seems to have trouble focusing, you might invite him or her to silently say "up" each time the breathing buddy moves up and silently say "down" each time the breathing buddy moves down. What did he or she notice about their breathing buddy as their breath went in and out?

Activity 19. Mindful Mountain Visualization

Time Requirement

10–15 minutes.

Theme

Feeling stable and steady, with a sense of peace and equanimity.

Background

Life has a way of throwing us unexpected challenges. Things may be constantly changing all around us; one day it's easy to be happy, the next it seems like everything is sad, stressful, or frustrating. People around us can be kind one day and cruel the next; classes change, friendships change, and change is difficult. But even with all the changes going on around us, we can remain calm and stable. Think about a mountain—it's always still and calm, despite the rain or shine, the fog or thunder, regardless of the seasons, it just sits—stable and calm—while the weather swirls around it.

This activity has been adapted from the "Mountain Meditation" for adults, developed by Jon Kabat-Zinn (2014), with imagery inspired by Thich Nhat Hanh (2009, pp. 35–36).

Materials Needed

None.

Mindfulness Activity

The group can be seated in chairs with both feet on the floor, preferably sitting up straight, like a mountain; or sitting cross-legged directly on the floor or on cushions. Invite the children to close their eyes if they wish, or to let their eyes take a soft gaze at the floor in front of them.

"Begin by finding a comfortable posture, sitting up straight and tall like a mountain. Now, take a moment and bring your attention to the sensations of your body settling into the chair beneath you [or the floor under you], and your head and torso rising upward toward the sky above. With each breath, you might even say to yourself, *'Breathing in, I see myself as a mountain, breathing out, I feel calm, stable, and still.'* Take a few breaths like this until you really start to feel like the mountain—calm, stable, and still . . .

"And now begin to imagine the mountain in the summertime. Perhaps there is snow at the peak, and green trees and meadows around its rocky sides. As each day goes on, the shadows change, and the mountain looks different in the different light of day. But through it all, the mountain remains calm, stable, and still.

"At night the mountain just rests in the moonlight or beneath the stars in the dark, remaining calm, stable, and still as the days slowly go by—each one different from the last. Some days clouds cover the top of the mountain, storms of thunder and lightning surround the mountain. But the mountain always remains calm, stable, and still.

"When autumn comes, the trees change colors and leaves fall away; the days grow shorter and colder, the nights longer. And through it all, the mountain remains calm, stable, and still. Gradually winter arrives, and snowstorms and blizzards blanket the mountain in snow, covering its rocky sides and meadows in white, trees sparkling with ice. And yet the mountain remains calm, stable, and still.

"Eventually winter fades, the snow melts into rivers and lakes, and waterfalls cascade down the sides of the calm, stable, and still mountain once again. Green trees appear, grass and flowers cover the meadows, and the days grow longer and warmer. Spring fog may arrive some days, sunshine or rain on others, but through all of these changes, the mountain is calm, stable, and still. As the seasons change, trees grow, shed their leaves, and then grow some more; flowers and grass sprout and fade, streams flow or dry up, and animals or people may visit. But through it all, the mountain watches, never moving or reacting to all the changes. The mountain sits calm, stable, and still, simply watching the big and small changes each season brings.

"And so while the outside world is always changing, those changes do not need to disturb the calm, stillness, and stability that the mountain always has. Can you find that stillness deep inside of yourself? Can you let your mind and body rest there at any time in the day, just repeating to yourself whenever you need to, 'Breathing in, I see myself as a mountain, breathing out, I feel calm, stable, and still?'"

Challenges and Tips

This practice is particularly helpful for kids who are living in stressful or challenging situations, or struggling with emotional reactivity.

Suggested Practice Activities

The mindful mountain takes some time (10–15 minutes), although the facilitator can stretch or shrink it according to the attention and engagement of the group. The simple statement, "Breathing in, I see myself as a mountain; breathing out, I feel calm, stable, and still" is inspired by the meditation master Thich Nhat Hanh (1991a), and can be used as a self-soothing mantra any time throughout the day when things begin to feel overwhelming or hectic for the kids. You might brainstorm when it would be helpful to sit up tall like a mountain and silently repeat the statement to themselves. You can even ask kids to come up with their own image (e.g., tree, lake, animal), or words (e.g., *strong, brave, calm*) that they might find helpful.

Activity 20. Mindfulness of My Feet

Time Requirement

5–10 minutes.

Theme

Bringing awareness from our minds down into our bodies can break the cycle of chattering thoughts and rumination that perpetuates anxiety and stress.

Background

When we feel overwhelmed with chattering thoughts, especially strong or uncomfortable thoughts, we want to bring our awareness out of our minds and somewhere outside of us or somewhere in our bodies. And what is the farthest place from our heads? Our feet, of course! Getting out of our thinking minds and into our feet disrupts the cycle of anxious or unpleasant thoughts, and calms us down pretty quickly.

Materials Needed

None.

Mindfulness Activity

The kids can be seated in chairs with both feet on the floor, or standing up if they could use a break from sitting. Invite them to close their eyes if they wish, or to let their eyes take a soft gaze at the floor in front of them. Begin by taking five long deep breaths in and exhaling five long deep breaths out. With each breath, they are to allow their bodies to relax more and more, and then on the fifth breath, they should follow their attention all the way down to their feet.

> "What sensations are you aware of in your feet? Are you feeling your socks and shoes? What textures are you noticing? Can you sense if the floor is hard or soft with carpet? Are your feet warm or dry? Are they cold or warm? Are your shoes tight or loose, itchy or cozy? Do the tops of your feet feel different from the bottom? What about the toes and the heels? Do the insides of your feet feel different from the outside? Does your left foot feel different from your right foot? Practice being detectives—using the mind's eye to explore all the different sensations of the feet."

Challenges and Tips

This activity is particularly helpful for kids who are emotionally overreactive or who struggle with impulse control. Although very useful with the "Pathway through Problems of Emotion Regulation and Impulse Control," a lot of kids with everyday stress or anxiety, or those living in demanding environments, find it a fun and useful way to manage their strong emotions and impulses by grounding themselves first before choosing what to do next.

Suggested Practice Activities

Encourage the kids to use this activity throughout the day:

> "You can practice Mindfulness of My Feet every day at various points in the day. It might be at regular intervals, or when you are feeling overwhelmed or stuck in your head with thoughts spinning, or when you are experiencing emotions or thoughts that feel intrusive or uncomfortable. You can feel your feet anywhere, any time, and the more you practice, the more quickly you will become friends with those pesky thoughts and feelings."

Activity 21. Body Scan

Time Requirement

5–15 minutes.

Themes

- Bringing awareness to sensations in the body can be a deeply relaxing and potentially healing mindfulness practice.
- By getting comfortable in our bodies, we can be more comfortable in our lives.
- By recognizing sensations and emotions in our bodies first, we can work with them more effectively than once they are in our minds.

Background

The body scan helps young people develop an ability to pay attention to how their bodies feel, moment by moment. Emotional reactivity is often preceded by physical sensations. They might feel a lump in their throats before anxiety is recognized as such, or tension in their shoulder muscles before anger arises. Paying attention to these sensations lets the child or teen tune into the warning signs of imminent mood shifts that might otherwise catch them unaware. Practicing body scans helps them identify—in real time—the warning signs of anxiety, upset, or irritation, which in turn gives them opportunities to choose a more skillful strategy to deal with whatever is happening more effectively. It's important to point out that it is perfectly okay to feel upset or annoyed. All emotions are real and valid. But we don't need to react thoughtlessly to these emotions with unhelpful words or behaviors. Practicing the body scan also enhances awareness of positive feelings.

In this practice, there is no physical movement. We systematically move our attention throughout the body, giving moment-by-moment attention to the various sensations in different parts of the body. Without ever moving a muscle, we bring our attention to different areas of the body—simply bringing what our friend Amy Saltzman (2014) calls the "flashlight of awareness" to whatever sensations are present in that place in that moment. When we practice the body scan, we begin by forming the intention to be present with our body sensations as best we can. When introducing this activity, it's best to keep the practice short (3–4 minutes) and be mindful of the level of attention in the room. If you notice the children becoming restless or fidgety, you can let them know that the activity will end in about another minute (or maybe six more breaths) and invite them to bring all their attention to the sensations of restlessness for that 1 minute. As children become more experienced mindfulness practitioners, the time can be extended up to 10 minutes (for adolescents, up to 15 minutes).

Materials Needed

Yoga mats (optional).

Mindfulness Activity

Children can be seated in chairs, sit in a circle on the floor, or lie on their backs on a rug or yoga mats. Invite them to close their eyes if they wish, or let their eyes take a soft gaze. Then, begin by forming the intention to be present (as best we can) while taking five long deep breaths in and exhaling five long deep breaths out. With each breath, we are letting the body relax and soften more and more. Assure them that if they sometimes find it hard to focus, that is perfectly normal. When they notice this, they should briefly shift their attention to the sensations in their chest as they breathe in and breathe out. Then, return their awareness to the sensations in the body.

"Staying as still as a mouse, bringing attention to the sensations at the top of your head and on your scalp. [long pause] Next, bringing your awareness to your face. Noticing what expression might be on your face in this moment, and what emotions your face might be expressing. What does that feel like from the inside? Focusing for a few moments on the sensations around your eyes. There's no need to try too hard, just letting your attention rest on different parts of the face. [long pause] Shifting your awareness to your mouth. In a barely noticeable way, maybe allowing a tiny smile to come to your face. Now shifting your attention to your jaw muscles. If they feel closed tight, softly loosen them. Letting your whole face relax. [long pause]

"Then slowly moving your awareness to your belly—feeling the small movements of your muscles as you breathe in and breathe out. Feeling calmness and lightness enter your body with each breath you take in. [long pause]. Gently bringing your attention to your back muscles. Their strength is what keeps you standing or sitting tall all day. Thank these muscles for their strength. Feeling your whole body becoming calm and balanced. [long pause] Now feeling your legs touching the chair [or floor, depending on where they are sitting or lying]. Finally, letting your awareness sweep down to the sensations in your feet and your toes. [long pause] Taking a moment to place your attention on any place in your body where you can feel your breath. This might be in your legs, in your belly or chest, or in your nostrils. Feeling (or imagining you feel) the air flowing in and out. Taking a moment to feel calmness and lightness fill up your entire body. [long pause] As we begin to end this practice, taking five more long deep breaths in and exhaling five long deep breaths out, and then gently bringing your awareness back to the room. Slowly opening your eyes but remaining still for a few breaths before you choose to move again."

Challenges and Tips

Although mindfulness of the body is relaxing and restful for most, it is important to be aware that the body scan (and other body-focused activities) can sometimes trigger extremely uncomfortable or emotionally distressing responses, which can occasionally rise to the level of requiring therapeutic attention. Children who have a history of trauma or abuse are the most vulnerable and the most likely to experience the body scan as distressing. This is particularly relevant if the abuse was of a physical or sexual nature. Many traumatized children are either completely desensitized or hypersensitive to their own body sensations. Please read the "Pathway through Trauma, Abuse, and Neglect" chapter before introducing the body scan to this population.

Suggested Practice Activities

Suggest several options to the children:

"You can practice body scans, short or long, every day. Many websites offer audio-guided body scans of different lengths. You can practice the body scan lying in bed at night or in the morning when you wake up. The body scan can be practiced sitting in a chair or even while standing up. The more you practice bringing awareness to body sensations, the more you will discover about your body and about all the different ways that your thoughts and emotions are related to your body sensations."

Activity 22. The Mindful HALT

Time Requirement

5–10 minutes.

Themes

- Bringing awareness to our basic bodily needs gives us information about what we *need* to stay healthy and happy in mind and body, more than just what we *want*.
- As we respond to and regulate our brain and body to think and see clearly, we make better decisions and more effectively regulate our impulses.

Background

When we practice awareness of our bodily needs, we can give our bodies and brains what they need to perform their best. In this practice, following the acronym HALT (hungry, angry or anxious, lonely, or tired), there is no movement; instead, we ask ourselves a series of questions and consider how to respond to them to be at our best. Without ever moving a muscle, we bring our attention to our needs in the moment and respond, instead of react, to the world around us.

Materials Needed

Yoga mats (optional).

Mindfulness Activity

The kids can be seated in chairs, sit in a circle on the floor, or lie on their backs on the carpet or on mats. Invite them to close their eyes if they wish, or let their eyes take a soft gaze. Have the kids begin by taking five long, mindful, deep breaths in and exhaling five long, mindful, deep breaths out—with each breath letting the body relax more and more.

> "Using the acronym HALT is a simple strategy that can help you remember to check in with your basic biological and emotional needs. When you're not aware of these needs (which we all have), they can be triggers for impulsive behaviors or interfere with making wholesome choices for yourself. By reminding yourself to HALT a few times during the day to ask yourself if you're feeling hungry, angry or anxious, lonely, or tired, you become more aware of what's going on inside yourself."

<u>H</u> Is for Hungry

> "Check in with your stomach, but also notice your overall energy. Are you feeling *hungry* at all? If you are hungry, your body and brain don't have the fuel they need to think and

see clearly, to regulate your emotions, and to control your impulses. Note this to yourself, and if you need to eat, plan a meal [depending on age] or ask for a snack."

A Is for Angry or Anxious

"Are you feeling *angry* or *anxious*? These two emotions can really affect your sense of danger and safety, and your ability to think things through clearly. If your body and brain are experiencing strong anger or anxiety, a few long mindful breaths or belly breaths can help you quiet down, let you look clearly to see what is fueling the emotions, which then allows you to make more skillful choices in how you want to respond to them."

L Is for Lonely

"Are you *lonely* right now, feeling isolated or disconnected? The emotion of loneliness is different from the state of being alone; you might be surrounded by people but still feel lonely. Reaching out to others to check in with how you are doing and what's going on can give you some perspective and help you feel better really quickly. There is an old saying that suggests 'If your mind is a dangerous neighborhood, don't go there alone.' Who could you reach out to in this moment that would feel safe to you?"

T Is for Tired

"Are you *tired* in this moment? Maybe from lack of sleep, or maybe you are just worn out from school, work, exercise, or relationship or family issues. When you are tired, it's almost like you aren't as smart as when you are well rested, and it's much harder to manage your emotions and impulses. What can you do to rest or relax, and if not now, then soon?"

Challenges and Tips

This activity is particularly helpful for kids who struggle with impulses or acting-out behaviors that may be associated with mental health issues. While its most useful for the Pathway through Problems of Emotion Regulation and Impulsive Behaviors, a lot of kids with stress and anxiety find it a fun and useful way to check in with what might be happening physiologically. When they remember to do this activity, some kids will even "freeze" in the middle of taking a step for a brief Mindful HALT.

Suggested Practice Activities

"You can practice the Mindful HALT every day at various points in the day to get to know your body's needs, especially at moments that are stressful or challenging. You can HALT anywhere, anytime, and the more you practice bringing awareness to your basic needs, the more you can be aware of your thoughts, emotions, and body sensations, while skillfully tending to your body's needs throughout your day."

Activity 23. Mindful Body Relaxation

Time Requirement

10–15 minutes, adaptable.

Themes

- Becoming aware of stress, anxiety, and emotions in the body.
- Managing emotions in the body.
- Teaching our bodies how to relax.

Background

When our bodies are tense, stressed, or anxious, it is impossible for our minds to also feel relaxed, open, and clear. This exercise will teach children how to be aware and mindful of their bodies, and also practice relaxing on purpose when they are getting tense. Ideally kids can lie down for this practice, but they can be seated as well. You may also want to keep an eye on kids as they can sometimes fall asleep during this practice. Adjust the time to what you have available and what the kids can tolerate.

Materials Needed

- A yoga mat or soft surface on which to lie down.
- A mindfulness journal for each child.

Mindfulness Activity

"Let's begin by lying down on your back, and just noticing the sensations of your body making contact with the surface underneath you. Bringing your awareness to your breathing, taking a deep breath in and feeling your belly rise and then fall as you exhale your breath and sink deeper into the surface underneath you.

"On the next breath, observing the sensations of your breath, then moving your attention slowly, all the way down into your feet. Noticing sensations there, then squeezing all the muscles in your feet and pointing your toes. Noticing what all that tension feels like running through your muscles, and how your breathing becomes tighter as you squeeze. Keep squeezing just a bit harder . . . and then let go. Feeling the tension flow away and the relaxation flowing into your feet and toes. Taking a moment to breathe and appreciate the difference before and after you released the tension.

"Now pulling [flexing] your feet toward the tops of your calves and stretching [flexing] the toes upward . . . holding . . . then releasing. As the tension flows away, feeling the new sensations of relaxation through your feet and toes, and just enjoy that for a few more breaths.

"Now, on the next breath, bringing your attention to the sensations in your ankles and calves, then clenching these muscles for a breath or two, noticing all the tightness and tension before relaxing and releasing, aware once more of the contrast between the sensations as you let go, completely relaxed, enjoying the sensations for a few breaths.

"Whenever you feel ready, taking a deep breath in and noticing the sensations in your knees and thighs, then squeezing and tensing those muscles for a moment or two, before just letting go and allowing the relaxation to wash over your whole lower body . . . letting go completely of the tension in your thighs and knees.

"Now, sweeping your attention across your hips, stomach, and lower back, bringing your awareness to all the pleasant or even unpleasant sensations, and then squeezing, holding tight all those muscles across your middle, and then once more releasing the tension and enjoying the relaxation.

"Now breathing in and turning your attention to the rest of your back, noticing any comfort or discomfort or tension already there. Feel the tension as your shoulders pull back and the muscles along your spine tighten . . . and then letting go . . . letting the relaxation flow through your body for a few more breaths.

"Now turning your attention to sensations in your chest, feeling your heartbeat and maybe noting the breath there, then clenching the muscles for a few moments and now relaxing your whole upper body.

"On the next breath, bringing your awareness to sensations in your hands, then slowly balling them into fists as tightly as you can and squeeze . . . and then just releasing and relaxing.

"Now following your awareness down into your forearms and wrists, tightening those muscles in your lower arms, then also tensing your biceps and triceps for a few breaths. Now letting go, enjoying the feeling of relaxation as it gently washes back into your arms. Whenever you are ready, first noticing sensations and tension in your shoulders and neck, then squeezing . . . holding . . . and then releasing, letting the relaxation flow into the space where the tension used to be.

"Last, bringing your awareness to the muscles of your face, noticing what expression is already resting on your face. Then furrowing your brow, squeezing your eyes and clenching your jaw, feeling the strain and stress in all of these facial muscles. Really feeling these sensations of tension and tightness in your face, and maybe even in your emotions. Then, just letting go, allowing the tension to flow out, and the relaxation to flow in. Resting with the flow, enjoying complete relaxation for the next few moments as you breathe in and breathe out.

"Taking a few minutes now to scan all the muscles of your body. Noticing any tension or relaxation in your feet and legs, your hips, and into your torso and back; noticing the sensations in your arms and hands, your neck and shoulders, then noticing the stillness in your face. Staying with those sensations for a few more moments as you lie there.

"[optional] If you feel like it, you may wish to shift to a comfortable sleeping position, focusing on the feelings of relaxation seeping into your mind, and allow yourself to drift softly off to sleep."

Variation: The CALM Reminder*

"Try using this simple acronym throughout your day as a CALM Reminder to check in with the different parts of your body, looking for tension, then squeeze and release. Close

---

* Based on Willard and Saltzman (2015, p. 13).

your eyes if you feel comfortable, taking one deep breath and exhaling slowly, then bring your attention into your body."

C Is for Chest

"What sensations do you notice in your chest and entire torso? Tight or relaxed? Hot or cool? Is your heart beating fast or slowly? Is your breath up in your chest or lower down in your belly? Try tensing all the muscles now in your chest and torso, and then just letting them go . . . letting the tension drain and the relaxation flow in."

A Is for Arms

"What sensations are you noticing in your arms? Are your hands warm or cold, sweaty or dry? Are your hands tensed up or relaxed? What about your forearms, biceps, and triceps? Now try clenching up all of these muscles, holding for a few breaths, and then on the outbreath, just releasing."

L Is for Legs

"What's happening in your legs, from the soles of your feet all the way up to your thighs? Are they tense or loose? Are they bouncing or still? Do the legs feel calm, or do they want to move or run? Now take a slow breath in and squeeze all of these muscles for a moment, and then breathing out, relax, letting the relaxation flow in."

M Is for Mind

"Finally, check in with your mind. What kinds of thoughts are you having there? Practice just noticing what is happening in your head, and then let the thoughts go as you return your awareness to your breath and body. Whenever you are ready, allow your eyes to slowly open and return your awareness to the world around you."

Additional Questions for Children/Teens

- "Where in your body did you notice the most tension?"
- "What are the times of day or events in your day that might make you more tense in those places?"
- "What happened to your breathing when you tensed, what happened when you released?"
- "What kinds of emotions and thoughts did you notice when you were tense or when you relaxed?"
- "Can you notice for the rest of the day and week where in your body (or mind) you are tense? Whenever you do, then try squeezing and releasing."

Mindful Awareness Activities

Group 4 activities, the mindful awareness practices, are generally fun, or aim to be, with an emphasis on greater internal and external awareness in daily living. These activities are meant to help kids practice mindful awareness in their everyday lives—outside of your group time. Once kids have developed the habit of engaging these practices informally and independently between sessions, consider moving on to the sensory-based activities.

Activity 24. Mindfulness in Everyday Life

Time Requirement

Very little additional time beyond the time necessary for the daily activity itself.

Themes

- In any moment of every day, we can remember to bring awareness to our thoughts, feelings, body sensations, and to the people or things around us.
- Doing this with intention and nonjudgmental awareness means that we aren't paying attention to decide if we like or don't like what's going on—we're paying attention to practice accepting *what is*.

Background

The intention underlying instruction in mindfulness is not that we just practice for a few minutes every day and then forget about it. Mindfulness is a way of being engaged in the world that we can practice in any moment of our lives. The time that we spend doing formal mindfulness practices certainly affects our moods and emotions, but remembering to practice mindfulness while we do the simple, ordinary activities that are part of each day can make a significant contribution to deepening our practice. We might sometimes see these ordinary everyday activities as getting in the way of practicing mindfulness. In fact, everything that we do in our lives can be part of our practice. No matter what we are doing, we can always remember to do it with mindful awareness.

So, we might choose eating or walking as our mindfulness practice. We can practice listening to others with mindful attention. No matter what we're doing, we can always choose do it with a little more kindness and compassion. We can be kind to ourselves by being attentive and noticing when we are shifting into autopilot mode. We can observe when we try to hold onto thoughts or feelings, and then practice letting them go. Living with mindfulness in this way is hugely empowering. We make the choice to live with awareness, with compassion, and with respect for ourselves and others—moment by moment.

Materials Needed

None.

Mindfulness Activity

Mindfulness involves bringing our awareness into the present moment. In this way, we learn to connect deeply with each moment of our lives.

"To be mindful is to be truly present and connected with yourself, with others around you, and with whatever you are doing in the moment. Pick one activity that you do every day and practice bringing mindful awareness to it each day for 5 days. It's not hard to do this, but it can sometimes be hard to remember to do it. You might find it helpful to place an object or a note where it will remind you to practice mindful awareness of that activity. For example, if you choose to practice mindfulness while brushing your teeth, you might put a sticky note that says *Breathe* on the bathroom mirror to remind you. You can choose to practice mindfulness with simple activities such as getting out of bed, eating breakfast, making your bed, getting dressed, combing your hair, or walking to school. Or you might try practicing mindfulness with something a little less pleasant, like a chore that you do every day. This could be setting the table, washing dishes, taking out the garbage, or any other chore that you do most days. Particularly if the chore is something you don't like to do, try doing it every day for 1 week while watching your thoughts and feelings carefully. Notice if your feelings change over the course of the week. Choose one activity—the same activity every day—and as best you can, practice being mindful of your thoughts, feelings, and body sensations as you are doing that activity. Record what you observe in your mindfulness journal."

Activity 25. Finding Five New Things

Time Requirement

10 minutes.

Theme

Looking clearly at the little things that surround us also teaches us to see the big things more clearly.

Background

Focusing and redirecting attention with intention, clarity, and awareness takes practice. In this activity, we invite children to bring mindful awareness to the ordinary things that are all around them—at school, at home, and elsewhere. When a child says, "Wow—I never noticed that before!," it signals that she has discovered that mindful awareness allows her to see more things with greater clarity. It might be something as mundane as seeing the textured pattern on her bedspread or the interesting carvings on the legs of the dining room chairs. Or it might be something more significant, such as noticing that her mother is feeling overwhelmed with household tasks and offering to help her. As Jon Kabat-Zinn has often observed, "The little things? The little moments? They aren't little."

Mindful awareness becomes a practice of slowing down just a little in order to see more of our world. The world is complex and ever changing. Sometimes we are on autopilot and may miss out on all the good things that are right in front of us. As we learn to see the world with greater clarity, we begin to realize that our own thoughts and feelings influence how we treat ourselves and others. We learn to see that we have choices. One big choice we might discover is that we can choose to relate to our thoughts in different ways. We discover that we don't need to believe everything we think, and that, with greater understanding, we can make better choices. With mindful awareness, we practice looking so that we can learn how to see—clearly—with acceptance and without judgments.

Materials Needed

Activity handout: *Finding Five New Things* for optional home practice activity.

Mindfulness Activity

Sitting in a circle will facilitate this activity. Start by practicing a few minutes of mindful breathing. Then look around the room you are in, select one ordinary object, and place it in the middle of the circle of children. If you are in a classroom, you might select a stapler, a book, a cup of pencils, or any other "ordinary" object. In a clinic setting, you might choose a box of toys, a vase of flowers, a figurine, or a sofa pillow.

> "When we look with mindful awareness, we see more clearly all the different thoughts that run around in our minds. We may see when our own self-critical or judgmental thoughts are making it harder to deal with whatever is happening in our lives. Being kind to ourselves when we become aware of those judging thoughts might make things a little easier. In this activity, we will continue giving our attention to the things we see around us and the things we see inside us to help cultivate greater clarity and awareness. Seeing clearly, we can see more choices. We might discover some great opportunities to make mindful choices."

Go around the circle and invite each child to describe one thing about what he or she sees. Each child should describe something unique about the object—something that no other child has already noted. Given that each child is seeing the object from a different angle, they are all actually seeing a slightly different object, so coming up with unique descriptors generally is not too difficult. If a child names the object without describing it, gently invite him or her to describe the color, texture, size, shape, or other quality. If the group has more than 8–10 children, you might prefer to break into two smaller groups for this activity.

Additional Questions for Children/Teens

- "Were you looking at this object in a different way than the way you normally look at things around you?"
- "If so, what was different?"
- "How could you bring this same quality of seeing into your everyday life?"
- "How might doing this be helpful to you?"

Challenges and Tips

- Select an object that is large enough for all the children to see easily.
- An object that has some complexity makes it easier to describe the activity.
- Be attentive should the children begin labeling, naming, or judging instead of describing.
- You might ask the kids to write their observations down as part of a writing assignment, or to draw or paint the details of what they see.

Suggested Practice Activities

- A similar seeing and describing activity can be done at home with family members.
- Children might try to notice at least one new thing each day.

Children can practice seeing new things in familiar settings using the *Finding Five New Things* handout.

Activity 26. Mindfulness of Pleasant Events

The world is full of magic things, patiently waiting for our senses to grow sharper.
—WILLIAM BUTLER YEATS

Time Requirement

Variable (home practice activity).

Theme

When we make a conscious choice to be present with our experiences, we open ourselves to opportunities to discover more pleasant events in our daily lives.

Background

A surprising number of pleasant events may be discovered each day just by looking for them. Noticing the small moments of daily pleasure that we often overlook allows us to enjoy the things that are right in our lives, instead of becoming stuck in what may not be going well. What's more, when we look for pleasant things on purpose for a while, we also start looking for them unintentionally too, eventually shifting our whole outlook.

Materials Needed

- Activity handout: *Mindfulness of Pleasant Events.*
- Mindfulness journal.

Mindfulness Activity

Invite the children to keep a "pleasant events record" that notes at least one pleasant event that happens each day for 1 week. Explore what these events might have in common. Practicing mindfulness of pleasant events is a practice of bringing awareness to how often we label and judge events, and understanding how all this judging changes what we experience.

Additional Questions for Children/Teens

- "Have you noticed the mind's tendency to label almost everything that happens as 'pleasant' or 'unpleasant,' 'good' or 'bad'?"
- "Have you noticed that we try to hang onto things we label as being 'pleasant,' and we try to get rid of things we decide are 'unpleasant'?"
- "What makes an event 'pleasant' or 'unpleasant'?"
- "Is it possible to experience pleasant moments even when we have difficulties in our lives?"
- "Can we feel sad or be in pain and still enjoy some pleasant events?"

Challenges and Tips

If you are working with children who are clinically depressed, you may see some resistance when suggesting that they look for pleasant events. Be aware that cognitive negativity is a symptom of depression and likely to color children's beliefs about themselves (e.g., "I don't deserve to be happy"), about their world (e.g., "Everything in my life is bad"), and about their expectations for the future (e.g., "Nothing good will ever happen to me"). One simple way to work with this cognitive negativity is to gently challenge children to schedule just one pleasant activity into their day. Brainstorm with them to help them select a specific activity, with a definite time and date to do this activity: for example, "On Saturday morning, I will watch my favorite cartoons with my best friend." Before the activity begins, they should rate how good they expect their mood to be after the activity, and then compare that to how they actually feel afterwards (10 = feels very good; 1 = feels very bad). Almost inevitably, they will underestimate their expected mood, which gives you an opportunity to explore with them the relationship between anticipatory thoughts and what actually happens.

You might make the activity playful for younger kids by suggesting they become detectives in their own lives, searching for pleasant and positive things. You might use a prop such as sunglasses to show how seeing things through smudged or dirty lenses compares to seeing them through clear lenses, which allows them to discover the positive.

Suggested Practice Activities

- After introducing children to vocabulary words associated with happiness (see Activity 43, Mindfulness of Happiness [Part I], pp. 124–125), you might ask them to rank the words in ascending order. For example, the list may start with *satisfied* and end with *ecstatic* or *on cloud nine*. There is no single correct ordering to the words. The purpose of this activity is to help children understand that emotions exist on a continuum and that words correspond to a range of emotional states.

- Ask children to label the type of happiness and to rate the amount of happiness (on a scale of 1–10) they might feel if they:
  - Overheard their best friend telling other children that they are kind and caring person.
  - Were given the new phone for which they had been wishing.
  - Found a dollar on the street.
  - Got to meet their favorite movie star, musician, author, or sports hero.
  - Received a compliment from a teacher or coach whom they really liked.
  - Gave a piece of gum to a friend.
  - Watched their favorite television show.
  - Bicycled in the park.
  - Helped their friend figure out his or her math homework.
  - Went to the movies.
  - Got a hug and a kiss from their mom, dad, or another adult caregiver.
  - Visited a cousin or friend whom they really liked.

Ask children to assign a happiness word to each event. As children offer responses, elicit additional answers from other children. Point out that the same event might be experienced differently by different people. In fact, some events, like "gave a piece of gum" or "went to the movies" might not even be pleasant for children who don't like gum or movies! As children begin to understand that multiple feelings and thoughts are possible in response to every event, the idea is planted that there is no hard and fixed event–thoughts–feelings link. It's different for everyone, and also different depending on each person's mood on any day. As their understanding of the subjectivity of personal experience deepens, children will be introduced to the idea that they might be able to adopt novel or alternative thoughts and feelings in response to events that may have triggered autopilot reactions in the past.

Activity 27. Mindfulness of Unpleasant Events

Time Requirement

Variable (home practice activity).

Theme

Mindful awareness of unpleasant events lets us see how our own thoughts contribute to our felt experiences.

Background

Mindfulness doesn't just mean paying attention to the sights and sounds or activities going on around us. Practicing mindful awareness teaches us to pay attention to what's going on in our own minds. Being mindful of unpleasant events is a practice of bringing awareness to our own thoughts, feelings, and body sensations. This mindful focus deepens children's understanding that judgments of events contribute to the nature of the experience of those events. Simply observing and noting an event often creates a very different experience than reactively judging what is going on and then wanting the experience to be something different from what it is.

Materials Needed

- Activity handout: *Mindfulness of Unpleasant Events*.
- Mindfulness journal.

Mindfulness Activity

Explain to children the relationship between our thoughts/judgments and how we feel throughout each day:

"What exactly is it that makes an unpleasant event unpleasant? Our own thoughts about what we *want* to be happening or what we think *should* be happening can make almost any experience less pleasant. Sometimes the mood we're in can make even a nice experience feel unpleasant. To see if we are creating more stress or unhappiness for ourselves, we first bring our attention to our thoughts, expectations, and beliefs about what is going on, and then check in with ourselves to note our emotional reactions to the event. For example, when you hear an "unpleasant" sound, what makes that sound unpleasant? Is it because the sound really hurts your ears? Or is it because you have decided that the sound is not what you expected? Or is it not what you believe should be happening right now? Or is it that you decided it's something you don't like? As we practice bringing mindful awareness to all events—pleasant and unpleasant—we learn to sort out what is really happening from what we think.

"What we think can make almost any event more pleasant or more unpleasant. Are your thoughts and feelings adding unneeded stress or anxiety to a situation over which you have no control? Open all your senses to become aware of what else might be going on in this moment. Notice all the sights, sounds, and smells around you. Notice your own body sensations. Notice the other people around you. Looking with mindful awareness, we often discover that something in the present is pleasant. Thoughts *about* what is happening are different from what really *is* happening. Thoughts are not facts, and we don't need to believe everything we think."

Activity 28. Mindfulness of Discomfort

Time Requirement

10–15 minutes.

Themes

- Pleasant and unpleasant sensations, emotions, urges, and thoughts all come and go.
- When we turn toward discomfort, sometimes it changes the experience.
- Our uncomfortable feelings may differ depending on the situation we are in.

Background

This group activity uses the discomfort of holding ice cubes to explore the impermanence of mental and physical discomfort. It also helps kids understand how their cognitive, emotional, and behavioral responses to discomfort can change their felt experiences.

Materials Needed

Cups, ice cubes, and napkins or paper towels for each participant.

Mindfulness Activity

Hand each child or teen a paper towel and a small paper cup containing an ice cube. Instruct the kids to just wait until every child receives a paper towel and an ice cube, practicing mindful awareness by noting their cognitive, emotional, and physical responses to wondering what activity is in store. Then explain the activity.

"For the next minute, we will just be mindfully aware of the sensations of holding this ice cube."

The children might giggle or look nervous. Feel free to ask them about their own reactions and to notice how those reactions might differ from the reactions of their classmates.

"Everyone, pick up your ice cube and hold it in your hand. Just noticing the sensations of holding the ice itself. What sensations are you noticing in your hand? What emotions are present? What actions do you feel like taking? What thoughts are you having? What are you doing with all of these thoughts and feelings and urges?"

After 1 minute (or other specified time), or once the ice has melted, allow the kids to dry their hands, clean up, and then reflect, working toward insights about impermanence, discomfort, and dislike.

Additional Questions for Children/Teens

- "What sensations did you experience? Just cold? Did it feel itchy or burning? Were the sensations constant or changing? Were they refreshing or uncomfortable?"
- "Did your feeling at the beginning (e.g., if you were hot or cold already) influence your reaction?"
- "What happened when you focused on the sensation directly? What is different from when you focused on something else, like your breath?"
- "How did you feel emotionally? Frustrated? Scared? Excited [if it's a hot day]? Irritated? Something completely different?"
- "What actions did you want to take? What urges did you notice? Did you want to show off, laugh, drop the ice, distract yourself?"
- "What thoughts did you have during the activity?"
- "How did you get through the discomfort? Did you ignore it? Did you focus on something else?"
- "What did you learn about how you deal with discomfort or dislike? What did you notice about how other people handled discomfort?"
- "Do you think you might feel or act differently if you were alone, if you were around different people, or if the temperature in the room were different? If so, why?"
- "Was it harder or easier to hold the ice when we told you it was for just 1 minute? Do you think that your feelings might have changed if we had told you to hold it as long as possible? Why do you think that?"

The central lessons that usually emerge include recognizing and tolerating feelings and urges, as well as recognizing that our own reactions to discomfort can actually change the experience. This exercise also offers lessons in impermanence, as whatever we wish and whatever we do, the ice cube will eventually melt anyway.

Activity 29. Mindfulness of Urges: Urge Surfing

> You can't stop the waves, but you can learn to surf.
> —JON KABAT-ZINN

Time Requirement

10–15 minutes.

Themes

- Strong urges can arise for just about anything—foods, substances, harmful or self-harming behaviors.
- We can locate these urges in the body and practice working through them, seeing that they don't actually last forever.

Background

All humans have basic urges and needs "wired" into us, like eating, sleeping, and self-protection. When we get into habits that may be abusive, such as self-harming or addictive behaviors, or using alcohol or drugs, these behaviors can become almost as compelling as our basic needs for food and sleep. The good news is that we can rewire our brains to *tolerate* and *respond,* rather than react, to these urges. We can locate urges first in our bodies and choose to manage them there, before they go up to our brains, where our thoughts can take over our behavior and get us into trouble. Here we practice by thinking about food, but any other urge could become the focus. In the addiction literature, this technique is known as *urge surfing* (Marlatt & Gordon, 1985).

Mindfulness Activity

"Allow your eyes to close (if you feel comfortable) and whenever you're ready, visualize yourself in front of a plate of your absolute most favorite food. Have you got something in mind? Pizza? Mac and cheese? Ice cream? Your favorite candy? Give a thumbs up when you have something clearly in mind. [Pause until everyone has raised a hand.]

"There it is on the plate, looking completely perfect, the exact amount you want to eat, and a fork and napkin are waiting for you to just begin digging in to this favorite meal. You can smell it, almost taste it, and you know exactly what the taste and sensations will be as you cut or scoop a bite, bring it into your mouth, and begin to enjoy the flavors filling your mouth.

"Now notice what happens in your body. Maybe your mouth waters and your stomach growls. What else is happening, and where? If there are a few spots, focus on the most intense place. Where in your body do you feel the physical urge for this food?

"In your mind's eye, don't try to smother the urge, just find where it is. It might take a moment, so just keep scanning through your body, looking for it. It might feel like movement in one spot, or perhaps tension somewhere, or a tugging feeling, a warmth or a tingling, or maybe something else entirely. Just explore, discover, and then focus on the urge sensations.

"If your mind begins to make a story or chatters about giving in to the urge, just go back to the body sensations. Maybe keeping your mind busy using descriptive words to describe the sensations as they rise and fall.

"Now, just try to continue to relax your body around the urge spot, breathing into it, as you watch yourself breathing in and breathing out.

"Staying with your breath, as you hold the image in your mind and the urge in your body. Just watching as the sensations rise and fall, change and shift, like a surfer on the waves, and eventually . . . slowly beginning to fade like a wave being drawn back into the ocean.

"When the sensations have faded, take a moment to thank yourself for getting through this urge."

Encourage the group members to identify and share where in their bodies they felt the urges and the sensations that accompanied them, while noting that everyone experiences urges differently. You may also wish to discuss the "life cycle" of an urge, explaining that even the strongest urges can never harm us, and only rarely do they ever last more than a few minutes.

If you feel comfortable doing so, you might lead a conversation about surfing through other urges, such as acting out anger, risky or self-harming behaviors, using drugs or alcohol, overeating, or any other challenging urges with which kids might struggle. You might also brainstorm other, more helpful, actions that can be taken when an urge strikes. Explore ways to manage the urge, distract from it, or simply wait for it to fade. Encourage the kids to identify times they might use this practice, emphasizing the importance of starting with smaller or less intense urges.

Additional Questions for Children/Teens

- "Where in the body does the urge start to grow? What does it feel like?"
- "As you keep watching the urge, notice how it changes. Did it feel different? If so, in what way?"
- "How can bringing awareness to body sensations of urges help us make different choices when we feel an urge?"
- "What things might make the urge stronger, or what might help it fade?"
- "How long did it take for the urge to start to lose its power?"
- "Do different urges feel different or come from different places?"
- "Do words or thoughts or emotions also come up with the urges?"

Challenges and Tips

We recommend not using food urges for this activity when working with children or teens struggling with restrictive eating disorders such as anorexia nervosa, as it could be misused to further restrict food intake. For therapists working with clients who are struggling with overeating, bulimia, or other binge-eating disorders, however, it could be very helpful.

Some kids may become too triggered if you encourage them to explore urges stronger than food (e.g., self-harming behaviors), so consult with a mental health professional and recommend that kids practice mindfulness around those urges with a professional. Before ending the session, you might invite the kids to do some breathing or walking to let go of any lingering feelings. You might ask the kids to imagine a peaceful calmness entering their bodies with each inbreath, and all the frustration and stress flowing out of their bodies with each outbreath. Remind them that they can always choose to tune into their breath or bodies when they find themselves being triggered by their urges.

Suggested Practice Activities

Help the children brainstorm and record in their mindfulness journals a list of thoughts or behaviors that they can use to calm themselves when they feel a strong urge. These choices might include the following:

- "Take a few deep, calming breaths."
- "Practice the mindful breath counting activity."
- "Look for more realistic or calming thoughts without adding more frustrating thoughts."
- "Check in with yourself to see if what you're telling yourself is totally true."
- "Ask yourself, 'Is what I'm telling myself right now really helpful to me?'"
- "Talk to a trusted friend or adult."
- "Remind yourself that no matter how triggered you feel, it will pass."
- "Burn off the urge with exercise."
- "Change locations, or even just add or change the music, lighting, clothing, or temperature; the change in the cues around you can reduce the urge."
- "Listen to music, comedy, or a podcast."
- "Ask yourself how you will feel in an hour, a day, or a week, or ask yourself more about the situation if you give in to the urge. How will you feel if you don't?"

Activity 30. The Mindful STOP

Time Requirement

5 minutes.

Themes

- Sitting in a mindful posture.
- Checking in with our experiences in the present moment.
- Making wise and skillful choices.

Background

For kids of all ages, we are introducing them to the idea of regularly pausing and making contact with the present moment—observing what is happening around and within them—then using that clear awareness to make a decision about what action to take. We call this activity the *Mindful STOP.**

Materials Needed

None.

Mindfulness Activity

We often find our thoughts racing to the past or the future, or wandering off somewhere else, distracted by the world around us and inside of us. Or we may get so caught up in strong emotions that we aren't thinking too clearly. At these times, we can choose to pause to observe

*Adapted from Stahl and Goldstein (2010) with permission from New Harbinger Publications.

what is happening in this moment and regain our mindful awareness. We can always find a few moments in our busy day to follow the acronym *STOP*.

<u>S</u> *is for STOP*

"Simply *stop* whatever it is that you are doing right now."

<u>T</u> *Is for Take a Breath*

"Allow yourself to *take one deep mindful breath*. Feeling the sensations of the breath going all the way in on the inhale and all the way out on the exhale. Or, just focus on the place in your body where you most feel the breath for one entire inhale and exhale."

<u>O</u> *Is for Observe*

"*Observe* what is happening right now. *Observe* your surroundings in the present moment. *Observe* what is happening in your body and mind in this present moment."

<u>P</u> *Is for Plan and Proceed*

"With a clear mind from stopping and taking a breath, and information from your observations about the present, what should be your *plan* for what to do next as you *proceed* with your day?"

Challenges and Tips

Children might want to write down or share aloud their observations and plans when they use the Mindful STOP, and discuss times they might find it useful.

Suggested Practice Activities

Encourage kids to take a mindful stop at transition times or at potentially triggering moments in the day and in their lives in and outside of school. You can even make it something of a game, holding up a stop sign at random, or put a stop sign reminder up in your classroom or office or around the school building, moving it occasionally, suggesting that the kids practice a Mindful STOP whenever their minds wander and their gazes fall on the sign.

Activity 31. Mindful Listening and Speaking

Time Requirement

10–20 minutes.

Themes

- Our minds are often filled with our own thoughts while we listen to others.
- Listening to others with mindful awareness increases understanding and connection.

Background

We often listen to others speak while also paying attention to a constant stream of our own internal commentary. This consists of thoughts, memories, beliefs, expectations, judgments, criticisms, analyses, or opinions about what we hear. We sometimes listen while planning what to say in response. We sometimes are thinking about how to interject our own ideas as quickly as possible. When this happens, we are not really listening. Truly *listening to* another person is more than just waiting for them to finish speaking. If we are not connected with the person speaking, we may miss a lot of what he or she is saying. We might misunderstand the feeling or the intention behind the words. When listening with mindful awareness, we practice being fully present to what we are hearing, without attending to our own mind chatter. We listen with spacious awareness, letting go of our assumptions or beliefs about what the other person is saying. We sit in our own still, quiet space, while opening our hearts and minds to really hearing everything that the other person is saying.

It is normal to see the world through the lens of our own experiences, personality, culture, and beliefs. When we listen with care and respect for what another is saying, it's easier to understand a situation from someone else's point of view. It does not mean we have to agree with him or her, just that we accept that someone else may have a different view of a situation than we do. To truly hear and remember, our minds need to be calm, open, alert, and receptive. Mindful listening is an active and engaged process that is cultivated with practice. It helps us be fully present with another person. When we practice mindful listening, we offer the gift of our attention, which moves us closer to each other.

Materials Needed

None.

Mindfulness Activity

For this activity, split the group into pairs, preferably creating dyads that will be comfortable with each other, but not so comfortable and close that they won't be able to focus. Give each pair as much space as the room allows. Invite the pairs to sit facing each other. Whoever is younger will be the first speaker. These roles will be switched in the second part of the activity, so everyone will have an opportunity to experience both perspectives. Select one question that everyone in the group will use. You might start with a clear and relatively simple question, such as "What is something that I probably don't know about you?," that can help them understand the activity. You can then dive into any age-appropriate topic that you think would be meaningful to the children. These questions should require more thought and care in order to answer. Some examples follow:

- "What qualities do you most like about yourself?"
- "If you could have a superpower, what would it be?"
- "What makes you feel good about yourself?"
- "What makes your life meaningful?"
- "What do you value?/What is important to you?"

- "What brings you great happiness?"
- "What are your hopes and dreams?"

You may want to point out that this is a practice of both mindful speaking and mindful listening. When you are speaking, you can practice being mindful of what you're saying, being open and honest with your partner. When you are listening, you can practice just listening and observing what it is like to listen with your full mindful attention.

Invite the first listener to look directly at his or her partner and ask the question. As the first speaker responds, the listener gives his or her mindful attention to the answer, and then responds by saying only, "Thank you." Nothing else. Then the listener asks the same question again, listens to the response, and again says only "Thank you." This process is repeated until the bell is rung. Make sure to be clear that one partner is repeatedly asking the *same* question and the other is repeatedly answering—this is not a back-and-forth dialogue. When the bell rings, the roles are switched so that the person who was the listener now becomes the speaker. The same question is asked for both parts of the activity.

Depending on the age of the children, each half of the activity should last from 1 to 5 or 6 minutes. If necessary, remind the listeners that they are not to respond to what the speakers are saying, but should simply listen with mindful attention. Time permitting, you can repeat this activity a few times, changing around the dyads and using different questions.

Additional Questions for Children/Teens

- "What was it like to be quiet and simply listen to your partner?"
- "Did you find that you got distracted while listening to him or her?"
- "Did you feel yourself wanting to respond to what he or she just said?"
- "What were your own thoughts doing while you were listening?"
- "How did it feel in your body to be still while listening to another person?"
- "What was it like to say something that is important to you when you know that the other person is listening very closely?"
- "Were you also conducting an internal dialogue with yourself, maybe even judging or criticizing yourself for what you said?"
- "What did you notice about your partner's body language, breath, tone of voice, listening, and speed of speaking? What might those communicate?"
- "Do you feel more connected to your partner? What does that feel like?"

Challenges and Tips

Although even very shy, socially anxious, or depressed children generally are fine participating in this paired listening activity, some may be less comfortable sharing their experiences with the larger group. For teachers, in particular, this may call for a mental shift from your usual classroom style; however, we encourage you to cultivate the habit of inviting children to speak, rather than calling on individual children to answer specific questions. In doing so, you help to create a sense of safety and model each child's freedom to choose his or her own level of participation.

Suggested Practice Activities

- "Early morning offers a wonderful opportunity to practice mindful listening. As you wake up, instead of checking your phone or turning on the TV, take a few minutes to lie still and just listen. In a rural setting, the sounds around you may be of birds or animals waking up, or the sounds of water from a nearby creek or waterfall. If you are in an apartment or condo in a city, you may hear a garbage truck, traffic sounds, or perhaps the sound of a lawnmower or building construction outside the building. In any setting, you may hear sounds inside the building—voices talking, footsteps in the hallway outside, or the sound of a door opening or closing. Listen carefully for the small sounds—a bee buzzing, a cat purring, wind rustling in the leaves through an open window; the quiet tap-tap of your dog's paws walking across the room. Practice bringing mindful awareness to one sound until it fades away, and then letting another sound enter your awareness. As best you can, observe when thoughts come into your mind, then just let them go and return to listening with your full attention.

- "You might try listening with mindful awareness to someone else's conversation—without focusing on the words or the content of what is being said. Maybe there are two people talking next to you on the school bus, for example. Listen for the emotion underneath the words. What is being communicated by the rhythm of the words? Or the person's inflection or tone of voice? We communicate so much without words.

- "Listen with mindfulness and compassion to the people in your life. Henry David Thoreau (1863) once said, 'The greatest compliment that was ever paid me was when one asked me what I thought and attended to my answer' (p. 484). Really listening to what is being said allows each of us to feel less vulnerable and freer to speak openly and authentically. Not listening to each other creates disagreement and disconnection, which is always unpleasant.

- "To listen mindfully to another person, stop whatever else you're doing, breathe naturally, and simply listen, without having your own agenda. Really listen to what is being said. When thoughts about other things arise, or the mind distracts you with its need to comment about what's being said, gently let the thoughts go and return your attention to the person speaking. Listen for the feelings being communicated too. And when you are speaking, if the person you're talking to doesn't seem to be listening attentively to you . . . well, it's a good opportunity to be kind. As Winnie the Pooh wisely said, 'It may simply be that he has a small piece of fluff in his ear.'"

ACTIVITY 25 HANDOUT. Finding Five New Things

When I'm at home, all the things around me feel very familiar because I see them every day. I may see these things so much that my mind goes onto autopilot mode, and then I'm not really seeing them anymore. When I practice bringing mindful awareness to the things around me, I may notice all kinds of things that I have never before seen. This week, I have discovered five new and interesting things in or around my home.

Example: I saw a bunch of wavy brown lines on the rug in my living room. I always saw the flowers pattern on it, but then I looked closer and saw these thin brown wavy lines. Each line is about 3 inches long and they go in all directions.

1. _____
   _____
   _____
   _____

2. _____
   _____
   _____
   _____

3. _____
   _____
   _____
   _____

4. _____
   _____
   _____
   _____

5. _____
   _____
   _____
   _____

Mindfulness of Pleasant Events

Name: _____ Date: _____

Practice bringing mindful awareness to one pleasant event each day makes each day pleasant.

Note your thoughts, feelings, and body sensations on this form.

The event	What were your thoughts?	What were you feeling?	What were your body sensations?
Example: Watched a girl playing in the park with her dog.	She's having a lot of fun. The dog is too.	Happy, cheerful.	I smiled and laughed.
Sunday			
Monday			
Tuesday			
Wednesday			
Thursday			
Friday			
Saturday			

ACTIVITY 27 HANDOUT. Mindfulness of Unpleasant Events

You are practicing bringing mindful awareness to an unpleasant event. Why did you choose this event? What about this event makes it unpleasant?

Day	Where you are, what you're doing, and what is happening right now?	What are you seeing, hearing, seeing, smelling, tasting, or touching?	What were the thoughts and feelings as you listened to the sounds around you?	How did your body feel during this experience?	How do your thoughts affect what you're feeling or doing?
Example: Saturday	Lying in bed in the early morning. A big garbage collection truck has stopped right outside my window.	Hearing loud clanging and banging sounds of cans being emptied. Bad smell of trash. Horribly loud grinding of the machine compacting garbage.	I'm angry! Why do they have to stop right in front of my window? Don't they know it's Saturday? This isn't fair. Everyone is trying to sleep. I wish they would go away.	Teeth clenched. My eyes are closed tight. Curled up in a ball with my fingers in my ears.	Angry thoughts aren't going to change what's happening. Just remembering that they'll go away soon could help me calm down and get back to sleep.

83

Sensory-Based Mindfulness Activities

Group 5 offers sensory-based practices that can an easier anchor of attention or focus than breathing or some of the other activities from earlier sections, especially when the mind feels dull or very agitated. Our five senses make for good anchors because sensations always happen in the present, even as thoughts or worries race to the past or future, or somewhere else altogether. What's more, short sensory-based practices can be grounding for kids who struggle with the breath or body activities because of intense anxiety or a traumatic history. Every child and teen can find at least one or two sensory practices that they can enjoy integrating into their lives as a way of getting out of their heads and returning to the present.

Activity 32. Mindful Eating (Part I)

Time Requirement

15–20 minutes.

Themes

- Mindfulness is a different way of engaging with the world.
- Thoughts, feelings, and body sensations combine with external events to create unique subjective experiences.

Background

Because eating is something that is done several times a day without much awareness, this activity is a particularly useful way to highlight how much of our time we spend on autopilot. Eating with mindful awareness helps young people understand what changes may emerge when a small, everyday act is done slowly and with careful attention to the experience. Understanding that mindfulness changes our perceptions and felt experiences is an essential first step to developing an experiential understanding of it. This mindful eating activity teaches children a new way of relating to their experiences.

The discussion that follows provides an opportunity to contrast mindful eating with their usual autopilot way of doing things. With all mindfulness activities, our goal is to foster an experiential understanding first and then to develop children's intellectual understandings afterward. Explanations of each activity should be kept very brief. It is generally better to say too little rather than too much. In the spirit of embodying mindfulness, we strive to convey an attitude of nonjudgmental acceptance and curiosity in our own speech, body language, and behaviors. We also encourage asking open-ended questions and inviting participation rather than calling on a specific child to respond. One of the biggest challenges for some teachers is to take off their "teacher hats," letting go of the idea that there are "right" and "wrong" answers. There are no "right" or "wrong" thoughts, emotions, or body sensations. Thoughts are thoughts. Emotions are emotions. Body sensations are body sensations. Our only task is to bring children's attention to these internal experiences, as best we can, while also helping them to describe whatever is present—with acceptance—whether they happen to like it or not.

Materials Needed

- A small box of raisins, enough for each child to have 3 or 4 raisins.
- Bowl and spoon (for hygiene).
- Chart paper and markers.
- Mindfulness journals.

Vocabulary

Observing or describing words: *sweet, spicy, salty, bland, crispy, sticky, chewy, crunchy, slimy, smooth, bitter, sour, chalky, juicy, dry, acidic, tender, tough, nutty, creamy, soft, hard, tart.*

Mindfulness Activity

Each child is given a few raisins to hold in his or her hand. Ask the kids not to eat the raisins just yet. Explain that this activity is conducted in complete silence, but there will be opportunities afterward to discuss their experiences.

> "Today, we explore mindfulness using the sense of taste. We will practice eating while using all five of our senses to increase our mindful awareness of the experience. Together, we will discover what might be different in our experiences when we bring mindfulness to the ordinary experience of eating.
>
> "Hold the raisins in your hands; look at them carefully. As best you can, watch for memories or images that may arise as I guide you through the activity. Observe when your thoughts are memories, not about what's here in your hand right now. Check in with your emotions and note the different sensations in your body."

Then verbally guide the children through the activity. The following script* can be read, but we encourage you instead to use this and the other sample scripts we offer as learning

---

* From Semple and Lee (2011, p. 129). Reprinted with permission from New Harbinger Publications.

tools. It's always better to use your own words, discover your own voice, and use your own experiences of mindful eating to guide your practices.

"What is your experience of holding this object in your hand? Looking at it very carefully . . . as if you are describing it to a Martian who has never seen one before. [pause] As best you can, note the thoughts or images that come up as you look at this object. [pause] Practice noting that they are just thoughts, and then gently return your attention to the object. [pause], Exploring it with your eyes, noting its colors . . . and any patterns. [pause] Exploring it with your fingers. [pause] Does the object feel dry or moist? Noting if it's bumpy or smooth . . . soft or hard. Is the texture the same all over the object? How heavy is it? [pause] Exploring the object with your nose and ears . . . Does this object have any smells? (pause) Does it make any sounds? [pause] With our senses, bringing all of your attention to this object lying in the palm of your hand.

Whenever you're ready, you may place the object in your mouth. I invite you to practice exploring it with your tongue. [pause] Does it taste or feel different in different parts of your mouth when you roll it around? [pause] Is your mouth watering in anticipation of eating the object? What are you tasting before you bite into it? What are you smelling? What are you hearing? Is the texture changing the longer it's in your mouth? [pause] As best you can, keep attending to this object while noting thoughts, feelings, and body sensations. Are the thoughts looking forward to swallowing this object and eating another? Are they attending to all the varied sensations of the one that is in your mouth? Are the thoughts somewhere else altogether?

Bringing your attention back . . . gently biting the object . . . tasting its flavors. [pause] Noting if the textures on the inside are different from the outside . . . bringing awareness to changes in the moistness or flavor. [pause] Slowly chewing the object while noting the sensations. [pause] As you swallow, bringing awareness to the sensations as it slides down your throat. Following the object all the way down to your stomach. [pause] Then, bringing attention back to the sensations in your mouth, noting what's there. Are there different tastes or flavors in your mouth now? Are your thoughts still here with this experience? [pause] Feeling now that your body is exactly one raisin heavier than it was a few minutes ago."

Discussion

Afterward, guide a discussion that focuses on describing the thoughts, feelings, and body sensations just experienced. Move the discussion away from an intellectualized evaluation of the experience. Children often describe differences between the way they ate the raisin during the activity and their normal ways of eating. They may comment on how much sweeter the flavor seemed. They share small, unexpected discoveries about raisins that they had never noticed. This theme can open up discussions about what else we might be missing when we are either on autopilot or are busy prejudging.

You may wish to look for opportunities to note that paying attention in this particular way (i.e., intentionally, in the present moment, and without judgment) might actually change the quality of the experience. Mindfulness can intensify our perceptions. Colors may appear more vivid, sounds clearer, flavors richer or sweeter, or scents and sensations more vibrant. Mindfulness helps us become more aware of things of which we were not previously aware. Look also for opportunities to emphasize the difference between describing an experience and evaluating or judging the experience: ruminating about, analyzing, or comparing the experience to other experiences. Gradually, children become aware that they modify much of their present-moment experiences by adding memories, beliefs, or expectations to the actual experience.

In addition to this verbal exploration of the experience, it can be helpful to chart thoughts, feelings, and body sensations on paper. As shown in this example, filling in the chart allows children to see clearly that each person brings his or her own subjectivity into every experience.

EXAMPLE CHART

Event	Description of taste	Thoughts	Feelings	Body sensations
Child A: Eating a raisin	Sweet, juicy, chewy, sugary	This is really good. I want more raisins.	Happy, excited	Mouth waters, lips curve up in smile, tongue licks lips, belly growls.
Child B: Eating a raisin	Sticky, mushy, bitter, dry	I don't like raisins at all. They taste nasty.	Disgusted, disappointed	Nose wrinkles, lips close, throat is tight, belly feels upset.

Additional Discussion Questions for Children/Teens

- "Was what you just did different from the way you usually eat? If so, what was different about it?"
- "That's really interesting that your mind kept wandering to other times you have eaten raisins. Did anyone else have a similar experience?"
- "What benefits might there be to practice eating every day with this same degree of mindful awareness?"
- "What did you learn about yourself or about the world around you by practicing mindful eating?"

Challenges and Tips

Sometimes a child might decide without tasting the raisin that he or she doesn't like raisins and doesn't want to eat even one of them. Requiring that he or she eat the raisin may backfire, but you definitely want to encourage the child to participate in the activity as best as he or she can. Invite the child to use each of their senses, watching the emotions and thoughts carefully as he or she considers eating the raisin—*before* deciding to taste or eat it. Help the child become aware of and better understand the tendency to mistake negative emotional prejudgments or expectations as being the actual experience. If the child ultimately does decide to eat the raisin, he or she may discover that the experience was not as bad as was expected.

As noted previously, we advise caution when conducting any activity involving food when working with children or teens struggling with restrictive eating disorders such as anorexia nervosa, as they could be misused to further restrict food intake. For therapists working with clients who are struggling with overeating, bulimia, or other binge-eating disorders, however, this and other mindful eating activities could be very helpful.

Suggested Practice Activities

- Mindful eating is about staying present, moment by moment, with each sensation that emerges—chewing, tasting, and swallowing—while we eat. When we begin to practice mindful eating, we try to remember not to judge ourselves when we notice our mind drifting away from the experience of eating. Instead, just keep returning to the sensations of the tastes, the textures, and the smells, involved in chewing and swallowing. Encourage the children to watch for when any autopilot judgments arise as they practice 5 or 10 minutes of mindful eating while they are at home or at school.

- Encourage the kids to share their experience of mindful eating with their family members and to invite them to join in eating one meal with full awareness. Mindful eating means eating with awareness; it means being aware not only of the food on the plate, but also of the full experience of eating.

Activity 33. Mindful Eating (Part II)

Time Requirement

10–20 minutes.

Theme

"Seasoning" our food with our own beliefs, judgments, and expectations can change what we experience when we eat.

Background

We continue to cultivate mindfulness by bringing attention to ordinary, everyday experiences that are often done on autopilot—habitually and with little awareness. We use experiential activities, dialogue, and Socratic questioning to provide opportunities to examine experiences of eating with mindful awareness, in contrast to similar activities that were done on autopilot. During the first mindful eating activity, we emphasized the subjectivity of experience by comparing different children's perceptions of eating one raisin—with each experience being seasoned with different judgments, beliefs, and expectations. In guiding this discussion of home-based experiences of mindful eating, we will explore how describing instead of judging might change how we interpret our experiences.

When a child notices differences between eating with mindfulness and his or her normal habit of eating, this new observation offers an excellent opportunity to reinforce the idea that just by intentionally bringing awareness to an experience, what is experienced may change. Mindfulness helps us become more aware of things that we had not previously noticed. In cultivating mindfulness, we become aware of both pleasant and unpleasant experiences that otherwise may just slip right by us. Letting the pleasant experiences pass by unnoticed means that our lives aren't as rich and happy as they might be. Being less aware of the unpleasant experiences means that we might miss opportunities to learn from those experiences.

Materials Needed

- Chart paper and markers.
- Mindfulness journals.
- One mandarin orange for each child (or other small food item).

Vocabulary

Judging words: *good, bad, tasty, nasty, delicious, terrible, stinky, yummy, yucky, disgusting, gross, nauseating, delightful, great, icky, horrible, awesome*

Mindfulness Activity

Start by eliciting several descriptions of children's experiences of mindful eating during the past few days. Help them identify and differentiate thoughts, feelings, and body sensations. The following example of a chart has an additional column (in relation to prior charts) for "judgments," which are now differentiated from descriptive thoughts. Explore how the judging thoughts might have influenced children's experiences. Help them explore what might change if they were simply to describe the experience instead of judging it.

EXAMPLE CHART

Event	Description	Thoughts	Feelings	Body sensations	Judgments
Child A: Chocolate cookie	Crunchy, dry, sweet, chocolaty, warm, sugary	This is a big cookie.	Happy, excited	Mouth waters, lips curve up in smile, licks lips with tongue, belly growls.	I love cookies. I want another one.
Child B: Chocolate cookie	Bitter, grainy, nutty, sticky	Chocolate is bitter. I don't know why anyone likes it.	Disgusted, disappointed	Nose wrinkles, throat is tight, belly queasy.	This cookie tastes nasty.

The next mindful eating practice can be done with a number of different food items. Make sure to check with parents or caregivers about food allergies before selecting any food item. If a child has any food allergies, you might ask the parent to provide a safe food item for that child. We often use mandarin oranges (sometimes called clementine oranges or cuties). These are small enough for children to hold and are complex enough to make them interesting to explore. We haven't yet had any issues with a child being allergic to them. Comparing the bitterness of the outer peel with the sweet flesh inside also offers opportunities to explore both positive and negative judgments. Offer verbal guidance similar to the script shown in the previous mindful eating activity, but with greater focus on observing when the mind is describing versus when it's evaluating or judging the experience, ruminating about or analyzing the experience, or comparing it to other similar experiences.

Additional Discussion Questions for Children/Teens

You can embody mindfulness simply in the way you word your questions and how you choose to respond to children's descriptions—with interest, curiosity, and nonjudgmental acceptance. *Why* questions are generally not as helpful as asking concrete, specific questions that begin with *what* or *how*. For example, asking, "Why didn't you like the orange?" moves the child out of describing the experience into an intellectualized thinking about the experience. These types of questions also implicitly accept the child's judgmental stance without encouraging exploration of what defined the experience as "unpleasant" rather than "pleasant." Alternatively, by asking questions such as "How did you know you didn't like it? How did your body and mind respond to that sour taste?," you invite the child to explore the discrete sensations and help him or her observe how the judgments and sensations interact to create the subjective experience.

As you frame your questions, it's helpful to be consistent in assuming that the act of experiencing and our judgments about that experience are not the same thing. Thoughts are not the experience. In this way, children begin to develop awareness of how they alter their present-moment experiences by adding their own beliefs, expectations, and judgments to the experience.

Continue to explore what benefits there might be to eating with mindful awareness. For example, when parents require them to eat something they don't like, they may discover that describing instead of judging actually makes the experience a little less unpleasant. You might even hear, "It wasn't as bad as I thought."

Suggested Practice Activities

- How many different things do we do every day while on autopilot? What other everyday activities might be done with greater mindfulness? And what might change? Ask the kids to pick one chore that they don't much like to do and practice doing it every day for the next 5 days with mindful awareness. They might discover that even mindfully washing dishes or mindfully taking out the trash can be interesting experiences. Encourage them to watch carefully to see what changes in their thoughts and to note their observations in their mindfulness journal.

- Facilitators can try using different foods aimed at eliciting different responses. Pleasant foods might include sweets or desserts. Unpleasant foods might be ones that are spicy, or bitter, or of the vegetable category. This can lead to discussions about liking and disliking, or to a focus on how to recognize and deal with food-related anxieties. Strong foods like spicy cinnamon candies or mints can stimulate conversations about tolerating temporary discomfort, and how we each might deal with it differently. Eating hard candy or a lollipop without biting it can help kids focus, delay gratification, and have something of a contest that can be fun. Slowing down the eating of pleasant foods enhances awareness of urges and teaches impulse control. Eating candy or cake very slowly, or instructing kids not to taste the food at all (maybe as a contest), also develops attentional skills.

Activity 34. Mindful Seeing (Part I)

Don't just see, observe.
—Sherlock Holmes

Time Requirement

20–25 minutes.

Themes

- Much of the time we are on autopilot and miss a lot of what is around us.
- Mindful seeing is a practice that lets us learn more about ourselves and the world.
- Observing is not the same as naming, labeling, or judging what we see.

Background

When we observe the world around us with mindfulness, we pay attention to what we see (as best we can). As with our other senses, it is easy to fall into the practice of leaping ahead to a judgment about what we see, while not really attending to what is actually in front of us. We might see a "beautiful" bouquet of flowers or an "ugly" factory building. But how often do we slow down long enough to actually observe in detail and see with clarity the features of what we are looking at—its lines, shapes, colors, and textures—before we leap to a judgment about it? With practice, we learn to let go of the thoughts and judgments that we normally use to make sense of what we see. With practice instead of seeing a "pretty" tree or an "ugly" car, we simply see things as patterns of color, shape, and movement—just as they are. An essential first step in helping children gain a firsthand understanding of what mindful seeing entails is to help them understand better how our visual perceptions, thoughts, and memories are connected.

Materials Needed

- Drawing paper and colored pencils.
- Written vignette (to be read aloud by the facilitator).
- Mindfulness journals.

Vocabulary

Observing Words

- **Shapes:** *straight, curvy, curly, wavy, square, triangular, circular, almond, heart-shaped, jagged, sharp, line, edge, solid.*
- **Colors:** *blue, black, green, red, yellow, purple, orange, violet, indigo, white.*
- **Textures:** *rough, smooth, bumpy, flat, bright, dull, shiny, soft, hard, silky.*
- **Other:** *deep, shallow, clear, clouded, fuzzy, light, dark, dim.*

Optional Vocabulary Words

- *Objective* means not based on, or influenced by, personal feelings, tastes, or opinions.
- *Subjective* means based on, or influenced by, personal feelings, tastes, or opinions.

If you choose to integrate these optional vocabulary words into the activity, you may want to invite the group to consider other words that were discussed in earlier activities: for example, *describing, observing, labeling,* and *judging.* This is an opportunity to deepen children's understanding of the relationship between the words they use to describe their experiences and those felt experiences.

Mindfulness Activity

If the room is large enough to support this arrangement, ask each child to sit where he or she cannot see what other children are drawing. If that's not possible, just ask them not to look at others' drawings. Pass out the drawing paper and colored pencils. Invite the children to bring their minds into the present by closing their eyes (if they are comfortable doing so) while taking a few slow breaths in and out.

> "Today we will explore mindfulness using our eyes and sense of sight. By observing things with mindful awareness, we have the chance to see things that may be very familiar to us, like our desks or the chairs we are sitting in right now, in very different ways. The eyes that we have in our minds can also see things in different ways."

Then slowly read aloud the following brief vignette. Instruct the children to simply listen carefully during the first reading.

> "She opened the door and squinted to adjust her eyes to the dim light in the small room. She saw a bed against the left wall and two small windows on the right-hand wall opposite the bed. Curtains printed with dainty pink flowers framed the windows. She could tell that someone had slept in the bed last night because the covers were crumpled and tossed back, hanging over the edge of the bed. There was a pillow lying on the bare wooden floor. Then she noticed a number of framed photographs that hung on the wall directly ahead of her."

Invite each child to clearly visualize the scene you have just described. Then explain that you will read the description aloud a second time, while the children simultaneously draw the image that they see in their "mind's eye" of the scene that you're describing. Allow 5–10 minutes for drawing. Partway through, you may read the vignette for a third time.

After the children have finished their sketches, guide a group discussion about the experience. First ask for descriptions of the children's thoughts, feelings, and body sensations that were present during the experience of picturing and drawing this scene. What parts of the image were the most vivid or clear as they listened? How is seeing with the mind's eye different from seeing with our actual eyes? Then invite them to share their drawings with each other. In what ways is each picture different? For example, the color of the bedspread wasn't specified. How did each of the children choose what color to make it? How big were the "small" windows to different children? Did they add things that weren't in the description? Did they see other things in their minds' eyes? What elements in the description did they not "see" or perhaps chose to leave out?

You may use opportunities during the discussion to repeat the main message of this activity, which is that seeing something and interpreting what we see are actually two separate activities. Thoughts, labels, and judgments, along with our emotional responses, influence how we interpret what our eyes see.

Additional Discussion Questions for Children/Teens

- "What does it mean to see with mindful awareness?"
- "How is doing this different from what we do every day when we are looking, seeing, and observing?"
- "Could practicing mindful seeing in everyday life be helpful? If so, in what ways?"

Challenges and Tips

For children with anxiety or who may have less confidence in their drawing skills, it can be helpful to reassure them that the skill or artistry of the drawing is not important at all. This activity is meant to illustrate that our thoughts work together with our eyes to interpret what we see. With our thoughts, we construct our individual experiences.

Suggested Practice Activities

- Invite the children to visualize in their minds an object in their homes that is very familiar to them, perhaps something that they see or even use everyday. This could be a picture that hangs on the wall, a piece of furniture, a TV, toaster, computer, etc. Ask them to draw that object in their notebooks as accurately as they can see it in their mind's eye, including every detail they remember, as best they can. Then they should take the picture home and compare it to the real object. How did the thoughts and memories in the mind's eye make the drawing different from the real object? Did some parts get moved to a different place or left off altogether? What was forgotten and what was remembered? What did they notice about what was left out? Were things added that weren't actually there? How many times had they looked at this familiar object without really seeing it, just as it is? How might looking at the world around them with mindful awareness change what they see or remember? Invite children to look around the room and select one object to observe with mindful attention for about 15–20 seconds. At the end of that time, ask them to close their eyes and describe what they were looking at. How many of the words used are objective observations (noting or describing words) and how many are subjective observations (labeling or judging words)?

  Read a poem that encourages the kids to look around them in a different way. Some examples include the poem "Looking" by Robert Kelly, the first stanza of "The Blue Between" by Kristine O'Connell George, or the first few lines of "Auguries of Innocence (to See a World in a Grain of Sand") by William Blake. After reading the poem, facilitate a discussion of how the poem relates to mindful seeing. How does their imagination change

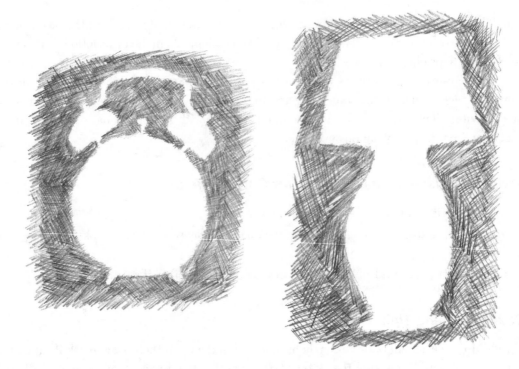

FIGURE II.1. Examples of negative space drawings.

the way they see the world? Why might two people see the same thing differently? Could their actual experience be different when they choose to see with mindful awareness?

Drawing negative space can be a challenging way to see objects with clarity by forcing us to look at them in a different way.

"Select any object that's in the room and then, without drawing an outline, fill in the space that surrounds that object using your pencil. It might be a chair, or a lamp, or a figurine sitting on a shelf. [Hold up the example in Figure II.1.] Or you might choose to draw the space around the scissors or stapler on your desk. Think of this activity as defining the boundaries of a shape using only what surrounds it. In other words, you aren't drawing the object but are simply creating an illusion of the object by filling in the space that surrounds it. Did you notice that the negative space changes its shape when you look at the object from a different vantage point?"

Activity 35. Mindful Seeing (Part II)

Time Requirement

20–25 minutes.

Themes

Without self-awareness, the chattering of the mind governs the way we see the world.

Background

The first aim of this activity is to demonstrate experientially that we can increase our awareness by bringing mindfulness to what we see. As we make the shift from autopilot to mindfulness, it is possible to see familiar objects as if we are seeing them for the first time. Mindfulness helps us learn to let go of labeling everything we see or trying to figure out if we like or dislike it. We learn to be more comfortable with what is actually happening. The second aim is to practice mindful seeing, while watching the judging thoughts that come into experience. Each time this happen, we simply note the act of judging and then gently return our awareness to describing the elements and characteristics of the form itself. In doing this, we practice seeing mindfully. This simple activity helps children understand the changes that can occur when an everyday act is performed with intention and with awareness of the experience. We practice *looking* so that we can learn how to *see*.

Materials Needed

- LCD projector (optional).
- Flip chart and markers.
- Mindfulness journals.
- Five to 10 color images (if you have a projector available) or paper prints of images of the facilitator's choice. It seems that, because the brain is such an efficient pattern detector (Siegel, 2007), the more realistic an image appears, the more difficult it can be to simply describe what is seen (e.g., shapes, colors, lines, textures). Instead, the brain puts together all those lines and colors and shapes, then labels what is seen as a specific object. The selected images can be shown in a sequence, from ones that are abstract expressionist to those that appear hyperreal, which creates an increasing level of difficulty to step back from labeling of the objects to simply describing what is seen. We suggest using the following images, in this order, to represent abstract expressionism to hyperrealism:

  1. Mark Rothko   *Saffron*
  2. Wassily Wassilyevich Kandinsky   *Dominant Curve*
  3. Lee Krasner   *Night Creatures*
  4. Pablo Picasso   *Three Musicians*
  5. Leonid Afremov   *Two Sisters*
  6. Edgar Degas   *Ballerina*
  7. Diego Rivera   *Delfina and Dimas*
  8. Michelangelo Merisi da Caravaggio   *Cardsharps*
  9. Edward Robert Hughes   *Oh, What's That in the Hollow?*
  10. Burt Monroy   *Lunch in Tiberon*

Vocabulary

- **Judging words:** *pretty, ugly, beautiful, gorgeous, fancy, unattractive, attractive, repulsive, gross, disgusting, cute, appealing, unappealing, crazy, scary, happy, etc.*

Review the optional vocabulary words:

- *Objective* means not based on, or influenced by, personal feelings, tastes, or opinions.
- *Subjective* means based on, or influenced by, personal feelings, tastes or opinions.

Mindfulness Activity

In this mindful seeing activity, children are asked to practice looking at a sequence of pictures purely as patterns of color, shapes, textures, and movement, rather than viewing the scene as a whole. You may need to help children to "see in the moment." By that we mean, reminding children that when they slip into labeling or naming the image as a whole, thinking about what is being seen (making inferences), or deciding if they like or don't like it, they can choose to gently bring their attention back to observing rather than judging, creating stories, or getting lost in memories, expectations, or emotions. This activity offers children the opportunity to view a series of paintings, practice describing them, and then discuss the thoughts, feelings, and body sensations that arose as they observed the paintings. For example:

"Today we will continue to explore mindfulness using our sense of sight. To practice mindful seeing, we're going to look at a number of different images."

Show the first slide or print (Rothko) and invite the children to silently observe it carefully for 1 minute (30 seconds is plenty for younger children). Then, leaving the image in sight, invite them to describe what their eyes are seeing. Encourage the children to use their observing words. Help them describe the colors, shapes, size, shadings, and textures that represent objective observations. Again, the intentions of the session can be shared: Seeing an object and judging an object are two different things. We can also emphasize that mindfulness increases the more we practice. You can complete a chart, as shown in the following example, while they share their comments.

EXAMPLE CHART

Image	Objective descriptions	Initial thought	Feelings	Bodily responses	Subjective judgments
1. Rothko	Orange, yellow, two rectangles with swirls, black dripping	It's simple.	Calm, quiet	Soft breath	I don't know why, but I really like this painting.
2. Kandinsky	Lots of colors, circles, boxes, curvy lines, busy	It looks cheerful.	Happy, energized	Smiling	This is weird, kind of crazy, but it's pretty.
3. Krasner	Black-and-white eyes with some splotches of brown	Those are eyes!	Nervous, scared	Frowning, teeth clenched	This is creepy. I don't like those eyes at all.

After the objective descriptions are shared, encourage the group to describe their subjective thoughts, feelings, body sensations, and then their judgments about the picture. Then show the next image (Kandinsky) and guide the children through the same process. Since each painting is progressively less abstract, it becomes more of a challenge for children to stick with descriptive, observational statements. Encourage them to be mindful of colors, shapes, the size and placement of the shapes, and even the width of the paint strokes. After objective observations (describing) are shared, then thoughts, feelings, and body sensations are elicited and recorded on the chart.

After repeating this with several pictures, invite the children to reflect on how mindful seeing might have been different with different images. What did it feel like to be restricted initially to sharing only objective observations? Was one of the paintings easier for them to view with mindful objectivity—that is, easier for them to use just their observing words? Did anyone notice that the mind jumped to labeling objects in the representational images before describing them? Is labeling another way of being on autopilot?

Variation for Younger Children

- The "peek through the holes" books by Tana Hoban include the *Look Book, Look Again, Look! Look! Look!, Just Look,* and *Take Another Look*. In these books, Hoban offers three chances to see ordinary objects in unusual ways. First, a cutout in a blacked-out page frames a detail on the next page. What is that wrinkled, hairy, gray thing? Turn the page and see the back end of an elephant; turn one more page and there it is in its entirety, nosing through some grass. An odd dingy square is really a lamb, and a geometrical object is the neck and frets of a guitar. Once children know what they are looking at, the book becomes a catalogue of familiar items. Using these books facilitates a discussion about seeing a part and seeing the whole of an object. What is happening in our mind as we try to make sense of what we see without having all the information?

Additional Discussion Questions for Children/Teens

- "Can our emotions influence the experience of seeing? If so, in what way?"
- "Can we see more when we practice mindful seeing?"
- "Can we respond to some things differently when we are practicing mindful seeing?"
- "Might there be things that we could learn about ourselves and the people around us by practicing mindful seeing?"

Suggested Practice Activities

- Invite children to bring a small item from home with which they have practiced mindful seeing to share with the other children. Place the item on a desk or chair and invite the child to share why they choose that item. Invite the other children to practice mindful seeing of this item. If the object is three dimensional, allow children to walk around and view the item from all directions. Remind them that the intention of this activity is to direct all of their attention to mindfully seeing the object—as if they have never seen it before and will later have to describe it to someone who has also never seen it before. If their minds become lost in other thoughts or they are drawn away by a sound, smell, movement, thought, or other distraction, just remind them to gently bring their attention back to seeing the object before them. Afterwards, invite a discussion about the experiences. How does mindful seeing differ from how they might usually look at the object? How does mindfully looking change the experience of seeing?

- Find an object that is relatively complex, perhaps a small piece of machinery or a visually complex picture. Ask children to mindfully observe the item for 30–60 seconds. Then put the item out of sight and ask children to draw the object or describe it with words. Then, bring the item back into view. Ask children how the object is different than what they remembered? Then spend another few moments observing the object with mindful attention.

- What differences do they notice from their "memory description"?
- What parts, if any, did they forget during their "memory description" of the item?
- Have they ever had the experience of remembering something differently than it actually is? If so, how do they think that happens?
- How do thoughts, memories, and feelings affect the way we see things?

• Encourage the practice of being mindful of surroundings. Ask the children to look around the room and find five things they noticed that are new to them—things that they never noticed before. For example:

"Did you notice that there is a red fire alarm box hanging on the wall by the door? . . . Did you notice what color my chair is? . . . How about the eye color of the person who is sitting next to you? . . . What is posted on the wall around you? . . . What color is the ceiling in this room?"

• Continue being mindful of the environment by asking the children to be explorers and look for new discoveries on their way home from the group.

"How many steps are there in one block? . . . Between two different houses that you walk past? . . . How many stops does the train or bus make before yours? . . . How many mailboxes can you find on your way home? . . . Can you discover flowers in five different colors along your route? . . . What is the most interesting thing you pass on your trip to school? . . . How does that thing change with the time of day, the weather, or the seasons?"

Activity 36. Mindful Touching

Time Requirement

20–25 minutes.

Themes

• We practice becoming aware of our tendencies to anticipate and judge all our experiences.
• Mindfulness helps us be better equipped to see the difference between our judgments about an experience and the experience itself.

Background

From a very early age, we all learn to make quick judgments about things for the purpose of avoiding pain or injury. Nearly all children have heard, "Don't touch that iron—it's hot and can burn you!" or "Stay away from the lawn mower—the blades are sharp and you might get hurt!" By getting hurt, we learn that it sometimes makes more sense to learn with our eyes rather than with our hands. Although these quick judgments are essential to our well-being and survival, they also strengthen the autopilot mode in which we function throughout much of the time. But the judgments we make are not only related to life-and-death experiences. We get goosebumps just thinking about what it will feel like to jump into a cold swimming pool. We learn to avoid things that might feel gooey or slimy or gross. The flip side is that we also tend to overlook many sensory experiences that can actually be really interesting. How often do we pay attention to the way the fabric of our clothes feels on our bodies? Or focus on feeling the breeze gently touching our faces? And, as with all the other senses, our present-moment experiences of touching are influenced by our memories and expectations.

Materials Needed

- Create five or six "feel boxes." Shoeboxes with lids work well for this activity. Cut a circle in the end of each box. Make the hole just large enough for each child to put his or her hand inside the box (about 3 inches in diameter). Label each box with only a letter or number. Opaque grab bags and gift bags can serve a similar purpose.
- Into the boxes place five or six small objects that have different textures. Examples include a wire scouring pad; a piece of velvet, silk, or fake fur; plastic bubble wrap; a smooth stone; sandpaper; a pumice rock or a pinecone. If there are washing facilities at hand, objects can be selected that are likely to elicit strong emotional responses: for example, peeled grapes, a bowl of cold spaghetti, or a bowl of gelatin pieces. Place one object in each box.
- Flip chart paper, markers.

Vocabulary

- **Observing words:** *sharp, smooth, prickly, pointy, rough, soft, hard, hot, cold, warm, slippery, gooey, spongy, springy, wet, dry, sticky, slick, slimy, furry, fuzzy.*
- **Judging words:** *relaxing, pleasant, nice, yucky, icky, disgusting, gross, messy, good, hurtful, painful, soothing, bad.*

Mindfulness Activity

During this activity, children will be touching various objects and exploring the tactile sensations as they bring their attention to the thoughts and feelings elicited when touching the objects. By exploring how each child subjectively experiences the same object, the children will deepen their understanding of how their own memories and expectations color their experiences. Line up the "feel boxes" on a long counter or table with enough space between them for a child to stand in front of each box. Explain that every box holds an object for everyone to feel with his or her hand. They should not try to look into the box. Line the children up and allow each child 30–60 seconds to explore what is in the box in front of him or her with his or her fingers. Then move to the next box and repeat, until every child has had an opportunity to explore every box. You might remind the children that there should be no talking during the activity. Following is an example of how to explain this activity to the group:

> "Today we will get to practice mindfulness using our sense of touch. Before we get started, let's look at our observing and judging vocabulary for touch. One thing I want to point out is that it is perfectly okay to judge whether something might be about to hurt you.

It's okay to use our judgments to keep ourselves safe. So, for example, it's important to observe mindfully and notice that a stove might really be hot without actually touching it. It's also helpful to think about how painful it might be to jump off a high ledge—before you jump. These kinds of judgments help keep us safe. Today, we are going to practice using describing words with safe objects.

"As you touch each object with your fingers, watch carefully to notice your first thoughts and emotional responses. Then bring your attention to the sensations in your fingers. Consider how you might describe the sensations you feel. Is the object soft? Hard? Spiky? Smooth? Rough? Do you feel warmth or cold or wetness or dryness when you touch the object? How heavy is it? How might you describe all the sensations? What describing words can we use? Notice that we all have a tendency to want to label or name the object instead of just describing it. Is your mind busily trying to figure out what the object is instead of focusing on describing the sensations? Once we figure out what it is, are we still attending to it mindfully or do our thoughts wander to something else? Bring your full attention to mindful touching. When thoughts, feelings, memories, fears, or judgments arise, just notice what they are, and then bring your attention back to the experience of touching."

Inquiry: Touching Our Experiences

After everyone has had an opportunity to mindfully touch each object, regroup and select one of the "feel boxes" to discuss. Pass the box around if you wish. Invite the kids to describe object A as if to a Martian or someone who has never touched or seen it. Encourage several children to describe the object. You might take a moment to restate one of the aims of the activity. As they touched each item, their minds might have been pulled away by thoughts and feelings about the object. Were they aware of their own memories or what expectations they might have had about the object? What emotions did they feel when they touched the object? Did they notice "liking" or "disliking" come up? What body sensations were experienced while touching the object?

As each child offers his or her response, the information about object A can be recorded on the sample chart. Help them sort their responses into each category shown on the chart. Randomly select another box. Pass object B around. What words could we use to describe object B so that someone else would know that it is different from object A? What information is not available to us using just one sense? Do we know how heavy or light the object is without picking it up? When it's hidden inside the box, can we tell what color is it? Can we tell if there are markings or lettering on the object?

EXAMPLE CHART

Object	Description	Thoughts	Feelings	Body sensations	Judgments
Object A (peeled grapes)	Slippery, gooey	My mom would never let me do this.	Excited	Hand feels slippery	This is fun, but it feels creepy.
Object B (pinecone)	Light, hard, sticky, bumpy	I know what this is. Reminds me of when we went camping.	Happy	Smiling, hand feels a little sticky	I really like pinecones.
Object C (piece of silk)	Smooth, soft	I wish all my clothes felt this nice.	Content	Feels cool and slippery on my fingers	I love the way this cloth feels.

"Now let's think *about* the items we touched. Let's see if we can identify some of the body sensations, thoughts, and feelings you might have had while you were touching the objects. Would someone like to share this with the class?"

As the facilitator guides the children in completing the chart, it is common for them to have some confusion distinguishing between the different categories. For example, children frequently offer their feelings when asked to identify their thoughts.

FACILITATOR: Okay, John. How would you describe the item in box *A*?

CHILD: It was kind of slippery and gooey.

FACILITATOR: Those are great describing words, so let's put them here. (*Writes the words in the description column.*) Now, what were some of the thoughts that you noticed as you were touching the item in box *A*?

CHILD: I was thinking this feels creepy.

FACILITATOR: (*Puts the word "creepy" in the judgment category.*) So it felt creepy to you, okay. So is that a judging word or a describing word? *Creepy* sounds like a judgment. Now let's see if you can share what you were thinking while you touched the item. What were some of the thoughts that went through your mind?

CHILD: I was thinking that I never stuck my hand in bunch of wet grapes before. That's what it was, right? It was grapes?

FACILITATOR: So you were thinking that these things are grapes? Thanks for sharing with us what your thoughts were. Did labeling the grapes do anything to make the experience of touching them any different? Now, how about for the feeling category? What other feelings came up as you touched the grapes?

CHILD: I guess excited, because it was fun to do it. It was creepy, but fun.

Additional Discussion Questions for Children/Teens

- "What does it mean to touch mindfully and how does that differ from how we normally touch things?"
- "Do our thoughts, feelings, or memories about objects influence the actual touching experience in the moment?"
- "Could mindful touching change the way we experience the world? If so, in what ways?"
- "If we imagine the objects or are told the objects are one thing, does that change our perception of them?"

Suggested Practice Activities

- In this activity, children can practice exploring two senses with mindful awareness: vision and touch. Have children work in pairs. Child *A* is given an object in a box (e.g., a hairbrush). Child *B* sits facing away from child *A*, with eyes closed. Using only observing words, child *A* must describe the object he is touching to child *B*. Child *B* is directed to use her "mind's eye" to visualize the object. Child *B* may ask questions to help figure out what the object might be, but the questions must be only about the touch sensations of the object. For example, one description might be, "It is oval-shaped, hard on one side, and has a round handle that is about 8 inches long. The hard part is smooth and cool. The end of the handle is flat and has a notch in it. On the other side, there are many soft bristles that stick out in lots of directions. They bend easily and are pointy on the ends. The bristles stop before the handle starts." Pick objects that lend themselves to fairly challenging descriptions. Take turns. Have children share their experiences of the activity in a class discussion. Invite them to notice when it was difficult to describe the object without using judging or labeling words.

- Read the parable of "The Blind Men and the Elephant" (readily available online). Discuss its meaning and what can be learned about mindful touching from this parable.
  - Do we sometimes think that our incomplete experiences are the whole truth?
  - Do we sometimes discount other people's experiences or perspectives?
  - Could we all be partially right?
- This is a home practice activity:

  "Choose an object from around your house. Hide the object in a box or bag and have several family members reach in and, without looking, describe the object. Write down their observations in your mindfulness journal. As best you can, record and categorize the observing and judging words that your family members used."

Activity 37. Mindful Humming

Time Requirement

5–10 minutes.

Theme

Becoming aware of our sounds, bodies, and intentions while having fun.

Materials Needed

None.

Mindfulness Activity

The group can stand or be seated in chairs. The idea is to using humming as an anchor, both the sound and vibration, and also to enjoy the anchoring and the practice. The sounds can help shift our focus off unhelpful thoughts, and bring awareness to the sound and its vibration. There may be some evidence to suggest that the vibrations can help calm down the nervous system (Oldenburg, 1984).

"Start by taking a breath in, and then just *hummmmmmmm* as you breathe out, maybe imagining yourself being a hummingbird. You might play with bringing the tone or volume up or down, finding the *hummmmmm* that feels just right for you, or that fits your mood. How does it sound? How does it feel in your mouth and the rest of your body? You can play with listening to everyone else humming too, seeing how long the group can go, or just tuning in and trying to maintain focus on your own *hum*."

Challenges and Tips

- A quiet, nondisruptive humming is a good way to disguise focusing on our own breath if we don't want others to notice that we are focused on or trying to manage our breathing. The trick is to hum so softly that we do not distract others or draw attention to ourselves.
- Humming can be a useful technique to downregulate strong emotions such as anxiety or fear. Simply shifting focus from thoughts to sounds and body sensations can cool down those hot thoughts that may be intensifying the emotions.

Suggested Practice Activities

"You might feel funny humming like this around other people, so try it on your own, or try humming a song and tuning into the vibrations and feelings at any time during the day that it's not a distraction or disruption to others."

Activity 38. Mindful Hearing

Time Requirement

10–15 minutes.

Themes

- Thoughts influence our emotions and responses to everyday events.
- When we blend our thoughts and emotions with the sounds we hear, we transform the felt experience in very subjective ways.

Background

We live in an ocean of varied and ever-changing sounds. Music is a particularly useful way to introduce children to the idea that our thoughts influence our emotions and that thoughts often dictate how we respond to everyday events. Sounds evoke clear images that are associated with specific thoughts, memories, feelings, and body sensations. By comparing the variety of images that different children associate with the same piece of music, kids deepen their understanding that felt experiences are subjective. What we call *our experience* is a combination of sensory input (seeing, hearing, touching, tasting, and smelling) combined with our thoughts, emotions, and body sensations. Bringing mindfulness to the exploration of sounds and our reactions to sounds brings mindfulness more into everyday life.

During the discussion that follows this activity, two core messages of mindfulness should be reiterated. First, thoughts, feelings, and body sensations are separate but related internal events. Second, our reactive thoughts and emotional responses to sounds combine with the external event (i.e., hearing the sound) to create a unique and subjective experience. Essentially, each of us lives in a unique world because we each have a unique history that underlies our habitual responses to events.

Your own openness and acceptance of each child's experience is essential to facilitating mindfulness in others. Your embodiment of mindfulness is conveyed in many small acts undertaken with intention and through words spoken thoughtfully and with attention to their meaning and appropriateness. Inviting children to share whatever thoughts, images, or emotional responses might emerge when listening to music is more helpful to cultivating mindful awareness than creating structured classroom lessons or providing information about each piece of music. Talking about music is an intellectual activity—very different from listening to music with full attention and mindful awareness. Comparing the wide variety of different images that the same piece of music can evoke in different children helps clarify the subjectivity of experiences. We move children toward seeing that their own emotional states, and the expectations or judgments that they bring into every experience, change the very nature of the experience.

Materials Needed

- Five to eight different short pieces of music (30–60 seconds each). It will be useful if your musical selections have no intelligible words, are highly variable, not familiar to the children, and seem likely to evoke an assortment of images and emotional responses. Examples include a Bach sonata, Noh chants, African drumming, mathcore, Tibetan chanting, Sufi dance music, Indian sitar, pan flute, soca or calypso, gamelan percussion music from Indonesia, reggae, minimalist (e.g., Philip Glass), or soukous dance music from Congo. You might also look for film soundtracks to evoke excitement, sadness, suspense, anxiety, anger, or other strong emotions. Free samples of audio music and sounds can be found on YouTube or streaming services.
- Music player (or a computer with speakers).
- Mindfulness journals.
- Chart paper and markers (optional).
- Yoga mats (optional).

Vocabulary

- **Observing words:** *loud, soft, sharp, clear, muted, faint, distant, near, tinny, deep, low-pitched, high-pitched, clanking, whining, whirring, squealing, humming, crying, thumping, grating, grinding, screeching, whistling, harsh, throaty, rippling, pounding, lilting.*
- **Judging words:** *annoying, horrible, irritating, bad, good, obnoxious, terrible, wonderful, lovely, beautiful, fantastic, grating, relaxing, soothing, melodic, harmonious.*
- **Emotional words:** *happy, joyful, elated, ecstatic, sad, depressed, lethargic, down, blue, angry, frustrated, annoyed, scared, fearful, afraid, terrified, nervous, bored.*

Mindfulness Activity

The ability to disengage from thoughts, emotions, and sensations is an essential first step in choosing more skillful responses to difficult thoughts, feelings, or situations that may arise. Mindful hearing can help children become more adept at identifying their thoughts as "just thoughts," their feelings as "just feelings," and their body sensations as "just body sensations." This mindful hearing activity can be done sitting in chairs or lying down on mats. To whatever extent possible, the room should be free from competing sounds. You may wish to dim the room lights.

"Today we will explore mindfulness using our sense of hearing. We will discover together how bringing mindfulness to the everyday activity of listening to music might influence how we experience the music. I will play several short pieces of music and invite you to bring your mindful attention to your thoughts, feelings, and body sensations while listening to each piece of music. After each piece of music stops, take a moment and check in with yourself. Note whether your emotional response to the music is positive (liking, attraction) or negative (disliking, aversion). In your mindfulness journal, jot down a 'plus' if you liked it or a 'minus' if you didn't like it. Then, checking in with your emotions, think of what would be a descriptive title for that piece of music. We will listen to the music clips without talking or sharing experiences, and then have a discussion at the end."

Begin by conducting a few minutes of mindful breathing practice. Then play short (30–60 seconds each) musical clips while the children listen with mindful attention. Each time you stop the music, repeat the instructions to note if there was a positive or negative response and to create a descriptive title for the piece. Repeat with at least three or four additional pieces of music.

Additional Discussion Questions for Children/Teens

Begin the group discussion by inviting children to share their emotional responses and titles for each piece of music. During the discussion, you might choose to chart each child's emotional response and title, as shown in the following example.

EXAMPLE CHART

Musical piece	Emotional response	Title
1	+ —	Summertime dancing under the stars Haunted house at midnight
2	— +	Car about to crash Sitting by a waterfall in the spring
3	+ +	Children playing in the snow School is out for the summer

You might direct attention to the fact that the same piece of music evokes a lot of different emotional responses and titles because everyone is different. The focus of this inquiry should first be to deepen children's understanding of the relationships between thoughts and feelings, and second to find opportunities to explore their understandings of how different people have such a wide variety of emotional responses and images to the same piece of music.

Judgments about any piece of music can be identified and labeled as judgments, and should be clearly differentiated from nonevaluative descriptions of the sounds themselves. Remember that labels (e.g., name of the artist or the type of music) are simply verbal communication shortcuts, and do not actually describe any individual's experience. As always, keep the discussion focused on the children's here-and-now experiences by discouraging them from making comparisons of the music they just heard with other things they may have heard in the past. You might gently observe that the habit we all have of comparing one experience to another is strong. Memories and images can be so strong that they sometimes get in the way of being mindful of the "here and now" experience of listening to the music.

Suggested Practice Activities

- We can practice mindfulness of sounds by discovering music in everyday things that are not usually considered music. We might even find music in discordant or strident sounds. For example, music of all sorts can be found by attending to the rich symphony of sounds heard on a busy city street, the sharp notes of dogs barking, the grinding of a garbage truck, the chirps of birds, or the daily choir of many voices talking at the same time on a subway platform or in a crowded room. These sounds can be demonstrated in the classroom (or in whatever room you are using) by playing a sound-effects CD or even a YouTube audio.

  "Can you hear the music in the honking of cars engaged in a dialogue at the intersection? Or perhaps you found music in the loud *whooosh* and squeal of brakes of a train coming to a stop. Note in your journal where you found music in ordinary sounds. How do your attitudes about sounds change when you stop judging them or expecting them to be different than they actually are? What is an obnoxious and annoying noise to one person may be music to the ears of another. Can you learn to hear music in all sounds simply by letting go of your expectations? How might that affect how you feel about yourselves and others?"

- To drive home the point that it is possible to transform our relationship to annoying sounds, we sometimes introduce the YouTube video "The Fly," about a meditating Samurai coping with an annoying, buzzing fly that is disrupting his practice (*www.youtube.com/watch?v=HZ1-Nj3vcXY*).

Activity 39. Mindfulness of Smells (Part I)

Time Requirement

20–25 minutes.

Themes

- Smelling with mindful awareness provides many opportunities to practice differentiating descriptive observations from judgments.

- Focusing on awareness of thoughts while smelling different scents lets us see how memories, beliefs, and expectations can alter the experience of smell.
- Practicing mindfulness through the sense of smell further develops awareness of things in our environment that often go unnoticed when we are running on autopilot.

Background

Events in our lives are often missed altogether or not fully experienced while we spend hours every day on autopilot. The experience of smelling is similar to that of hearing sounds, in that scents/aromas/odors are so pervasive in the environment that we tend to be aware of them only when they are extremely pleasant or extremely unpleasant. Milder scents frequently go unnoticed. When are we aware of the scent of the evening air? Or the smell of clothes in a laundry hamper? Or the smell of chalk in the classroom? Even at mealtimes, where smells tend to be stronger, how often do we notice all the scents coming from our plate or bowl before we start eating? Do we notice different smells not just at different places but at different times of day?

Smells stick in our memories and become strongly associated with emotions. These associations can be positive or negative. One child used to sit in her grandfather's workshop, playing with wood shavings. For her, freshly shaven wood carries a distinct smell of childhood happiness. For another child who suffered a bad car accident, the smell of burning rubber might trigger unpleasant and fearful memories. The sense of smell can often lead us to skip mindful observation and rush straight to judgment. Some scents are immediately labeled as *pleasant* or *good*, whereas others are labeled as *unpleasant* or *bad*.

The purpose of practicing mindfulness of smells is to slow down enough to experience a smell as it actually is, discover that judging the scent is not the same as experiencing it, and that our judgments strongly influence how we define our experiences. In this activity, we explore the distinction between the scent stimuli and the children's reactions to them, which in turn leads the children to a better understanding of how thoughts and emotions contribute to their felt experiences.

Materials Needed

Please note that this activity requires a little bit of advance preparation.

- Six small containers with tight lids. Glass baby food jars, spice jars, salt and pepper shakers, or single-serve jelly jars with metal lids work well for long-term use. (Plastic containers tend to absorb the scents and need to be replaced frequently.) You may want to label each jar with a letter or number for your own reference. Do not identify the name of the scent on the jars.
- Use a different jar for each scent sample. It is quite easy to source a variety of scents from around your own home. Examples include ground coffee beans, vinegar-soaked cotton balls, chocolate, cinnamon, ginger root, dill, camphor, cloves, garlic, perfumes, smoked paprika, aromatic soaps, and lotions. You may want to select some of the scents to be "pleasant" (e.g., chocolate) and some to be "unpleasant" (e.g., camphor). We recommend avoiding

scents that may trigger distress (e.g., ammonia and other cleaning solutions, rotten foods) or allergic reactions (e.g., turpentine, acetone, and other solvents).

- Flip chart paper and markers.
- Mindfulness journals.

Vocabulary

Observing or describing scent words: *sweet, sour, bitter, strong, mild, pungent, tangy, aromatic, fruity, spicy, acrid, sharp, musty,* or whatever else the kids come up with.

We have very little vocabulary that is specific to the sense of smell. Descriptions are most often made by comparison with another thing that has a distinctive odor—the smell is described as being "like" something else. Environmental examples include the smells of lavender, fresh-cut grass, ocean air, pine trees, and wood fires. Smells are sometimes described by comparison with a food that has a characteristic smell. Examples include strawberries, bananas, cooked cabbage, lemons, oranges, vanilla, cinnamon, bubble gum, roast beef, mint leaves, and warm bread. Describing a smell without resorting to comparing one thing to another is one reason that this activity is an advanced mindfulness practice. The tendency to judge a scent quickly, being almost instinctive, is another reason that this activity can be so challenging.

Mindfulness Activity

"Today we will explore mindfulness using our sense of smell. Each jar holds a different scent and will be passed around for you to smell. As you inhale, consider how you could describe the smell to someone else. Is it strong? Spicy? Sweet? What body sensations do you notice as you smell the scent? How does this smell 'show up' in your eyes, your mouth, or your cheeks? How might you describe those sensations? Pretend that you will have to describe the scent to a Martian who has never smelled it before. What words can you use?"

Pass the jars slowly around the circle, giving each child a long moment with each jar. This part of the activity is done in silence. After all the jars have been passed around, select one of the jars to discuss. Recirculate the jar, if necessary.

"How would you describe this mystery scent to your new Martian friend? What body sensations did you notice as you smelled it? [Pause for child's answer.] Does anyone else have other ways to describe this scent?"

As children offer their responses, record the information about scent X on an unlabeled T-chart by categorizing the responses into one of two columns: the "Descriptions" side or the "Judgments" side. Do not label the chart yet, and don't remark on how you are categorizing the responses. Select another scent jar. Pass scent Y around the group again. What words could they use to describe scent Y so that someone who didn't smell it would know that it is different from scent X? What thoughts or feelings come up for each child, as he or she smelled what was in the jar? Was the mind busy trying to figure out what that smell was? Was the emotion one of satisfaction when they figured it out (or one of frustration when they couldn't figure it out)?

"Did that effort to name what was in the jar change your experience? If so, how? What memories came into your mind as you smelled this? Do all of us have memories of smells? Do we have different memories? How might those memories influence how we responded to this scent today?"

As children offer their responses, the information about scent Y is recorded on the T-chart. Using different color markers can be useful to differentiate the responses. Compare and contrast the descriptions and judgments of scents X and Y. Time permitting, you can repeat this with additional scents.

Then, referring to the information on the T-chart, ask the children what they noticed about how the chart is organized. Point out specific words on the chart. For example, how are the words *sweet* and *strong* different from *yummy* and *icky*? Which words would be more useful to describe the scent to that Martian who does not know what it is? Does describing the smell with "judgment" words help our Martian understand what this smell is like?

Then, write in the headings on the T-chart (*Descriptions* and *Judgments*) and invite them to consider the words in both columns. Which side of the chart has more words for thoughts, feelings, and memories connected with the scent in it? Which side has more words that refer to the actual experience in the present moment? Referring again to the T-chart, you might explore further by pointing out when the list of descriptors is different for the same scent. Invite children to describe how their observations of scent X are different from scent Y.

"Did you notice any feelings that came up when you smelled scents X and Y? Describe the different feelings that these scents caused you to have. How are your thoughts and feelings about a scent different from the experience of smelling? How might your behavior change based on your thoughts and feelings about the smell?"

It is common for children to have intense visceral reactions to smells. If the smell is particularly strong, as with vinegar or strong cheese, children are most likely to label the smell with a judgment. For example:

CHILD A: (*Smells scent X, which is vinegar.*) Yuck, that's nasty.

FACILITATOR: That's interesting. Smell the jar one more time. Can you tell me what makes it smell *nasty* to you?

CHILD A: Well, it's really strong and it makes my eyes feel tingly and my nose too. It burns the inside of my nose a little.

FACILITATOR: Great job using your observing words. So really, a lot of body sensations were going on before you said, "That's nasty." That's what mindfulness can help us with—slowing things down so we are more aware of what's really going on. Thanks!

Another child may have completely different reactions to the same smell. For example:

CHILD *B*: I thought it smelled kind of good, like what my mom uses when she makes tangy chicken.

FACILITATOR: That's interesting. You both smelled the same thing, but to you [child *B*] it was "good," and to you [child *A*] it was "nasty." We have two different reactions to the same scent. How interesting that two people experience the same smell so differently. Why might that be? What were some of the sensations and thoughts you had while smelling this?

CHILD *B*: It kind of makes my mouth water and tingle.

FACILITATOR: Great job observing your body's reaction to this smell.

Additional Discussion Questions for Children/Teens

- "How might we describe two related smells, such as two different flowers, so that someone else could understand how they are different?"
- "We've learned that memories or associations can be evoked by smells. Then our thoughts are more on the memory than on what is happening right now. Could this focus on the memories make us less mindful of the present experience?"

Challenges and Tips

We have found that this activity is one of the most interesting and challenging for both children and adults. Although we have never seen anyone experience a significantly adverse reaction to any scents, keep your eyes open for signs of distress, and be aware of allergies.

Suggested Practice Activities

- If you are in a classroom, draw a large chart and place an assortment of unidentified scent jars on a side table for your students to smell during the week. Invite them to smell the scents carefully and record their descriptions, thoughts, feelings, and body sensations on sticky notes and add them to a class chart. As the chart fills up, the children will see that each person brings his or her own perceptions and expectations to the same scent stimulus and, in doing so, creates very different experiences.

EXAMPLE CHART

Scent	Description of amell	Thoughts	Feelings	Body sensations and reactions
Scent A (bubble gum)	Sweet, fruity, sugary	I want to eat this gum right now.	Happy, excited	Mouth is watering, lips curve up in smile
Scent B (lavender soap)	Flowery, smooth	This smells like my grandmother.	Warm, contented	Relaxed and smiling

- Invite children to discover times during the day to engage in mindful smelling. Possible times include during lunch, on the playground, or walking home from school. Provide opportunities for them to share their observations. Continue to point out the distinction between observing words and judging words.

- For home practice you might suggest that the children engage in mindful smelling during one meal at home. Before eating their meal, they should take a moment to mindfully smell the different foods on their plates.

  "What smells do you notice that you might have overlooked in the past? What kinds of body sensations go along with mindfully smelling the various foods you have in front of you? As you begin to eat the food, continue to practice mindful smelling."

- Suggest to the kids that they consider how the senses of smell and taste are linked together and to write down their observations in their mindfulness journals.

- To make a game of mindful smelling, prepare pairs of bottles with the same scent and ask the kids to match the smells to each other.

Activity 40. Mindfulness of Smells (Part II)

Time Requirement

20–25 minutes.

Themes

- Smells stimulate strong memories and their associated emotions.
- Smelling with mindful awareness helps us differentiate our own thoughts and feelings from the actual scent that is reaching our senses in this moment.
- Becoming more aware of how we blend our own memories into current experiences helps us understand the subjectivity of all our experiences.

Background

As discussed in Part I of Mindfulness of Smells, the experience of smell is a powerful in evoking thoughts, judgments, memories, and sometimes even strong emotions. The sense of smell is our most primitive sense, and scents easily bring up memories that pull us away from being fully present in the moment. Warm bread in the oven reminds us of our family kitchen. A certain cologne or perfume may remind us of a person we know or knew, for better or for worse. Rather than being experienced just as it is—maybe as flowery or sweet or spicy—the scent of the perfume blends with our thoughts and feelings about the person with whom we associate it. We slip into judgments about the smell without noticing the qualities of the scent that triggered these judgments in the first place. In a manner of speaking, we smell the trees, but not the forest.

This activity seeks to deepen children's awareness of the interaction between external stimuli (in this case, scents) and the internal experiences of thoughts, feelings, and body sensations. The main message is that the act of smelling and the process of interpreting and judging what we smell are actually two different activities. As noted with other activities that often occur on autopilot, the process of mindful smelling enhances and changes our actual experience.

Materials Needed

- Completed extension chart from the first mindful smell activity.
- A second set of four to six unlabeled scent jars prepared as described in Part I.
- Flip chart paper and colored markers.
- Mindfulness journals.

Vocabulary

Judging scent words: *disgusting, stinky, wonderful, smelly, gross, yucky, putrid, delicious, beautiful, delightful, lovely, icky, nasty, sick, repulsive, yummy, fresh, fragrant, rotten, pleasant,* and any words the kids may come up with.

Mindfulness Activity

This activity is similar to the previous one. In Part I, we focused on differentiating descriptive thoughts from judging thoughts. The inquiry that guides this activity is focused on separating our thoughts, feelings, and body sensations from the sensory perception.

> "Today, I'm going to pass around some more containers with different scents in them. As you describe your experiences, I invite you to help me fill out our mindfulness of smells chart."

EXAMPLE CHART

Perceptions	Judgments	Thoughts	Feelings	Body sensations
Sweet, fruity, sugary	Smells great!	I want to chew this gum right now.	Happy, excited	Mouth is watering, lips curve up in smile
Minty, sweet	Yummy smell.	I know this is bubblegum. I wish I had some.	Frustrated, grumpy	Frowning, tight feeling in belly
Flowery, smooth,	This smells like my grandmother.	I love my grandmother.	Warm, contented	Relaxed and smiling
Strong, acrid	This smells like that lady in the store.	She was dressed funny.	Uncomfortable, repulsed	Nose wrinkles, tingling in nostrils

Select one of the scents represented on the chart (but not marked on the container, so the children do not know which scent it is) and pass it around to each child. As children volunteer to share their experiences, elicit descriptions, thoughts or judgments, memories, feelings, and body sensations, and then add their contributions to the chart in the appropriate columns. Then invite them to reflect upon the differences between the categories. The distinction between smelling bubble gum and judging its appeal can be challenging for young children—and adults too. This chart offers a concrete way for children to differentiate between the experience of smelling the scent versus thinking about or making judgments about it. In an open and exploratory manner, help children direct their observations, thoughts, feelings, and body sensations into the appropriate spaces on the chart. If the smell is particularly strong, children might offer their judgments of the smell before using describing words. The dialogue might go this way:

FACILITATOR: Who would like to share their experience of smelling scent *X*?

CHILD: Ughhh, it's nasty.

FACILITATOR: That's interesting. Where would you place that comment on this chart?

CHILD: I guess in the judgment category.

FACILITATOR: Okay, let's write it down here. Now, can you find some describing words to tell us exactly what you notice about this smell?

CHILD: It's strong. And it's also a little sour.

FACILITATOR: Okay. What were some of the thoughts you had when you smelled it?

CHILD: I thought, "Get this thing away from me."

FACILITATOR: And what were some of your body sensations as you smelled it?

CHILD: It made my eyes water and I got that little funny feeling you get when you smell a pickle. Like when something is going to make my lips pucker.

Continue in this way until child has completed the charting. Then present another scent jar to the class and pass it around, asking several children to note the judgments, thoughts, feelings, and body sensations elicited by the scent. Record each of the comments on the chart in the appropriate column. Invite the children to explore what causes each child to have a different reaction to the same scent. What makes each child's experience subjective?

Inquiry: Describing versus Judging

Guide a Socratic inquiry directed at identifying the ways in which judgments of an experience are different from the experience itself. Using the flip chart, bring attention to the relationship between the scent stimulus and the child's internal responses to that stimulus. Questions should be consistently based on the assumption that the judgment of the experience is not the same as the experience itself. In particular, look for opportunities to observe and note what happens when describing the experience in a moment-by-moment way, versus what it feels like to be evaluating or judging the experience, ruminating about or analyzing the experience, or comparing it to other experiences. In this way, children start to develop awareness of how often they transform their present-moment experiences by adding memories (i.e., living in the past) or expectations (i.e., anticipating the future) to the actual experience.

Additional Discussion Questions for Children/Teens

- "The first reaction we often have to a lot of smells is simply that we like them or we don't like them. Did you notice the judging thoughts when they showed up as you smelled the scent? Were the judgments the same throughout the entire experience, or did they change as you continued to practice mindful smelling? Did your emotional experience change when the judgment changed? If so, how?"

- "Why do we each have different judgments about the same scent?"
- "How might we feel if we were to spend more time describing instead of making judgments about everything that happens in our life? Or if we were to stop judging other people . . . or foods . . . or events . . . or the tasks we are required to do? Do you think that anything might change? If so, what?"

Suggested Practice Activities

- If you are in a classroom, keep the collection of scent jars on a table for children to smell during the next few days. Invite them to smell the different scents and record their body sensations, thoughts, and associated feelings on sticky notes to add to the class chart. Adding a column for "Judgments" can help make more explicit the differences between observing and describing the actual experience, identifying subjective responses to the sensations, and thinking about or drawing conclusions about the experience.

EXAMPLE CHART

Descriptive experience		Subjective responses			Evaluative responses
Event	Description of smells	Thoughts	Feelings	Body sensations	Judgments
Scent A (clove)	Child 1: Spicy, orange-like	Smells like pumpkin pie	Pleased, excited	Mouth waters, lips curve up in smile, tongue licks lips, belly growls	This smells yummy.
	Child 2: Pungent, strong, musty	What is this stuff?	Unhappy, agitated	Nose wrinkles, nose tickles, lips close	This smells gross.
Scent B (camphor)	Child 3: Sharp, kind of like medicine	Reminds me of when I was really sick.	Sad, nervous	Frowns, moves away	I hate this smell.

- Encourage the kids to consider how their thoughts and judgments might affect the experiences they have when they notice the smells around them. What happens to their emotions or mood when those judgments don't match what is really happening right now? Suggest that they write down their observations in their mindfulness notebook.
- Provide suggestions for home practice:

"Continue to practice mindful smelling of your meals at home. Before eating your dinner, take a moment to mindfully smell the different foods on your plate. What smells do you notice that you might have overlooked in the past? What kinds of body sensations go along with mindfully smelling the various foods you have in front of you? As you begin to eat the food, continue to smell mindfully. Think about how the senses of smell and taste are linked together. Write down your observations in your mindfulness journal."

Mindfulness of Thoughts

Group 6 practices begin to explore mindfulness of thoughts, an important skill for children and teens to become comfortable with as they cultivate greater self-awareness. In recognizing thoughts as thoughts, we are better equipped to skillfully weigh whether to believe them, ignore them as being inaccurate, or restructure them to create more accurate or helpful thoughts. Then we can choose a skillful response, which helps us become happier and more effective in daily life. Lastly, thoughts begin to lose their power to control emotions and behaviors. Therefore, kids can grow up more resilient, having a healthier relationship to their own thoughts when they encounter stresses or difficulties later in life. The basic intention of these practices is to cultivate awareness of thoughts and the process of thinking, while conveying the idea that the thoughts are not necessarily true.

Activity 41. Mindfulness of Thoughts

Time Requirement

10–15 minutes.

Themes

- No matter how hard we try, we can't control our thoughts.
- However, we don't need to believe everything we think.

Background

Humans didn't evolve to have the fastest legs or sharpest claws; we survived because we evolved with the smartest brains. Our brains developed to think carefully, and we do this very well. One of the first things we learn when we begin practicing mindfulness is that we can't control what goes on in our minds. Most of us discover very quickly that the mind seems to have a mind of its own. It's important to validate and normalize this "monkey mind" so that children don't feel that they are practicing mindfulness in the "wrong" way when they discover that they can't control their thoughts and feelings. Mindfulness practices are not to stop our thinking or even change what we think. Instead, mindfulness helps us know *what* we're thinking, *when* we're thinking it.

Thoughts appear and bring feelings along with them. Those thoughts and feelings influence our speech and behaviors. A lot of times, we're not even aware that this process is happening. We call this being on *autopilot,* as we've noted previously. When we practice watching our thoughts, we discover a lot of habituated patterns. We see when thoughts emerge and how they develop. We may also learn to see how accurate, helpful, or not so helpful those patterns of thinking might be.

Although we can't stop our thoughts, we can change how we relate to them. By simply taking a few mindful breaths, we may discover a space between the thing that happens to us and our reactions to it. We learn that we don't have to react the same old ways that we have done in the past. We also learn that thoughts often don't have much relationship to whatever is actually happening right here, right now. We learn to step back for just a moment—long enough to say to ourselves, "That's just a thought or a feeling, not a fact." Thoughts become like clouds floating across the sky. They may look big and solid and unmoving, but they're not. Instead of seeing thoughts as being solid and permanent, we practice just watching and letting them pass by, like clouds in the sky. Thoughts only control us if we believe they are facts. In reality, all thoughts are just thoughts. Even the ones that tell you otherwise.

Materials Needed

- Activity handout: *Thoughts Are Just Thoughts* (for use with the suggested practice activity).
- Mindfulness journal.

Mindfulness Activity

This visualization activity helps kids decenter from their thoughts by using the metaphor of thoughts being like leaves floating in a stream.

"Sit in a comfortable, alert posture. If you are comfortable doing so, close your eyes, or if you prefer, softly gaze at a spot 2 or 3 feet in front of you. Take a few deep breaths. In your mind's eye, see yourself sitting next to a softly flowing stream under colorful autumn trees. The sun is shining, and there are red, orange, and yellow leaves falling gently off the trees and floating downstream on the water. Rest your attention on the leaves as they slowly move by. [long pause] "Now, take each thought that comes into your mind and carefully place it on a leaf. You watch each thought sitting on its leaf, slowly floating by. Whenever another thought comes up, just place it on another leaf and let it float downstream. [long pause] It doesn't matter what the thought is. Each thought just gets placed on a leaf and goes floating away. Some of the leaves might swirl around for a moment, but then they too float downstream. Happy and sad and angry and scared thoughts are all put onto leaves and float quietly away. All thoughts are just thoughts—even thoughts like, 'I'm hungry,' 'This is stupid,' 'I'm bored,' or 'I'm really bad at this' are just more thoughts to place on leaves and watch drifting downstream. [long pause]

"If you don't notice any thoughts for a while, just breathe and watch the leaves and the water flow by. More thoughts will certainly show up soon. [long pause] Let the stream flow at its own pace—not trying to speed it up to rush the thoughts away or to slow it down to hold onto the thoughts longer. Let the thoughts come and go at their own pace. [long pause]

"If a difficult or painful thought shows up, take a moment to acknowledge that it's there. You might want to say to yourself, 'I'm aware that a painful thought is here to visit.' Then place the painful thought on a leaf, too. [long pause]

"At times, you might discover that your mind has gotten caught up in a thought and you have forgotten to put it on a leaf. This is okay—it happens to everyone. As soon as you notice that, congratulate yourself for being in the present again, and then place that thought onto another leaf."

Additional Discussion Questions for Children/Teens

- "What patterns of thinking did you notice?"
- "Were the thoughts strong and intense or a little milder?"
- "Were they excited and jumping around all over the place, or were they slow, plodding thoughts?"
- "Were the thoughts about what we are doing, here and now, or were they running off somewhere else altogether?"
- "As best you can, describe what your thoughts were *doing*, not the content of the thoughts."

Suggested Practice Activities

"Read the activity handout, *Thoughts Are Just Thoughts*. Then think about a time when your thinking about a situation changed. It might be when you had a disagreement with your best friend and later found a way to agree . . . or when you thought a homework assignment was impossible and later decided that it wasn't as hard as you had thought. Practice mindful breathing as you remember that situation. Look carefully at what changed in your thoughts. How did your thinking change? Did your emotions change too? Write in your mindfulness journal what you think changed and why."

Activity 42. Mindfulness of Judgments

Time Requirement

20 minutes.

Themes

- We all judge our experiences.
- Judgments fit into one of three categories: positive (e.g., *like, approve, want, appreciate*), negative (e.g., *don't like, disapprove, don't want, don't appreciate*), or neutral (e.g., *indifferent*).
- When we look closely, we discover that it's the judgments about experiences that create unhappiness, not the experiences themselves.

Background

Practicing mindfulness requires that we see and let go of our attachments to all the judg-ments on which we habitually rely to make sense of the world around us. When we shift out of autopilot and practice mindful awareness, we suspend our reactive habits (mostly unnoticed by us) to decide whether we like or dislike the events and the people that fill our worlds. We become more practiced in choosing to accept what happens with fewer judgments, without wanting something to be different than it is, and without relating everything that happens to other experiences. As we practice being more mindful of our own judgments, we simply note all the judging thoughts that arise and let them go as best we can. Over and over again, our task is simply to bring our attention back to what we observe—in our thoughts, in our feelings, and in our body sensations. Two visualization scripts are offered that can facilitate a mindful exploration of judgments. Feel free to use one of these scripts or make up your own.

Materials Needed

- Visualization script.
- Activity handout: *Mindfulness of Judgments*.

Mindfulness Activity

Prepare the children for this activity by explaining the concept of mindful acceptance and linking the judgments they make with the emotions they subsequently feel about their daily experiences. Acceptance can be a challenging concept to convey. Acceptance is active. It's not passive resignation to whatever happens. Tara Brach (2004) defined the term *radical accep-tance* as "the willingness to experience ourselves and our life as it is" (p. 4). Wholehearted willingness to accept that which cannot be changed is an essential component of emotional and psychological well-being.

"In practicing mindfulness of judgments, we might see how living with mindfulness can make our lives a little bit easier. As we become more aware of all the things that we judge so quickly, we discover that the judging, even more than the experience, is what affects our emotions. We see how expecting things to be different than they really are, or even pushing away things that have already happened, actually increases our unhappiness. Learning to accept our experiences *just as they are* allows us to let go of worried, sad, mean, or angry thoughts and feelings more easily. Accepting our experiences doesn't mean that we will like everything that happens in our lives. Acceptance means simply that we acknowledge that this event did happen—even if we really wish it hadn't. It doesn't mean that we won't experience unpleasant events or difficult thoughts or feel-ings, but rather that we become better equipped to step back from them and observe them more clearly before deciding how to skillfully respond. Trying to resist or reject our experiences doesn't change the reality; it just creates more suffering for ourselves. Just as we can look carefully at a vase, noticing its angles, lines, textures, and colors, by look-ing carefully, we can become more aware of our thoughts–judgments as they arise. In this way, those judgments may not take on exaggerated importance or take control of our behaviors. Practicing mindful awareness allows us to better observe all the ways that we judge our experiences—with an attitude of self-kindness and acceptance."

Begin by inviting the children to take a mindful posture and close their eyes (if they wish). Then have the children take three long breaths in and out. Prompt the children to listen carefully to the story, making it feel as real and vivid in their heads as they can.

Visualization 1

"A new student walked into your classroom. She looked around the room and then asked the teacher where she should sit. The teacher told her to sit at the desk that was in front of her. The girl walked right into the desk and dropped her books. Along with the other children, you laughed at her because she was so clumsy."

Pause and invite the children to visualize this experience, and then check in with themselves to note what sensations, thoughts, and feelings are present right now. Now finish the story:

"Then you discover that the new student is blind."

Pause again and then invite the children to check in with themselves once more, noting the current sensations, thoughts, and feelings.

Visualization 2

"Your grandmother just told you that she was taking you to Disney World next summer. Really excited, you called your friend to share this wonderful news. Your friend just said, 'Sure, that's great,' and then hung up on you. Thinking that was rude, you got angry. So, you called him back, told him how angry you were, and then hung up on him."

Pause and invite the children to visualize this experience, and then check in with themselves to note what thoughts are present right now. Now finish the story:

"You saw your friend the next day and he apologized for making you angry. Then he tells you that his grandmother had passed away just before you called."

Pause again, and then invite the children to check in with themselves once more, noting the new experiences, sensations, thoughts, and feelings.

Discussion and Inquiry

With this activity, like many of the other activities described, the postactivity inquiry is an important component of the learning process. It is essential to allow sufficient time for the children to reflect on their experiences. Facilitating the discussion provides an opportunity for you to model mindful attention, compassion, and nonjudgmental curiosity. First, invite exploration of the experience itself—what were the thoughts, emotions, and body sensations that came up during the visualization. You might use the acronym SEAT that we describe in Activity 6 (pp. 27–28), or use the acronym SIFT to explore Sensations, Images, Feelings, and Thoughts (Siegel, 2007). What changed as the visualization progressed? How did the judgments that arose color their experiences? How did the judgments affect their emotions? Next, inquire as to how this experience was similar to how they might react in everyday life. Do these quick judgments help us feel happier? Or do these judgments make our lives less happy? Highlight the distinction between observing and noting an event versus judging, criticizing, or analyzing it. Last, explore how what the kids discovered today might be applied in everyday life. Help them identify choices that might be more helpful than engaging in a knee-jerk, autopilot reaction to the thoughts–judgments. As you guide the discussion, remember to invite participation rather than calling on children to respond.

Suggested Practice Activities

Every day, we all swim in an ocean of judgments. This is normal, but sometimes those judgments can create unhappiness or can even prompt us to act without thinking in ways that we might later regret. Instead of trying to stop all this judging, we learn to look carefully at all the judgments and make conscious choices in how to respond to them. Use Activity 42 Handout at the end of the chapter to guide the students through the exercise of writing down three judgments that they made during the past week and explore how the judgments affected how they felt. The handout can also be used as a home practice activity for the upcoming week.

Mindfulness of Thoughts

When we are on automatic pilot, our thoughts and feelings can take over without even knowing that it happened. By bringing awareness to our thoughts, feelings, and body sensations, we may discover some things that we have not seen before. When we are more mindful and aware, we are less likely to be carried away by our thoughts. We may not even be aware of some of the thoughts we have, but they still have a powerful effect on our emotions. However, thoughts always come and go, and our thoughts and feelings are not facts.

Sometimes, the same event can bring up many different thoughts. For example, the way we understand a situation can change over time or what we think about it might change depending on how happy or sad we feel. Just because we usually think a certain way does not mean we must continue to think that way. We can't control our thoughts, but we have choices in how we respond to them. Instead of being pushed into an emotional knee-jerk reaction, we can choose to first look, see clearly, and then respond in a more conscious way. We can sometimes find helpful ways to manage difficult situations just by bringing our awareness to the fact that we have choices.

Using our breath is one way to bring awareness to the present moment. Our breath is always with us and it can help us feel stable and strong enough to look clearly at our thoughts and feelings. With practice, we learn to choose our own responses, not just reacting as if we were on automatic pilot. With mindful awareness, we have the freedom to choose how to respond. Thoughts are just thoughts. We don't have to believe everything we think.

ACTIVITY 42 HANDOUT. Mindfulness of Judgments

Something happened today that made me feel bad, unhappy, mad, or scared.

Now, I'll practice mindfully looking at how my own thoughts–judgments contributed to this experience.

Event	Thoughts–Judgments	Emotional Response	Describing Thoughts	More Helpful Thoughts
Example: My mom made me eat asparagus for dinner.	Yuck! I hate asparagus. It's not fair that I have to eat this stuff.	Upset, angry, frustrated	Stringy, earthy, salty, a little like green beans	Well, I only had to eat three of them. Mom thinks they're good for me.

Mindfulness of Emotions

Group 7 activities encourage exploration and acceptance of emotions, along with the thoughts and bodily sensations that accompany them. Emotional awareness and the ability to self-manage our behavioral responses to our feelings are essential to our overall well-being. The extent to which we can identify and modulate our feelings greatly affects our ability to function effectively in a wide range of settings. This is particularly true for children. Kids who are easily overwhelmed by emotions are ill-equipped to self-manage behaviors induced by strong feelings, and are at a decided disadvantage when it comes to attending and succeeding in the classroom and other environments. Mindfulness brings increased awareness to the connections between the events in our lives; our thoughts, feelings, and body sensations; and our behavioral responses. Just as we often function on autopilot when it comes to our sense perceptions, habituated or overconditioned reactions are common when strong feelings arise.

Across a range of activities, we can teach children to become more aware of the choices they have when responding to events in their lives. This is particularly important for children or teens who habitually react impulsively to emotional triggers and also for those who experience difficult environments over which they have little or no control. Children will gain practice in slowing down their automatic reactions in an effort to consider a wider repertoire of emotional and behavioral choices. Essentially, with mindfulness practice, kids learn that events don't automatically translate into a single feeling, response, or behavior. Once that autopilot mode has been disengaged and children become more mindful of their emotional states, more choices emerge for them.

As we move into the mindfulness of emotions activities, we offer a friendly reminder that kids need to feel safe when expressing their emotions and emotional experiences. They need to feel that their disclosures will remain confidential within the group, and that other kids won't laugh at them or put them down for discussing their feelings or any different things that come up during practice. So, as you begin this group of activities, it might be useful to again remind the children of the guidelines for mindful behaviors discussed on page 8. And, of course, if any child appears to experience a high degree of distress during or after any classroom activity, referral to a therapist might be warranted.

Activity 43. Mindfulness of Happiness (Part I)

Time Requirement

30 minutes.

Themes

- Learning to apply mindful attention to our feelings (emotional events) and moods (emotional states) allows us to connect more deeply with our own experiences.
- In exploring our own emotions, we may also develop a clearer understanding that emotions are transient events and that they exist on a continuum.

Background

Although we have all experienced happiness, how often do we bring our full awareness to various aspects of that feeling, including the thoughts, body sensations, and judgments that often determine our state of happiness? In this activity, children will be given a gift and asked to observe the thoughts that accompany their feelings of happiness. This includes noticing memories (past) and anticipations (future) associated with the present event. We also explore the body sensations that are associated with feeling happy. Is there a variety of happy feelings? Do people experience different intensities of happiness, even about the same thing? All of these questions provide children with opportunities to develop greater attunement with their emotional states in general, as well as understanding of others' emotional experiences.

During this activity, children will better understand which thoughts and body sensations are associated with happy feelings. They will gain practice identifying a variety of "happy" feelings. As we continue to explore our emotions, we learn to observe the connections between personal experiences and emotional expectations and responses. As our awareness of these connections grow, we begin to see that we have personal choices in terms of how we respond to our experiences—both emotionally and behaviorally.

Materials Needed

- One large box wrapped festively as a present. The box contains envelopes that each has a "happy announcement" inside. Make sure there are enough envelopes for each child to receive one. Examples of "happy announcements" might include:
  - "Today we will have an extra-long recess."
  - "There will be no homework tonight."
  - "A very nice surprise is coming your way."
  - "Your generosity to others is noticed and valued."
  - "Your smile warms the hearts of your friends."
  - "Something good may happen to your best friend today."
  - "You will be attending an exciting event soon."
  - "Someone is saying very nice things about you."
  - "Never underestimate yourself—you have boundless potential."

- ○ "Your friends appreciate your kindness."
- ○ "You are creative and have great ideas."
- Activity handout: *Being Present*, one for each child.
- A sheet of small, colorful emoji-style stickers to use as markers on the *Being Present* handout.

Vocabulary for Grades 4–8

Happiness words: *content, blissful, joyous/joyful, "over the moon," wonderful, overjoyed, psyched, gleeful, elated, ecstatic, satisfied, sunny, grateful, jubilant, wonderful, thrilled, pumped, jazzed, exultant, "on cloud nine."*

Vocabulary for Grades K–3

Happiness words: *happy, glad, pleased/pleasing, cheery/cheerful, excited, great, thankful, delighted, sunny.*

Mindfulness Activity

The facilitator brings out the wrapped box while expressing great excitement. "Today everyone in our class will receive a present! Take a look at it, so beautifully wrapped! So festive!" Don't open the box yet, but take a few moments to simply look at the box together. Ask the group not to speak out loud, but to simply look at this wonderful gift. After a minute or so has passed, invite children to bring awareness to their thoughts, feelings, and body sensations as they look at the box. You might invite inner exploration by asking:

- "What thoughts did you notice right after the box was displayed and the announcement was made? What feelings did you have? How did those feelings change over time?"
- "What body sensations did you experience when you saw the box and heard the announcement?"
- "What thoughts are you having right now, after you received your present?"
- "What feelings are you experiencing right now?"

Then record the children's comments on a chart like the following sample.

EXAMPLE CHART

	Event	Thoughts	Feelings	Body sensations	Judgments
Child 1	Wrapped box	Wow! But why are we getting a present?	Curious, surprised, happy	Tingling, feel lighter, clap hands together	I love presents.
Child 2	Wrapped box	I'm confused. What is this about?	Puzzled, worried	Scowling forehead, hands sweaty	Surprises freak me out.
Child 3	Wrapped box	Great, I love presents!	Elated, excited	Eyes brighten, mouth open in smile, giggling	This is the best class ever!

Referring back to the chart, bring attention to the range of internal experiences triggered by this announcement. You may guide the kids in identifying how their expectations about an experience may be different from the experience itself. Using this chart, bring attention to the relationship between experiencing events and anticipating or judging events. Questions should be consistently based on observations that the judgment of the experience is not the same as the experience itself. In particular, you may want to look for opportunities to observe and notice the difference between describing the experience in a moment-by-moment way compared to judging, comparing, or analyzing the experience. In this way, children develop awareness of how often they transform their present-moment experiences by adding memories or beliefs (drawn from past experiences) and judgments or expectations (anticipations of the future) to the actual experience.

Before the box is opened, children are invited to become aware of their thoughts, feelings, and body sensations, watching closely as the contents of the box are revealed. Each child selects one wrapped "happy announcement." For example, this announcement might be "Everyone appreciates all the nice things you do," or "There will be no homework tonight." It is important that each announcement be something that the teacher or clinician can and does deliver.

Invite the children to observe their feelings after opening their gift. Ask them to pay special attention to their thoughts and feelings before they opened the gift and how these might change after. The kids may reflect on whether they were happier anticipating the gift or after finding out what the gift was. In a welcoming and inquisitive way, guide an exploration of how their thoughts about the gift may have influenced their feelings.

Additional Discussion Questions for Children/Teens

- "What does it mean to be mindful observers of our feelings?"
- "How might our lives change when we observe our feelings more mindfully?"
- "How do you know when you are happy? What does it feel like in your body?"
- "How do you know when other people are feeling happy?"
- "How do other people know when you are feeling happy?"

At the very end of this activity, ask each child to rate (from 1 to 7) how happy he or she is about the gift on the *Being Present* handout. Collect and save these ratings. They will be used during the second Mindfulness of Happiness activity.

Challenges and Tips

We do not recommend using food rewards as happy announcements.

Suggested Practice Activities

"During the next few days, observe a happy experience at the time it is happening. Record this event in your journal, taking note of your thoughts, feelings, and body sensations. How did you decide that this was a happy event?"

Activity 44. Mindfulness of Happiness (Part II)

Time Requirement

30 minutes.

Themes

• This activity reminds children of the idea that all feelings pass and none lasts forever.
• The relationships between internal events (thoughts and feeling) and subsequent behaviors are explored.

Background

One of the most important lessons inherent in teaching children to be mindful observers of their emotions is the understanding that no feelings last forever. All feelings change. Euphoria turns into elation, which fades into joy, which moves into happiness, which ends in satisfaction or some other more euthymic or "baseline" feeling. The path of change is different from person to person and/or from event to event. But the fundamental notion that all feelings change applies to everyone. We might use the ever-changing nature of the weather as a metaphor.

With the present activity, children are introduced to the concept of the transience of emotions by observing how their feelings and responses to the same event shift over time. Rating their feelings and responses to the same event at two points in time makes this clear. Through this experience, children gain greater awareness of how their feelings change. When we are in an emotional autopilot reaction, we tend to deal with our own strong feelings in one of three ways:

1. By zoning out or spacing out; becoming numb or habituated to the experience, and not fully taking part in it; or
2. By wanting to hold onto pleasant experiences longer in order to continue feeling happiness, joy, or contentment; or
3. By attempting to move away from or get rid of the experience to avoid the unpleasant feelings associated with it.

Understanding that all feelings are temporary allows us to be better able to experience whatever feelings arise without grasping onto or avoiding what is happening inside of us. We can become more mindful observers of our feelings when we understand that feelings are temporary. By watching our feelings in this more objective way, we practice "stepping back" and simply observing rather than becoming swept up in every surge of emotion.

Attempting to avoid uncomfortable or unpleasant experiences is not the only way we function on autopilot with our feelings. Sometimes we try to hold on to pleasant feelings, but this impossible task often creates even more unhappiness in our lives. Mindfulness helps us appreciate and savor the happy moments in our lives, and bringing mindful awareness to our thoughts, feelings, and body sensations also helps us to better regulate our emotions and behaviors. True happiness comes from recognizing the value of moderation as opposed to overattachment or overindulgence in pleasurable activities. Learning to fully enjoy the happiness of the moment and then move on to the next moment is as important a part of mindfulness as facing those feelings that are less pleasant.

Materials Needed

- Completed chart from Mindfulness of Happiness (Part I).
- *Being Present* handout that was rated and collected at the end of the first Mindfulness of Happiness activity.
- Flip chart, paper, markers.

Mindfulness Activity

Take a few minutes to review the previous happiness activity. Then guide a discussion in which children describe their experience of pleasant events during the past few days, either at home or during the daily class practices. Help the children identify thoughts, feelings, and body sensations as they share their experiences. You might conclude by asking, "What did you learn when you mindfully looked at a pleasant event?" Then review the chart created during the last group.

> "During our mindfulness lessons over the past weeks, we've talked about feelings. Mostly we've talked about how feelings relate to our thoughts and body sensations. Today we are going to continue to talk about happiness. Let's look at the chart from our previous group."

EXAMPLE CHART

	Event	Thoughts	Feelings	Body sensations	Judgments
Child 1	Wrapped box	Wow! But why are we getting a present?	Curious, surprised, happy	Tingling, feel lighter, clap hands together	I love presents.
Child 2	Wrapped box	I'm confused. What is this about?	Puzzled, worried	Scowling forehead, hands sweaty	Surprises freak me out.
Child 3	Wrapped box	Great, I love presents!	Elated, excited	Eyes brighten, mouth open in smile, giggling	This is the best class ever!

Inquiry: Thoughts and Feelings

Encourage children to continue making connections between their thoughts, feelings, and body sensations, particularly as they relate to events that bring them happiness. Make explicit the observation that different children experience different thoughts, feelings, and body sensations in response to similar events. You might then point out that children who feel similar emotions (e.g., happiness) may respond in very different ways to the same event. Note the different responses of students 1 and 3 in the preceding chart, for example, and explore what made the experience different for each child.

Invite the children once again to rate, on a scale of 1–7, how they feel right now about the present they received during the last group. Encourage them to focus on their present-moment emotional experience as they each remember their gift—rather than thinking back to how they felt at the time they received the box. Ask them to pay special attention to their thoughts, feelings, and body sensations in the present moment. Take few minutes to offer the children opportunities to share their observations with the group. Next, give back the *Being Present* handout that each child completed during the last session, when the gifts were initially distributed. Allow children to look at and reflect upon the differences (if there are any) between the two sets of ratings. Did their emotions change over time? Maintaining a curious stance, open a conversation as to how children might explain these differences. Ask them to consider the ways in which their feelings of happiness about the box may have shifted from when the present was received to this moment, several days later. How do they account for these "feeling differences"?

Additional Discussion Questions for Children/Teens

- "What is different about observing our feelings and being caught up in, or overwhelmed by, them?"
- "Might we find different ways to respond to our emotions?"
- "To what extent do we need to act on our feelings?"
- "How might we better appreciate moments of happiness?"
- "Can practicing mindfulness help us to be happier with ourselves and with other people?"

Challenges and Tips

The major teaching point of this activity is simply that no feelings remain the same. All feelings change over time. Pleasant emotions fade away, just as do the painful or difficult ones. This is just a fact about feelings. We may try to hold onto them to keep them longer or we may try to push them away faster, but they all change, inevitably. No feeling lasts forever. Most of us are fine with this idea when the feelings are unpleasant ones. For many kids, the idea of letting pleasant feelings go may be harder to accept.

Supplemental Group Activity

This activity can be useful to help children understand that trying to hold onto pleasant emotions might also bring about unhappiness:

"Enjoying feelings of happiness is a wonderful thing! And being mindful of our happiness is one way to really appreciate those feelings. But sometimes, trying to hold onto these feelings might cause us problems. For this activity, think of a time that you did something to try to keep or hold onto a happy or pleasant feeling and it turned out to be a problem for you."

EXAMPLE CHART

Enjoyable event	How I felt while doing the activity	What I did to hold onto the feeling	How this became a problem for me	What I could do next time to avoid the problem
Swimming at the pool	Happy	Didn't leave when my mom told me to.	Couldn't go back to the pool for a week.	Enjoy swimming until it's time to leave.
Playing tag during recess	Excited, having fun	Pretended I couldn't hear my teacher calling us back to class.	Missed the next outdoor recess.	Remind myself that there's another recess tomorrow.
Eating ice cream	Content, cheerful	Kept eating more and more ice cream.	Got a stomachache.	Next time, eat one bowl instead of four!
Playing video games	Entertained, really psyched because I was winning	Played for 4 hours.	I got in trouble the next day because I didn't do my homework.	Play a few games, then turn it off.

Suggested Practice Activities

• "During the next few days, notice a pleasant experience at the time it is happening. Record this event in your journal, making notes describing your thoughts, feelings, and body sensations. See if you can bring back this happy feeling later in the day or the next day. By remembering the event in as much detail as possible, try to reexperience the happy or joyful feeling. Can you mindfully reexperience exactly the same thoughts, feelings, and body sensations? Why or why not, do you think?

• "Practice mindfully smiling while you wake up each morning. Hang a happy face sign on the ceiling or wall near your bed so that you can see it when you open your eyes. This sign is your reminder. Give yourself a gift even before you get out of bed. Inhale and exhale 15 slow breaths while keeping a half-smile on your face. Watch each inbreath and each outbreath with mindful awareness. Write down your observations in your mindfulness journal."

Activity 45. Mindfulness of Worry and Anxiety (Part I)

Time Requirement

10–30 minutes (with optional charting and discussion).

Themes

• Worried thoughts and anxious body sensations contribute to feelings of worry and anxiety.

• Learning to bring awareness to the thoughts and body sensations that are associated with worry and anxiety, and then learning that the thoughts and body sensations don't need to control our emotions, is one way to help manage these uncomfortable emotions.

• Choices are never available anywhere but in the present moment. Learning to see what choices exist in each moment is another way to help manage worry and anxiety.

Background

It's normal to experience anxiety—and often helpful. Anxiety helps us focus in challenging situations, prepare for the future, study harder for an exam, play better for that important game, and keep our attention on important tasks. Anxiety also helps to protect us in dangerous situations. Some anxiety motivates us to do things that support our success. Too much anxiety, however, is not helpful and tends to happen when we think about things in the future rather than focusing on the present. Children might think about next Monday's exam and become anxious. "Will it be hard?" "Will I do well?" "What if I don't know the answers and do poorly and get a bad grade and fail Spanish?" Left unchecked, worries can spiral out of control—turning anticipated events into certain catastrophes.

Practicing mindfulness can be helpful in many settings: while preparing a class presentation, studying for a test, rehearsing for the school play, or practicing for the big game. Including mindfulness as part of our overall preparation can help manage anxiety in two ways. First, it relieves our anxiety in the moment, which allows us to focus and be more effective in what we do. Second, staying calm and focused also helps us perform better when the big moment arrives.

During the next activity, you will guide a visualization activity in which the kids imagine an anxiety-provoking situation, while carefully observing their subjective experiences of anxiety. Through this activity, children learn to bring awareness to body sensations and thoughts associated with anxiety. They will then share their experiences and what they learned about worry and anxiety. By becoming more aware of the thoughts and body sensations associated with anxiety, they develop choices and skills to better manage these uncomfortable feelings.

Materials Needed

- Visualization script (included below). This vignette describes one child who didn't complete his or her part of a group project that is scheduled to be presented to the whole class today. This child's classmates expect that everyone did their part of the work and are prepared. The unprepared student is anxious and worried about how the teacher and classmates will respond.
- Flip chart paper and markers.
- Activity handout: *Things We Can Learn from a Dog* (for the suggested practice activity).

Vocabulary for All Grades

- *Worry* means thoughts that are uneasy, troubled, or concerned; it is usually directed toward oneself, another person, or some event. Worry is thinking too much about problems and often imagining the worst possible consequences of an event.
- *Anxiety* is a combination of thoughts and expectations about an unknown or uncertain danger, mixed with feelings of worry, apprehension, or fear. Anxiety may increase when we think about an upcoming stressful event, anticipate a situation that has a risky or uncertain outcome, or have a fear of being judged negatively.

Mindfulness Activity

You might begin by offering age-appropriate definitions of worry and anxiety and ask kids to think about times they have experienced either one. Explain that mindfulness can help us be more aware of when worry and anxiety might be interfering with our well-being or with things that we really want to be doing. With older children and teens, you might discuss how we can't always control what happens to us, but we can choose how we respond to our own worries and anxiety. When we're lost in worry, it's easy to mistake our fears and worries for facts, instead of remembering that they are just thoughts. We know that some situations can feel very stressful. What's more, when we become anxious, we often do things that make us feel worse and end up creating even more anxiety. But, with mindful awareness, we can choose to pay attention to our anxiety—just as it is in the moment, and see things how they really are. Seeing more clearly, moment by moment, we discover that we have choices.

Visualization Script

"Please sit comfortably, relaxing with your eyes closed, if you wish, or with a soft gaze in front of you. Listen closely and pretend that you are living through the event that I will describe. See the scene in your mind's eye as clearly as you can—almost as if you are really experiencing it.

"Imagine that you are doing a group project with three of your classmates. Your assignment was to prepare one part of the project that the group is presenting to the class today. Last night, you got distracted talking with your friend and watching a video, and you did not work on your part of the project. All morning, you were too scared to tell the teacher or your group partners, so everyone thinks that you are ready. Now, your group is getting ready to make its presentation to the class, and you are the only one not prepared. It's time to stand up in front of the class in a group with your three classmates. Your teacher is watching. You see your classmates looking at you. They are all prepared and they think that you are, too. Now imagine getting up from your seat and slowly walking up to the front of the room, standing there with your teacher and group partners, and all your other classmates watching you and waiting for you to speak. See the scene clearly. [long pause]

"Now bring your attention to your thoughts. What is happening in your head right now? Are your thoughts racing around in circles or jumpy like ping-pong balls? Are your thoughts slow and dull? Are you thinking about all the unpleasant events that might happen next? Or maybe remembering another time when you weren't prepared for an assignment? Checking in with what's happening in your thoughts. Just noting and describing what is there. There's no need to judge your thoughts. With mindfulness, we learn to simply observe our thoughts. [long pause]

"Now shift attention to your feelings. Can you find and label what you are feeling right now? Inside, you might be feeling anxious, fearful, scared, nervous, angry, or embarrassed. You might even feel some of all of these. Checking in with yourself and noting what you are feeling right now. [long pause]

"Last, turn your attention to your body sensations. What is happening in your body right now as you imagine standing in front of the class not prepared for this assignment? Noticing how your belly feels. Noticing the feelings in your chest. What is happening in your throat? Your hands? Noticing if your breathing has changed. Do you feel hotter or colder? Are you feeling sensations of pressure or tightness anywhere? Do you feel like tears might be coming up? Checking in with yourself and observing how anxiety feels in your body. [long pause].

"Now relax and let go of this picture. Remember that it is just a story, and it didn't really happen. Let go of the worried thoughts and anxious feelings; instead feel relaxation flow through you as you remember it's just a story. Take a moment to focus on your breath, maybe using a favorite mindful breathing activity. Feel your belly moving out as you breathe in and your belly relaxing as you breathe out. As best as you can, bring your attention to the sensations of air moving in and moving out of your body, washing away the story. [long pause] Whenever you feel ready, you can open your eyes."

Now invite the children to observe, and if they choose, to share what just happened in their thoughts, feelings, and body sensations. Guide a discussion focused on the relationships between thoughts, feelings, and body sensations and ways in which strong feelings like anxiety might affect their behaviors.

If you have time, you may want to create a chart and record key elements of the discussion, as shown in this example.

EXAMPLE CHART

Thoughts	Feelings	Body sensations	Choices
I don't want to be here. I wish I could just run away.	Anxious and scared.	Butterflies in my stomach, heart beating fast, feels hard to breathe.	Tell myself that I am here now and I can cope with this. Focus on my breathing and practice noting how my thoughts are running away on autopilot.
I'm a terrible student. I let my group down.	Afraid they will be angry with me.	Hot feeling behind my eyes, throat tight, lips closed together hard.	Recognize that I'm not a bad student all the time; I just made a mistake this time. I can admit my mistake and apologize. My friends will still like me.
This class is horrible. I hate school.	Mad and worried.	Hands clenched, feel like crying, sick in my belly.	I'm making things worse by telling myself these things. I can calm down by relaxing my hands and taking a few deep breaths.

Referring to the chart, elicit children's ideas about the many points at which a different choice could have been made. Can choices be made that could help manage anxiety in other difficult situations? Although mention can certainly be made of the various things that one might do to anticipate and minimize difficult situations (e.g., prepare for the class presentation), for the purpose of this activity, focus the discussion on strategies that might help manage stress *in the moment*, as opposed to increasing stress with catastrophic thinking and misinterpretations of physical sensations related to anxiety.

You might want to explore the variety of memories and associations evoked by just imagining a stressful event and how those associations might interfere with seeing our choices. Help children understand that judgmental thoughts intensify an experience and how often we make our anxiety worse by creating unrealistic, unhappy stories about the future. Use the chart to bring attention to the relationship between experiencing an event and the subjective responses to that event. The aim is to elicit observations that thoughts and judgments about the experience are different from the experience itself. Observe and notice the distinction between describing the experience in a moment-by-moment way versus ruminating about, overanalyzing, or anticipating unknown outcomes to the experience. You might even point out that the physical sensations of anxiety are actually pretty similar to excitement—the difference is that we decide one is positive and the other is not.

Children can begin to develop greater awareness of how often they transform their present-moment experiences by adding memories (i.e., living in the past) or expectations (i.e., anticipating the future) to their actual experiences. Being mindful of thoughts as "just thoughts," feelings as "just feelings," and body sensations as "just body sensations" makes more choices become clear. When we can see our choices, we can make better decisions about how to handle challenging situations.

Additional Discussion Questions for Children/Teens

- "How do we know when we are feeling anxious or worried?"
  - "What are your sensations, emotions, actions, and thoughts at those times?"
  - "What part of the experience of anxiety is most upsetting to you? The thoughts? The feelings? The body sensations? What about the uncertainties?"
- "Can our thoughts make a situation worse than it really is? How does that happen?"
- "How do our bodies trick us into autopilot mode and into thinking lots of worried thoughts? How can we tell when other people are feeling anxious or worried?"
- "How might mindful awareness help us to learn more about our own feelings of anxiety or worry? How might this be helpful in our everyday lives?"
- "How might mindfulness help us to see more clearly what the actual situation is when we are feeling anxious?"
- "How can we practice finding the most skillful choices to help us manage stressful situations?"

Challenges and Tips

During this activity, keep an eye out for any child who shows indications of having experienced an unusually vivid or lucid imagery accompanied by intense anxiety, or who is experiencing any residual anxiety following the activity. Soothing the child can be done by reminding him or her that the imagery in this activity is just a story and did not really happen, and by taking a few minutes to practice mindful belly breathing or slow walking.

Suggested Practice Activities

- Read the handout *Things We Can Learn from a Dog*. After reading, discuss the points together. Key points might include how dogs are present-focused, rarely worry about the future, and tend to experience life joyfully, with enthusiasm, and without remorse or regrets.
- While focusing attention on body sensations, you can play recorded sounds that may

provoke anxiety or a startle response in resilient children who wouldn't be overwhelmed. Examples include ambulance, fire engine, or police car siren;, large animal sounds; and people screaming or having a loud argument. Several websites offer free or inexpensive downloadable sounds (e.g., *www.zapsplat.com* or *www.sounddogs.com*). You might also play music that provokes anxiety—for example, suspenseful movie soundtracks. Music with surprise changes in it can have a similar effect. Observe how being startled by an unexpected sound can create body sensations that mimic anxiety. When conducting this activity, stay attentive to any kids who might be getting overly anxious, and stop the activity if this occurs.

- Over the next few days, invite children to observe those moments when they might be worrying or experiencing anxiety. They may choose to record each trigger event, along with their thoughts, feelings, and body sensations in their journal. Questions for them might include:
  - "How many times each day do you feel worried or anxious?"
  - "How often do you get scared or anxious before anything actually happens?"
  - "Have your worries or expectations about something negative that might happen ever turned out to be worse than the actual event?"
  - "Does anxiety ever interfere with doing some things that you really wanted to do?"
  - "What might happen to your anxiety if you were to practice finding the space between thoughts, feelings, body sensations, and your behaviors where choices might be made?"
  - "What kinds of things can you do to help manage your anxiety?"

Activity 46. Mindfulness of Worry and Anxiety (Part II)

Time Requirement

20 minutes.

Themes

- Everyone experiences some worries, anxieties, or fears. Sometimes these emotions can get in the way of our doing the things we would like to do.
- We do have choices in how we respond to our own thoughts and emotions.

Background

In the first Mindfulness of Worry and Anxiety activity, the kids described thoughts, feelings, and body sensations related to feelings of anxiety. The first step in coping with anxiety is to identify and describe the thoughts, feelings, urges, and body sensations that we habitually bring into play when anxious thoughts and feelings arise, and then take positive action. For example, if we study, plan ahead, and pace ourselves, we can generally avoid the anxiety of not being prepared for a test. Sometimes, however, there may be stressful situations over which we have little or no control. For example, accidentally noting an upcoming test on the wrong week of your calendar might lead you to plan differently and be unpleasantly surprised when the test occurs a week earlier than you had expected. So, we can never avoid all stressful situations, and it just creates a lot more anxiety to try to accomplish this impossible task. Throughout our lives, we will face large and small challenges, and there will be times when we experience anxiety. This is part of what it means to be human. Mindfulness offers us a set of skills that can be used to more skillfully manage the challenges in our lives.

For this activity, children are divided into pairs. One child is the team recorder and the other is the team reporter. The recorder has the job of writing down strategic choices, and the reporter shares the information with the group. Each pair of children is given a worksheet that lists a number of anxiety-provoking experiences. After reading the scenarios, children will select two and together develop strategies to manage the stressful situation. Once they have developed their strategies, the group will reconvene for a general discussion in which the facilitator can highlight selected mindfulness-related strategies that can help manage stressful situations.

Materials Needed

- Activity handout: *Managing Worries and Anxieties*.
- Pens or pencils.
- Chart paper and marking pens.

Vocabulary for Grades 4–8

Stressed, nervous, concerned, troubled, bothered, apprehensive, uneasy, fearful, agonized, startled, alarmed, tense, jittery, jumpy, edgy, and any other words that the kids suggest.

Vocabulary for Grades K–3

Worried, scared, upset.

Mindfulness Activity

This activity is conducted in pairs. After sorting the children into pairs, pass out pencils and the *Managing Worries and Anxieties* handout. Then describe the activity as follows.

"During the last activity, we discussed feelings associated with worry and anxiety. We practiced exploring and describing our thoughts, feelings, and body sensations. Today, we are going to work in pairs to better understand situations that may bring about anxiety and fear, and develop strategies that may help us manage these difficult feelings when they arise. On the *Managing Worries and Anxieties* worksheet is a list of stressful events—things that can make some people anxious. Your job is to pick two events from this list that you worry about and develop three strategies for each event that could help manage those worries and anxieties.

"Each pair is a team, and each person in that pair has a role to play. One child will be the team recorder. It is the recorder's job to record all the interesting ideas developed by your partner and yourself. The other child will be the team reporter. It is the reporter's job to share the team's ideas with the rest of the class."

Children can self-designate their roles, be assigned roles by the facilitator, or be assigned roles by some random factor (e.g., the recorder is determined by coin toss, or is the child whose birthday is earliest in the month, or the child who is wearing the darkest color shoes). As soon as children have a worksheet and understand the instructions, they can begin working. Allow about 10 minutes to complete the task, and then invite the children to regroup for a discussion. On the chart paper, create the following chart:

EXAMPLE CHART

Stressful event	Strategies that help manage stressful events (these are "before-the-fact" preparations and behaviors)	Strategies that help manage worries and anxiety (these include mindfulness activities that focus attention on the actual events, thoughts, feelings, or body sensations occurring in the present moment)
Math test	Plan to study for 2 evenings.	Remind myself that I know the material very well.

As each reporter shares the choices that he or she and the partner developed, record them on the chart in the correct column. Be attentive to strategies that use mindfulness. Examples include:

- "Take several deep breaths."
- "Relax my body by practicing mindful slow walking."
- "Notice that my thoughts are thinking about something that hasn't even happened yet."
- "Recognize that my thoughts are probably worse than what is actually happening right now."
- "Stop and ask myself if I'm on autopilot right now."
- "Look for my choices."

You might wish to emphasize the benefits of bringing attention to all of one's thoughts, feelings, body sensations—even the more challenging or difficult ones. Help children articulate their understanding that bringing mindful awareness to stressful experiences may help make those experiences more manageable. Encourage reflections about ways to use their awareness of body sensations (particularly the breath) to be more present with all of their emotional experiences—the more difficult ones as well as the more pleasant ones. Increasing awareness of body sensations can help us let go of chronic autopilot worry thoughts and be more mindful of what is really happening in the present moment.

Additional Discussion Questions for Children/Teens

- "What does it feel like to be *mindful* of anxiety?"
- "Is it different from just being anxious?"
- "How does this differ from being mindful of more positive or pleasant emotions?"
- "How do you respond when you feel worried or anxious? Is this what you clearly choose to do or do you feel pushed and pulled by your emotions?"
- "Could mindfulness help you create space between your thoughts, feelings, and behaviors so that you respond less impulsively and more skillfully."
- "Does practicing mindfulness even when you're not worried help you worry less?"
- "Can practicing mindfulness protect you from being hijacked by your own thoughts?"
- "When you are anxious, how might you remember to look for choices?"

Challenges and Tips

Because worries and anxieties are so common with children and adolescents, we offer more extended guidance and a number of additional practice activities that can be helpful for working with intense anxiety (and other strong emotions). Any of the activities described next can be done in additional group sessions or as individual home-based practices.

Suggested Practice Activities

- Digging deeper: Ask children to practice mindful breathing for a few minutes, and then bring their attention to their own patterns of worry or anxiety. For example, some children may notice that taking tests or speaking to strangers makes them very nervous. Others may worry when they are required to speak in front of the class. Still others may get excessively anxious around transitions or beginnings (e.g., entering a new grade or going to camp for the first time). In a nonjudgmental way, invite the children to look—gently and with kindness for themselves—to see if they observe a worry pattern in their lives. What feelings do they recognize underneath the worry? What fears are there? Are there concerns about disappointing others? Fears of failing? Ask the kids to dig deeper underneath the worry to see what else might be there. They might take a few minutes to note their observations and thoughts about these worry patterns in their mindfulness journals.
- Ask children to spend a few moments thinking of a recent stressful event or something that they are currently worried about, preferably something small. Paying close attention to the thoughts that may increase feelings of stress, invite them to consider how they might relate differently to those thoughts in a way that reduces the worries and anxiety. They might want to list specific strategies in their journals that could help them manage that particular stressor, both before the fact and while the stressor is happening.
- Suggest that the kids practice using a body-focused activity (e.g., body scan, mindful movements, mindful slow walking) to bring awareness to what anxiety feels like in their bodies. Invite the children to explore how those body sensations might be related to thoughts and emotions. Encourage them to focus their attention on body sensations and explore how those sensations might be related to their thoughts and feelings.

- No matter how hard we try to avoid it, anxiety is a part of all of our lives. Suggest that the kids record one stressful event that they experienced this week in their mindfulness journal. Invite them to describe the event or situation, the thoughts, feelings, and the body sensations that they experienced, the choices that they identified, and how they chose to respond to the stressful event. As they observed their own thoughts, feelings, and body sensations, did they notice themselves thinking or feeling any differently than they usually do in similar situations? After finding their choices, did they choose to respond in a way that is different than they normally do?

Activity 47. Mindfulness of Sadness and Loss (Part I)

Time Requirement

15–20 minutes.

Themes

- We can practice identifying thoughts and body sensations that are associated with feelings of sadness and loss.
- We can recognize sadness in others.
- Sadness (like all emotions) is often mixed with a variety of other emotions.
- Sadness changes over time, and usually becomes less intense as time passes.

Background

For many of us, experiences of loss, grieving, and sorrow are among the most difficult emotions to face. Sadness can be particularly powerful or painful when it is linked with memories of other sad experiences that reinforce and intensify the emotional impact of the current experience. Sadness is a hard emotion just to sit with, and we can spend considerable energy trying to avoid sadness by distracting or distancing ourselves from the feelings. We might attempt to mask our distress with other emotions such as denial, indifference, or sometimes anger. Only rarely do we allow ourselves to just sit and be present with our sadness, compassionately, without trying to push it away or becoming numb to it. When practicing mindfulness, we can practice getting to know our sadness. It's like giving our sad feelings permission to exist. We learn to accept that sadness is a part of ourselves—a part of who we are. Sadness, like other emotions, exists on a continuum. It may be as slight as feeling disappointment at breaking your favorite mug or as intense as the grief of divorce, moving houses, or the death of a loved one. But, like all emotions, the intensity of loss, grieving, and sorrow is not permanent.

Unlike other emotions such as happiness, social norms can tell us how sadness "should" be expressed. Some children may be more embarrassed to cry in front of a group of classmates than they would be to express anger. Especially for boys, openly displaying sadness carries risks of being socially ostracized or censured—labeled by peers as being weak or effeminate. Different cultures may also display and process grief in different ways. It may be helpful to reflect upon how the children respond to sadness both in experiencing and expressing their own sadness, and how comfortable they are when another person expresses sadness. How comfortable are the kids when a child displays sadness? Can they simply be present with another person when he or she experiences a significant loss—without trying to "fix" the grief? Creating a supportive classroom environment, or a mindful and compassionate community, where all of the kids feel free to express sadness is fundamental to helping children cultivate self-compassion and mindful acceptance of these feelings when they emerge.

In this activity, children will practice bringing mindful awareness to feelings of sadness by identifying the thoughts and body sensations that accompany the feelings. We will reinforce the idea that the same events can affect different people in different ways. Feelings of sadness can be experienced and expressed in many ways. There is no right or wrong way to feel or express sadness. We will look carefully to see how we may incorporate memories of our previous experiences of sadness or expectations of future sadness with our present-moment experiences. We may even discover that just by looking clearly, we change the very nature of the experience.

Materials Needed

- *Charlotte's Web* by E. B. White (the last two paragraphs of Chapter 21: The Last Day) or another passage of your choice that involves loss and grief. Particularly for children in grades 4–6, we might suggest *Old Yeller* by Fred Gipson or *Where the Red Fern Grows* by Wilson Rawls. Teens may respond to a sad love story such as *Beneath the Tree That Wept Flowers* by Michael Anderson. Alternatively, you might choose to have the teens watch a poignant scene from a sad movie—for example, *Love Story*, *Titanic*, *Me before You*, or the opening sequence of the animated film *Up*. You may have better, more contemporary examples at your disposal.
- Activity 43 handout: *Being Present* (one for each child) and stickers.
- Chart paper and markers.
- Mindfulness journals.
- Activity 47 handout: *Child Figure (Boy or Girl)*. This is an optional drawing activity that can be done in session or as a home-based activity. With younger children (5–7 years old), it is best to do this activity in session. If this activity is done in the group, you will also need crayons, colored pencils, or markers.

Vocabulary for Grades 4–8

Grieving, miserable, heartbroken, down in the dumps, disturbed, gloomy, dejected, sorrowful, woeful, melancholy, depressed, desolate, tearful, despondent, glum, grief-stricken, or whatever creative words the kids come up with.

Vocabulary for Grades K–3

Sad, unhappy, feeling low, blue, down

Mindfulness Activity

Before beginning this activity, you may wish to guide a few minutes of mindful breathing practice. You can then describe today's activity, as suggested here.

> "Today we are going to continue our practice of becoming mindful observers of our feelings. I am going to read a passage to you from E. B. White's *Charlotte's Web*. As I read, you may want to close your eyes so that you can see the story better. As best you can, keep your complete attention on the story. As you listen, your mind might wander. When this happens, just notice that your thoughts have wandered, and then gently bring your attention back to the story. Listen closely, bringing mindful awareness to being in the story, while also bringing attention to any thoughts, feelings, and body sensations that may arise."

As you finish reading, pause to let them reflect on the story. Then pass out the *Being Present* handout and stickers. Ask children to rate on their scale from 1 to 7 how sad they felt as they listened to the story. Some children will be more moved than others, so you will probably discover variability within the responses. Invite the children to share other feelings they might have experienced in response to the story as well. If a child says that he or she didn't feel sad about the story, invite him or her to share whatever emotions were experienced as he or she listened to the story. Encourage exploration of thoughts that might have influenced the child's emotions. For example, "I felt relieved because she was going to die anyway and at least she was peaceful." Or perhaps, "I felt okay because I knew she was going to die, like my turtle did, but she would go to heaven, where it's better." You may want to write down some of the expressed thoughts, emotions, and body sensations on a chart as the discussion unfolds.

EXAMPLE CHART

Thoughts	Emotions	Body sensations
Charlotte must have felt horribly alone in the last few hours of her life.	Depressed and angry when I realized that Charlotte was going to die.	Wet eyes, face is hot, lump in my throat
Wilbur is really lonely. He misses his best friend.	I am heartbroken for poor little Wilbur.	Heart feels soft and open.
Charlotte is in heaven now.	I feel bad that Charlotte died, but also kind of peaceful because she went to heaven.	My whole body feels empty but heavy.

It is not unusual for children to say that they feel "bad" after hearing a story that involves loss. If this happens, gently probe further for additional descriptive words that express the feelings that the child might have experienced. You might want to write some alternative descriptive words for *sadness* on the chart to expand their vocabulary. It is also important (no matter how tempting) to not put your words into their mouths. Part of cultivating mindfulness of emotions is for each person to practice identifying what is present. Being provided with labels can interfere with their practice of attending to those feelings. However, to help increase their vocabulary, responding to child descriptors with a synonym can be helpful. For example, if a child says, "I felt really, really bad," you might respond by saying something like, "Wow—that sounds like a whole lot of sad—were there some feelings of grief or loneliness mixed in there, too?" As the chart is filled in, help each child identify where in the body he or she feels the sadness. Where did children feel the sadness in their bodies when they learned that Charlotte was dying? Where did they feel the sadness in their bodies after she died? You might also explore if people ever feel sadness in the body in other ways (e.g., stomach upsets or headaches). The story might not have generated strong body sensations, and that's okay too. For example, some people may cry when they are sad, but will only do so when they are alone. Or they may have felt anger at Charlotte's death, but not be willing to express this to others. Only rarely does the story elicit no emotional reactions at all. Some kids may have emotional reactions, but be less willing to express them outwardly. At the end of this part of the discussion, invite the children to check in with themselves and again rate how sad they feel at that moment on their *Being Present* handout.

After exploring their own sad thoughts, feelings, and body sensations, invite the kids to reflect on how they know when people around them are sad. How does sadness show on other people's faces? In their bodies? In their words? What about the tone of voice? Is it possible to detect sadness in how someone moves or gestures? Have them think of one person in their lives who they know very well and with whom they feel emotionally close. It might be a parent, a sibling, or a close friend. How does this person look, sound, and act when he or she is sad? Can you detect sadness in the sound of the person's voice or the words he or she uses? How about through facial expressions or posture? How does this person act? And is this different from how he or she normally acts? How do other people in your family express sadness?

Before ending this session, you may want to conduct another short breathing practice or a letting go practice such as mindfulness while lying down. Give the kids permission to let go of any sadness that they might have felt in response to the story. You might say, "Imagine the sadness gently flowing out of your bodies with each breath."

Additional Discussion Questions for Children/Teens

- "What are some of the ways that sadness is experienced and expressed differently by different people?"
- "How do you know when you are sad? What does sadness feel like in your body? In your thoughts and mind?"
- "Does the way you think and the kind of thoughts you have change when you are sad?"
- "How do you know when other people are feeling sad?"
- "Does what you see or the way you see the world change when you are feeling sad? How?"

Challenges and Tips

During this activity, be attentive to any teasing, unkind, or invalidating behaviors among the children. This kind of response could manifest in a number of ways: for example, a child being teased for crying or admitting to sleeping with a teddy bear when he or she is sad.

Although it rarely happens, when teasing or unkindness does emerge in a mindfulness group, the first step is to recognize that there may be a lot of pain present, both in the child who said the unkind words and in the child on the receiving end of those words.

The most effective response to meanness is compassion. Model mindful compassion and empathy in your own speech and behaviors. Before you respond to either child, let yourself feel what is going on. Check in with yourself and acknowledge your own emotional state. Validate the experiences of both children. You might say to the recipient of the unkind remark, "It is normal to feel bad when someone says something that feels hurtful." You might suggest to the child that made the remark, "Sometimes when we get angry or don't feel great about ourselves, it can seem easier to put those unpleasant feelings onto someone else." The key is not to deny the feelings in the room, but rather to model acceptance of the entire experience by inviting both children to take a moment to breathe and reconnect with their own feelings. Then you might invite all the children to do a short breathing practice together with you.

Suggested Practice Activities

- "Take the *Being Present* handout home with you. Tomorrow morning, take a moment and think back to the story we just read. Ask yourself how sad you feel right then (not how you felt when the story was read). What, if anything, about your feelings has changed? Are you thinking differently about the sadness now than you were thinking yesterday? Do you feel more or less sadness? If you are experiencing sadness because of some other event in your life today, how might that affect what you feel about the story? Explore how your feelings have changed over the short time from yesterday to today. Note your observations in your mindfulness journal.

- "Think about a sad event that happened to you a long time ago, something that was somewhat difficult for you when it happened, but has become a little less sad over time. Spend a few minutes relaxing with a mindful breathing practice, and then bring that sad event into your mind as vividly as you can. Be like a detective and explore what emotions come up. Where in your body do you feel them? What do you notice about these feelings? What other memories, if any, are connected to this sad event? Stay with the feelings as best you can. What words might you use to describe them? How long do the feelings last? Do you notice changes as time passes? Remind yourself that feeling sad is okay. You do not have to push it away. You can handle sadness. You are bigger than sadness. Just like each breath comes and goes, so too does sadness come and go. When the intensity of the memory fades, just rest in the stillness. Breathe in and breathe out for another 15 slow breaths."

This activity can be done in session or at home, in appropriate doses. Distribute copies of Activity 47 handout, *Child Figure (Boy or Girl)*, to children. Ask the children to think of a time when they were sad and invite them to draw what this sadness felt like in their bodies. If you are doing this in a group, you might want to play some sad music or music that has a melancholy or reflective quality while they draw. This can be a powerful way for children who are not comfortable discussing their emotions verbally to express and process strong emotions.

Activity 48. Mindfulness of Sadness and Loss (Part II)

Time Requirement

Each of the two activities described below will take about 15–20 minutes. They do not need to be done at the same time, but we do recommend doing them in the sequence shown here.

Themes

- Sadness is experienced and expressed in different ways.
- Recognizing when others are feeling sad and offering support to them is one way we cultivate compassion.
- Being more aware of the consequences of our choices, we can speak and act with more skillfulness.
- Developing the skill of staying present with difficult emotions supports the healing process.

Background

With this mindfulness activity, we build on the groundwork from the first Mindfulness of Sadness and Loss activity about the natural human desire to avoid painful or unpleasant emotions. This activity focuses on getting to know our experiences of sadness in a fuller way. When we are on autopilot, we push away sadness, but this can create more challenges down the road. We may fear or avoid sadness so much that we engage in behaviors that are harmful in the long run. We might find ourselves engaged in activities that deny or numb our feelings of sadness. We might try to cover up the sadness with feelings of fear or anger. We do many things to push sadness out of our awareness. Kids might write or share about ways that they or others do this. It takes determination to be willing to simply "sit with" these feelings of distress, face the difficult emotions directly, and let them be within us—just as they are. Learning to live with sadness, loss, and grief with mindful awareness and skill is essential to emotional self-regulation. Further, mindfulness skills offer simple and positive alternatives to risky coping skills that older kids might choose to adopt, from substance use, sexual acting out, to self-injury, and other self-harming behaviors.

Materials Needed

- Chart paper and markers.
- Mindfulness journals.

Vocabulary

The same vocabulary that was used during the previous activity.

First Mindfulness Activity

We recognize the importance of a cohesive group—whether in the classroom or in the community. To support this, we help children bring compassionate awareness to their feelings and to engage in compassionate behaviors toward others. This activity provides opportunities to consider ways in which we might support others during their sad times. As we build a mindful community, we invite children to give as much compassionate attention to the emotions of those around them as they do to their own experiences of sadness. Children will gain practice in recognizing mindful choices about their own sadness and in how they relate to the sadness of others. Finally, we encourage the kids to explore possible consequences that may emerge from their own choices.

"During our last mindfulness activity about sadness, we became mindful of the thoughts, feelings, and body sensations that came up as we listened to a sad story. We noticed how our thoughts can help us *be with* sadness a little easier, or make it feel even harder. We explored what sadness feels like in our bodies and how those feelings might change over time. Now, we will explore how we know when other people are feeling sad. What are some of the signs we might look for in others?

"Today we are going to explore a time in your lives during which someone close to you felt sad. It might be something that just happened or it might have happened a while ago. It could be a family member or a friend. It could be a really big event, but it may be more helpful if it's something a little smaller. The important thing is that you remember the experience clearly. I invite you to describe this sad event with as many details as you can remember. Who would like to begin?"

Questions to facilitate the discussion might include:

- "What happened? Who did this happen to?"
- "How did this person respond? What did he [or she] say? What did he [or she] do?"
- "As best you can remember, what were the thoughts, feelings, and body sensations you experienced when this event happened?"
- "How did you respond to this person's sadness? What, if anything, did you actually say or do? Was there anything you wanted to say or do at the time that you didn't? What stopped you?"
- "Looking back, would you say or do anything different from what you did at the time?"
- "How did being present with this person's sadness affect your own mood?"
- "What helped you cope with your own feelings?"

It is not always easy to think or talk about sadness. In fact, a lot of times we try to get away from those sad feelings as fast as we can. But, as we practice mindfulness of sadness, we discover that we are strong enough to look closely at our sadness and the sadness of others. We can pay attention to sadness without pushing it away. As you encourage several children to share their stories, you might want to note the main points on a chart, as shown in the following example.

EXAMPLE CHART

Trigger event	How I know he/she was sad	How I felt	What I did or said
My brother's girlfriend broke up with him.	He kept talking about how much he missed her. He cried a lot and was angry. He stayed in his room all day listening to sad songs.	At first, I was a little sad for him, but I didn't like his girlfriend and was secretly glad they broke up. Later, I was annoyed. I wished he would just get over it and stop moping around.	I told my brother that his ex-girlfriend was not a very nice person and he should be glad that she broke up with him.
My best friend told me that she flunked an important exam.	Her face got red. She looked like she was going to cry. She said, "I don't know what happened. I really do know this stuff. I studied hard, but my mind just went blank." She walked home alone after school. Her head was down and she walked slowly.	I was sad and felt sorry for her. I know she really works hard to get good grades.	I didn't know what to say so I just patted her on the back. My eyes got wet when I saw she was trying not to cry. I left her alone and went to talk to another friend.

Second Mindfulness Activity

By practicing mindfulness of emotions, we gain the freedom to make choices about how to respond to others in helpful and compassionate ways. We always have choices in how to respond to our own feelings and how we respond to the emotions of those around us. We might visualize the present moment as being like a giant mat that is laid out for us to stand on while we choose what to do. While we are standing on the mat, we can make decisions about how to respond to our own feelings and how to respond to the feelings of others. By getting out of autopilot mode, that mat gets much bigger, so we can see more choices and pick the best one. Choices happen in the moment *before* we act. At any moment, we can look at all the different options we have, and then choose the best one for ourselves and for the people around us. It is important to be mindful of the potential consequences of each choice as well. Sometimes the most skillful choice may simply to be present and feel compassion for the feelings of others.

> "Let's explore choices by brainstorming some behaviors with which we might compassionately respond to sadness. What are some things we might do to help ourselves be more compassionate of others who might be feeling sad? As we come up with mindful choices for how to deal with sadness, let's also think about the consequences of these choices, and how we might feel after making them."

Brainstorm possible choices on a chart like the one shown here. When the choice seems to be a way of pushing away the sadness, it might be helpful to point out that it's certainly okay to want to feel better right away, but it's also important to find ways to experience the sadness without avoiding it or doing something that might result in negative consequences. When we try to avoid sadness, we sometimes make choices that aren't the best for others or for ourselves. Practicing being mindful of sadness, we can make choices that don't ignore the sadness or push it away.

EXAMPLE CHART

Choices I might make to manage sadness (for myself or another person)	Possible consequences	How I might feel afterward
Listen to my brother talk about his ex-girlfriend and tell him that I'm sorry he feels so bad.	That might make him feel a little better.	I would probably feel better because I do love him and don't want him to be so upset.
Talk to my parents or a teacher that I trust.	Someone safe will listen to me.	I would feel more connected with that person and not as sad.
Eat two bags of chips. When I feel sad, I sometimes eat too much junk food.	Get a stomachache.	Still feel the same sad feelings, plus I might feel kind of sick to my stomach.
Go play outside with my friends.	Have fun with my friends so that I feel better.	Had fun, but the sad feelings came right back when I went home.
Sit with my friend and tell her it's okay to cry. Help her see that flunking one test isn't going to ruin her life.	My friend would probably feel like I really care about her and that might make her feel better.	It would feel good to be able to help my friend even a little bit.
Steal some of my parents' alcohol and go out drinking with my friends.	If my parents notice the missing bottle of alcohol, I'll probably get grounded for life.	When I drink, I always feel terrible the next day. I'll also be afraid that my parents will find out. And the sadness will come back.

Other ways to experience sadness (our own or in others) with mindful compassion include the following:

- Talk to a friend whom I trust.
- Write about it in my journal.
- Give my friend a hug and let her know it's okay to cry.
- Cry together with my friend.
- Spend time just hanging out with my friend.
- Sit with my sad feelings.
- Take my friend for a walk.
- Take some deep breaths.
- Make a card for my friend.
- Tell my friend that I really care about him.
- Tell myself kind and comforting thoughts.
- Remind myself or my friend that that it's okay to feel sad.
- Remind myself that sadness doesn't last forever.
- If I've been sad for a long time, like if someone dies, remind myself that it's okay to laugh and be happy and still be sad too.
- Remind my friend of all the other things that she's done very well.
- Cuddle with my dog or cat.
- Tell my pet how I'm feeling.
- Listen to my friend.
- Share a story with my friend about when a similar thing happened to me.
- Do something he loves to do, like riding bikes or playing a game together.

- When I can, let the feelings go.
- Listen to music.

Suggested Practice Activities

We highly recommend providing kids with a number of possible activities from which to choose when they are attempting to handle sad feelings. For example:

- "It is important to be able to help ourselves when we are feeling sad. And it is also important to help those around us if they are feeling sad or upset. Imagine that your best friend comes to school and tells you that his or her pet died last night (or something else sad). Your friend is feeling very sad about his or her pet's death. In your mindfulness journal, write down some of the things you might choose to say or do that might help your friend be okay with his or her sadness. How could you help your friend be more compassionate and mindful of his or her own sadness?

- "During the next few days, be attentive and see if you can notice when someone you know is experiencing sadness. Record this event in your mindfulness journal. How do you know that this person is feeling sad? Was it through words? His or her expressions? Behaviors? What helpful choice could you make now? Make a point of saying something or doing something for your friend that you think might be helpful. Remember that sometimes, the best choice may be to just *be with* that person . . . sit with him or her and just listen, without doing anything else. Sometimes just giving people the space they need to feel sad is the most compassionate thing we can do."

Activity 49. Mindfulness of Frustration and Anger (Part I)

Time Requirement

Each of these activities will take 15–20 minutes. They do not need to be done at the same time, but we do recommend doing them in the sequence shown here.

Themes

- Feelings of frustration and anger can emerge when we think that we have not gotten what we want or deserve.
- Our thoughts contribute to creating or worsening strong emotions—but our thoughts can also help us manage those emotions with greater skill and compassion.

Background

Anger and related emotions (including annoyance, frustration, irritability, rage, and wrath) can be deeply embedded in our emotional memories. For the most part, children learn what they see. If the adults who influence children as they grow are modeling constructive behaviors by managing their own anger skillfully, demonstrating effective de-escalation of conflict, and are able to calm themselves after experiencing irritation or frustration, children are likely to learn these skills too. Unfortunately, many adults do not provide ideal role modeling when it comes to management of anger and frustration. Whether or not children arrive in a classroom or a therapy group with appropriate anger management models or skills in place, they can benefit from mindfulness to manage these big emotions. One factor that contributes to how well children can cope with anger is how clearly they observe events. This ability includes noting their own thoughts and feelings (e.g., frustration, embarrassment, guilt, shame, or disrespect) before they escalate into damaging anger or rage. Approaching these events and the accompanying thoughts and feelings from the stance of a "neutral observer" is a fundamental tenet of mindfulness approaches to emotion self-regulation. How much pain, aggravation, and remorse might we spare others and ourselves if we could just step back and observe a potentially frustrating interpersonal interaction objectively, rather than being swept away by habituated reactive thoughts and emotions?

Frustration is a feeling of being upset or annoyed that can come from a feeling of powerlessness. Something or someone is blocking our progress or keeping us from achieving a desired goal. We can think of frustration as the emotional response when expectations and reality don't align—and that can fuel anger. When people are emotionally "flooded" with full-blown anger, they cannot step back to be an objective observer of their own thoughts and emotions. Never in the entire history of the world has anyone in a rage been told to calm down and actually had that advice calm him or her down. Anger is too visceral—too deeply embedded in our primitive brain—to respond to reason.

The aim of the next two activities is to help children bring greater awareness to feelings of frustration, which if unchecked, can develop into full-blown anger. These activities provide practice in identifying thoughts and body sensations that typically accompany these feelings. We look at the physical experience of frustration in the body and we explore thoughts that might increase or decrease that frustration. Part II continues the mindful exploration of frustration and anger by helping children find effective ways to manage more extreme feelings along the annoyance–frustration–anger continuum.

Materials Needed

- Paper copies of a crossword puzzle that is well beyond the children's expected ability level. We intend the puzzle to be too difficult (and therefore frustrating) for the children to complete in the allotted time.
- Flip chart paper and markers.
- Activity handout: *Feelings Thermometer* (optional).
- Supplement: "Transforming Feelings" by Thich Nhat Hanh (optional).
- Mindfulness journals.

Vocabulary for Grades 4–8

Irritated, infuriated, annoyed, fuming, livid, cross, outraged, heated, ripped, flipped out, steamed, irate, aggravated, perturbed, bothered, exasperated, enraged, pissed off, and whatever other words the kids might come up with.

Vocabulary for Grades K–3

Angry, mad, frustrated.

First Mindfulness Activity

Rather than beginning the activity by informing children that the focus today is on feelings of frustration, simply give them these instructions:

> "Today we are each going to complete a crossword puzzle. The person who finishes first will get a special reward. [Offer a highly desirable reward.] Once we start, you may not ask any questions or speak to others in the group. You aren't allowed to use a dictionary or other reference materials. Are there any questions?"

Take a moment to answer any questions they might have, and then begin. After a few minutes, and without any advance notice, stop them from continuing. Then gather together to discuss the experience. Invite a volunteer to share his or her experience of this activity. It is not uncommon for children to confuse thoughts and feelings. That is why the use of a chart can be helpful. In an open and nonjudgmental manner, complete the chart as shown in the following example, eliciting the children's responses and then guiding them to identify into which box each part of their response fits.

EXAMPLE CHART

Thoughts	Feelings	Body sensations	Judgments
This looks really hard.	Nervous, annoyed, angry	Tense shoulders, teeth clenched, fidgety	None of us can do this. It's so unfair that she's making us do this.
I've never done a crossword puzzle before.	Puzzled, scared, frustrated	Scowling forehead, sweaty palms	This is stupid.
Oh boy, I like doing crossword puzzles.	Excited, eager	Heart racing, smile on face	This is not fair. She should never give us anything this hard.

Some are likely to express very clear and visible frustration—which provides a key opportunity to help kids identify and stay present with what may be relatively strong thoughts and body sensations associated with the emotions.

FACILITATOR: (*to a child who raised his hand*) Would you like to share your experiences of this activity?

CHILD: I thought it was stupid.

FACILITATOR: Okay, I'll go ahead and write *It was stupid* over here in the judgment column. As you were working on it, what feelings did you notice in your body?

CHILD: My head started to hurt and I felt angry that we had to do this.

FACILITATOR: That's really careful observing of what was going on for you as you worked on this difficult puzzle. I'll go ahead and put *head hurt* under the column for body sensations, and I'll put *angry* under the feelings column. Did you notice any other body sensations? Were you aware of what your breath was doing?

Encourage children to share anything they may have noticed about their breath, and then invite discussion about the connection between the breath and how we feel.

> "Think about what your breathing was like during and after this activity. Have you ever noticed that our breath changes with our mood? It can be short and shallow when we are tense or angry, and faster when we get excited. Is it slow and full when we are happy or contented? Almost disappearing when we are afraid? When we get frustrated or upset, our breath can also be used as an anchor—to bring calmness back to the body. The nice part is that we don't need to remember to bring our breath with us—it's always right here."

Elicit descriptions of the experience from several children, using the chart as guidance. Then refer back to the chart to note and explore the variety of feelings that arose for different people. Using separate columns for thoughts and judgments helps children identify the differences between describing an experience and judging it. Look for opportunities to make that distinction. One is describing the event in a moment-by-moment, nonjudgmental, accepting way. The other is criticizing, evaluating, or judging the event, ruminating about or analyzing what happened, comparing it to other experiences, and/or anticipating what may follow the event. In this way, children are learning how often they transform their present-moment experiences by adding memories (i.e., living in the past) or expectations (i.e., anticipating the future) to the actual experience.

> "Since we started practicing mindfulness, we have explored how our thoughts and feelings are connected. This may be especially true when it comes to stronger emotions such as frustration and anger. There are thoughts we can tell ourselves that help manage our frustrations and thoughts that we can tell ourselves that may make the frustration more difficult to tolerate. Sometimes we are not even aware of all the thoughts that are running around in our heads when we get frustrated or angry. But thoughts are always there, and our challenge is to remember to be aware of those thoughts as *just thoughts*, not facts. In real life, we can't always control what happens to us, but we can always choose how we respond to our own thoughts. And this choice can change the way we feel."

Second Mindfulness Activity

This is a journaling activity aimed at building skills to better manage difficult emotions. Because we are human beings, challenging events will happen. Sometimes we will have feelings that are not comfortable or pleasant. This is just part of what it means to be human. Mindful acceptance of our feelings means that when we get frustrated or angry, it is perfectly okay to allow ourselves—in that moment—to feel frustrated. Nevertheless, we then also have choices as to how we will respond. Will we hold on tight to the frustration and maybe let it grow into anger or rage? Or will we choose to let the feelings of frustration fade away? The thoughts we choose to focus on can determine which way our emotions go. We can choose thoughts that might increase frustration or thoughts that might decrease frustration. What happens to us is not always our choice, but how we deal with it is.

> "I would like each of you to think of a time recently when you got really frustrated about something. Take a minute and think back to what happened, how you felt in your body

and mind, and what you did. Maybe think about your mindful SEAT. Write in your mindfulness journal some of the thoughts that might have made you feel more frustrated in that situation and some thoughts that might have helped you feel less frustrated."

This activity may be challenging for younger children and require some assistance to identify the two types of thoughts. Even distinguishing between thoughts and feelings is not always easy. It can take further practice to differentiate judging thoughts from describing thoughts.

EXAMPLE CHART

Trigger event	Judging thoughts (that might increase frustration)	Describing thoughts (that might decrease frustration)
Missed the school bus because I couldn't find my shoes.	I'm in huge trouble; this is the third time this has happened. I'm going to be suspended from school if I'm late again.	I can practice being more organized, but freaking out isn't going to help now. I'll ask my mom for a ride to school and tell her that I'll try to be more organized so this doesn't happen again.
Having trouble figuring out the math homework.	This stinks. It's so unfair. This is way too hard. I'll never be able to do this.	This is hard for me, but I will learn it. I'll call my friend and see if she understands it. It's not the end of the world, I guess. If I can't figure it out with my friend, I'll just ask my teacher for help.

Additional Discussion Questions for Children/Teens

- "Where in the body does your frustration start to grow? What does it feel like?"
- "How can bringing awareness to your body sensations help you move away from frustration and anger?"
- "What happens when you try to focus on the sensations rather than on the thoughts or emotions?"
- "What types of thoughts fuel your anger and what cools it down?"
- "Could separating thoughts from feelings be a way to better manage some of these strong emotions? If so, how?"

Challenges and Tips

- Some children will get more frustrated than others and have to struggle to let go of their frustration. Before finishing, you might invite the children to make a choice to let go of any feelings of frustration that might still be hanging around, perhaps sharing with each other some self-talk, mindfulness, or relaxation skills that can help. This could be a few minutes of mindful breath counting. Or you might suggest the image of a peaceful calmness entering their bodies with each inbreath, and all the frustration and stress flowing out of their bodies with each outbreath. Remind them that they can always choose to tune into their breath when they find themselves feeling frustrated or angry.
- The second tip is to monitor your own reactions carefully when a child expresses frustration or anger. The most common response is to jump to soothing or calming, usually by offering false reassurances or platitudes. This is precisely what we do *not* want to do during

this activity. Although strong emotions can feel uncomfortable, their emergence represents an opportunity to help the child simply *sit with* those emotions, not acting on them, but rather getting curious about his or her own emotions. In doing so, the child strengthens his or her ability to sit with strong emotions and learn that acting on them is not inevitable. The experience of sitting with emotions opens the children to the important understanding that *feelings are not facts* and never last forever.

- Angry pop music, from punk to rap to film soundtracks, can also trigger mild feelings of anger and frustration with which to work and explore.

Suggested Practice Activities

- The Activity 49 handout, *Feelings Thermometer*, can be a useful tool to help kids differentiate the intensity of their anger or any other strong or uncomfortable emotion. It also serves as a reminder to stop and check in with themselves before reacting without thinking. For older children, you might want to use the *Feelings Thermometer* handout instead of the *Being Present* handout that was introduced in Activity 43, Mindfulness of Happiness.

- For older kids or teens, working more deeply with strong emotions can help manage their intensity and decrease the urge to react with thoughtless speech or behaviors. We included this practice in the frustration and anger module because managing these emotions is difficult for many teens. However, this activity can be practiced with other strong emotions such as fear, anxiety, shame, or grief. Start by reading the short passage by Thich Nhat Hanh, "Transforming Feelings," from his book *Peace Is in Every Step: The Path of Mindfulness in Everyday Life* (1991b, pp. 53–55), which is reprinted on page 183. Discuss the five steps to transforming emotions. Using examples from the teens' personal experiences, explore how these steps might look in practice, and then consider potentially challenging situations in which using these steps might be helpful:
  - Step 1. Use your mindful awareness to *recognize* your feelings as they come up.
  - Step 2. *Connect* with your feelings—get to know them and become friends.
  - Step 3. *Calm* down the feelings using your breath.
  - Step 4. *Let go* of the feelings—remember that feelings won't overwhelm you.
  - Step 5. Then, *look deeply* at the feelings. Discovering what is causing the suffering will help you transform the feelings.
- Brainstorm with the kids the thoughts or behaviors they can choose to use to calm themselves when they feel frustrated or angry. Invite them to make their lists in their mindfulness journals. These choices might include:
  - Taking a few deep calming breaths.
  - Giving themselves a hug or placing a hand on their hearts.
  - Practicing the mindful breath-counting activity.
  - Looking for more realistic or calming thoughts, and not adding more frustrating thoughts.
  - Checking in with themselves to see if what they are telling themselves is totally true.
  - Asking themselves, "Is what I'm telling myself right now really helpful to me?"
  - Getting help if they can, especially with frustrating schoolwork.
  - Talking to a trusted friend or adult.
  - Reminding themselves that no matter how frustrated they feel, it will pass.

- ○ Burning off frustration with exercise or play.
- ○ Asking to be excused from the room to get a drink of water until they calm down, or maybe splashing some cool water on their faces or hands.
- ○ After mindfully observing the frustration, take steps to calm down and let the feelings go.
- ○ Listening to soothing music.
- ○ Finding something funny about the situation and letting themselves laugh.
- ○ Asking themselves "How big a deal is this, really? Is it worth getting really frustrated over? Will I even care about this in an hour or a week?"

Activity 50. Mindfulness of Frustration and Anger (Part II)

Time Requirement

15–20 minutes.

Themes

- We certainly can't always control what happens to us, but we can always choose how to respond to the events of our lives. Or as Jon Kabat-Zinn (1994) has observed, "You can't stop the waves, but you can learn to surf!" (p. 32).
- Learning to observe, tolerate, and accept uncomfortable emotions such as frustration and anger can make it easier to act with mindfulness and compassion for others and ourselves.

Background

It can be particularly important to bring mindful attention to feelings of anger and related emotions such as annoyance, irritation, and frustration for several reasons. First, these emotions can be triggered very quickly. Ingrained memories, fears, and snap judgments about someone's intentions can fuel knee-jerk reactions. Strong emotions make it harder to think clearly and objectively. When we react on autopilot to a trigger event, we are reacting from habit—in sensations, emotions, thoughts, and actions. Sometime our reactive thoughts and behaviors happen so fast that we regret them later. By bringing mindful awareness to our body sensations, thoughts, feelings, and urges in the moment, we are slowing the reactivity down long enough to take a look inside—and examine how our thoughts and emotions might influence how we interpret events. Slowing down creates opportunities to make more conscious choices about how we want to respond, which in turn makes it less likely that we will be swept away by our own emotions and act in ways that we later regret.

Second, practicing mindfulness helps us see that emotions are indeed real. However, they are real *emotions*—not real facts. Anger is a strong emotion that sometimes provokes strong reactions. We might sometimes see ourselves as victims of events. "This happened *to* me." "That person did such and such *to* me." "It wasn't my fault, *she* started it." It is true that we rarely have control over what other people say or do. But, in regarding ourselves as victims of happenstance, we also give away control of our own emotions. What we hear is, "He *made* me mad" rather than, "He said something to me and I chose to respond from a place of anger." Bringing mindful attention to our anger empowers us to see that we do have choices in how we respond to our own emotions.

Viktor Frankl is credited with saying, "Between stimulus and response there is a space. In that space is our power to choose our response. In our response lies our growth and our freedom." Choices live in that brief moment between the triggering event and our reaction to the event, and choices can only be made in this moment, never in a past or future moment. Mindfulness helps us become more attuned to that space between stimulus and response, perhaps slowing us down just a little, and gives us the gift of clarity in that one moment in which conscious choices can be made.

When practicing mindful awareness, we pause, observe, and describe the triggering event—all this before we let reactive emotions drive our speech and behaviors. We check in with our own thoughts and feelings, and then we choose to respond. In that moment, we likely will respond with greater clarity, intention, and wisdom. This is the basis for understanding that, regardless of what happens to us, we are empowered to choose how to respond in our thoughts, in our feelings, and in our speech and behaviors.

An autopilot reaction to anger is quick and often unintentional. A mindful response is made with clarity, thoughtfulness, and intention. Choices are platforms from which children have the freedom to choose to make mindful versus thoughtless choices about how to respond to feelings of anger or frustration. In this activity, children learn to identify skillful ways to manage their anger, and they explore ways to remember to use those skills when they are most needed.

Materials Needed

- Flip chart and markers.
- Mindfulness journals.
- Activity 50 handout: *Exploring My Own Trigger Events* (optional; for use with suggested practice activity).

Vocabulary for All Grades

- *Reactions:* Knee-jerk or autopilot types of speech and behaviors can emerge with little or no consideration in response to a trigger event. Reactions are often fueled by strong emotions, are not skillful, and may lead to unintended negative consequences.
- *Responses:* Freely and consciously chosen speech and behaviors after mindfully attending to all aspects of an event. Responses are more likely to be situationally appropriate, more skillful, and less likely to lead to unintended negative consequences.

Mindfulness Activity

Start by conducting a few minutes of mindful breathing. As you're ending the practice, invite the children to keep their eyes closed or to gaze softly at the floor and rest in the still, quiet space with their breath.

"Today we are going to continue looking mindfully at feelings of anger and frustration. I am going to describe a story to you. I'd like you to sit quietly with your eyes closed or gazing softly at the floor so that you can visualize the story as clearly as you can. Picture what is happening with your mind's eye.

"Imagine that your school is having a contest to see who can come up with the best name for the school's new cafeteria. The person who comes up with the winning name will get a sign in the cafeteria with his or her name on it and will get to be first in the lunch line for a month. You think of a great name—'Hungry for Knowledge: Learning to Lunch'—which you are sure will be the winner. You tell your best friend the name, and he promises that he won't tell anyone.

"Everyone places his or her nomination for a name into a sealed box. On Friday morning, the principal will open the box. The naming committee will look at all of the different suggestions and select the winner. You wait anxiously for the big day. On Friday morning, the principal calls you and your best friend into her office. To your astonishment, she tells you that you both have submitted the same name! When she reads it, you are furious. 'Hungry for Knowledge: Learning to Lunch' is the name *you* thought of and told to your friend. The principal asks who thought up the name first. Both of you say you did. She says, "It's a great name and the committee would like it to be the winner, but only one person can win, so if you can't work it out between you two by this afternoon, we will have to pick another winner." You get into a shouting match with your friend and call him a liar, but he refuses to admit that he got the name from you, so you both lose the contest."

Encourage the children to visualize this story really happening to them. Ask them to check inside themselves to see what is happening right now—in their thoughts, feelings, and body sensations. Then invite them to let go of the story and slowly return awareness to the room while opening their eyes. Begin a discussion by inquiring about the thoughts, feelings, and body sensations they had while they listened to the story. Encourage them to share how they would be likely to think and feel, and what they would be likely to do, if this had really happened to them. What might they think about their friend's behavior?

"We have discussed how we can't always control what happens to us, just like the child in the story couldn't control whether or not his or her friend cheated. The only thing we do have choices about is how we respond to the anger—in the moment and afterward. When we are angry, we sometimes do things that make us feel worse or end up causing even more grief and pain for others and for ourselves.

"There is always a moment before we choose to say or do something we might later regret. In that moment, we can choose to calm ourselves down as best we can, so that we can make better choices about what to do. The moment *before* you act out of anger (or any emotion) becomes an opportunity to make a choice. You might think of that space as a giant mat that is laid out for you to stand on while you choose what to do. While you are standing on this mat, you can make a decision about how to respond to whatever you're thinking and feeling. It is sometimes helpful to think about what the consequences might be before you act.

"Mindfulness might make it easier to make better choices. When we practice mindfulness, we make our mat bigger so that we can see more choices. With mindfulness, we can stop from slipping into autopilot so that we can make the best choice for ourselves in that moment. When you find yourself standing on that mat of choices, you might choose to respond in many different ways."

Elicit suggestions about some ways they might manage their anger in a way that would make it a little easier for themselves. Encourage children to think about the consequences and results of each possible choice. This is part of making mindful choices. As you fill in the chart that follows the list here, help each child who shares his or her responses to identify at least one mindful choice. Some mindful choices might be:

- Practice mindful breathing or mindful breath counting.
- Talk to someone you can trust, like a parent or teacher, about what is happening.
- Take a break from the person with whom you're angry so that you can clear your head and try to figure out what's really going on.
- Count to ten, especially ten breaths, ten sensations, ten sounds, or something more concrete.
- Visualize being in your favorite calm, peaceful place.
- Observe and note how the anger feels in your body without having to respond at all.
- Run around and burn off energy to clear your head.
- Write down your feelings in your mindfulness journal.
- Listen to relaxing music.
- Take a walk.
- Write a letter to the person with whom you are angry, but *don't* send it.
- Help your thoughts become more realistic about what may happen.
- Observe your body sensations and then let the angry feelings flow away like water.

EXAMPLE CHART

Thoughts	Feelings	Body sensations	Mindful choices	Possible outcomes
I can't believe he did that to me.	Anger, betrayed	Flushed face, body tense all over	Take 10 deep breaths.	I would feel calmer and might be able to talk to my friend.
I'll never trust him again.	Outraged	Tearful, heart racing, stomach hurts	Excuse yourself to go spend a few minutes practicing mindful breath counting to calm down.	Wouldn't shout at my friend and get into more trouble.
That was really a rotten thing to do.	Irritated, upset	Head hurts	Talk to a trusted teacher or friend about what happened.	Try to let go of the anger so that we can still be friends.
Winning the contest must be really important for him to ruin our friendship like this.	Sad, sorry for my friend, compassionate	Heavy feeling in heart, tightness in throat	Tell the principal that you thought of the name first, but that your friend is more important than winning the contest. Ask if you can share the prize together or give it to your friend rather than let it go to another child.	Friend apologizes for his behavior, and you both get to share the prize.

Additional Discussion Questions for Children/Teens

- "Is it possible to experience strong feelings without acting upon them?"
- "What thoughts make the anger worse? What thoughts might calm the anger?"
- "Could being mindful observers of your thoughts and feeling help you feel better about yourselves? If so, in what ways?"

Suggested Practice Activities

- Like all feelings, anger exists along a continuum. Some incidents may trigger minor irritation or annoyance inside us. Others might result in stronger anger reactions. Often we don't bring our full awareness to the true intensity of our feelings. We say we are "so mad," when in truth we are just annoyed or a little irritated. On a scale from 1 to 10, have the children rank how angry they think they might feel in response to the following different events (10 being the angriest and 1 being the least angry). Kids might also appreciate a visual metaphor like a thermometer for rating their anger or other strong emotions.
  - Someone cuts in front of you in line.
  - You get blamed for something you didn't do.
  - Someone says something bad about you or your family.
  - You team loses to a team you don't like.
  - Your best friend yells at you.
  - Someone steals something from your desk.
  - You lose your iPhone or tablet on the bus.
  - Your mom makes you do homework when you don't want to do it.
  - Someone pushes you on purpose.

Discuss why different events might be rated as more or less intense by different people. For a follow-up activity, using the same list, have the kids practice creating a list of mindful choices. Ask:

- "What might you do if this happened to you?"
- "What might you suggest to a friend?"
- "What might the consequences of different choices be?"

In the story described above, what other feelings might be hiding beneath the anger— for example, disappointment, loss, sadness, confusion, hatred, anxiety, guilt, shame, betrayal? If we pay close attention, we often find that underneath anger is a whole mix of other feelings that can get ignored, especially if the anger is quite strong. Suggest to the children that "the next time you find yourself feeling angry, look deeper. What other feelings might be living underneath the anger?"

Distribute the *Exploring My Own Trigger Events* handout to the kids. Invite them to notice small events that might happen in the next week or so during which frustration or anger is triggered. Suggest that they complete the worksheet for each event and notice if they were able to use their mindfulness skills to attend to their thoughts, feelings, and body sensations. How did they select their kinder choice? Did this choice change the expected outcome?

Activity 51. Mindfulness of Embarrassment

Time Requirement

20–30 minutes. To reduce in-session time, the writing portion of this activity can be assigned as homework in advance. This will allow more time for reflection and discussion.

Themes

- Embarrassment is an emotion that happens when we fear ridicule or rejection.
- Some thoughts reduce the intensity of difficult emotions (such as embarrassment), whereas other thoughts maintain or make it worse.
- Cultivating compassion for ourselves and empathy for others is one way to help manage the discomfort of embarrassment.

Background

Embarrassment is an emotion that we feel when we are being seen by others in an uncomfortable way. By and large, embarrassment strikes when we feel we did something bad or wrong, or made a visible error, or feel deficient—with fear of being judged or ridiculed by those watching us. To some, fears of embarrassment can be significantly impairing or completely debilitating. The desire to avoid real or perceived social humiliation influences our behavior considerably. This can be especially true for children in the classroom or other group settings. Fear of being embarrassed often prevents children from trying new challenges. The embarrassment may be focused on feeling "less than" others (e.g., less wealthy, smart, attractive, athletic, popular) or on fears of failing in front of peers. When the emotional safety of a social setting increases, feelings of embarrassment tend to decline. We encourage children to see themselves as interconnected and meaningful members of their classrooms and their larger communities. Cultivating compassionate intentions toward oneself and others is essential to this perspective.

The mindfulness of embarrassment activity has two aims. The first involves helping children become more aware of their own emotions, along with thoughts and body sensations that may accompany feelings of embarrassment. Children practice identifying thoughts that create, maintain, or increase feelings of embarrassment. We also help them identify thoughts that may calm the embarrassment. By bringing mindful attention to the thoughts, feelings, and body sensations that accompany moments of embarrassment, children begin to see that they can "survive" those moments and that the uncomfortable feelings will pass. A sense of mastery and competency develops as children learn to recognize and accept the full range of human emotions.

The second aim involves bringing mindful awareness to other people's experiences of embarrassment. The development of empathic compassion—learning, for example, what we might say or do to help another person who is feeling embarrassed—is an essential step toward building a mindful classroom or community group. How might we recognize when that kind of helping is warranted and appropriate? How might we address our own feelings of inadequacy or embarrassment so that we can be more empathic and compassionate of the suffering of another person? These are big questions with no clear answers. The first step, however, is to bring awareness and attention to our own fears and difficult emotions. Empathic compassion begins with self-compassion and then the recognition that others might feel the same difficult emotions and suffering that we do.

Materials Needed

- Flip chart paper, markers.
- Mindfulness journals.

Vocabulary for Grades 4–8

Embarrassed, ashamed, humiliated, bashful, chagrined, mortified, demeaned, awkward, self-conscious.

Vocabulary for Grades K–3

Uncomfortable, shy, guilty, uneasy.

Mindfulness Activity

Before starting, you might want to remind children of their commitment to speak and act toward others with care and kindness. Depending on the group dynamics, being very explicit can be helpful. We sometimes say:

"Today we are going to practice bringing mindful awareness to feelings of embarrassment. When we began learning mindfulness, we each agreed that we would speak and act toward others with care and kindness. Today, this means that when someone chooses to share a difficult or embarrassing experience, we listen with mindful attention and do not make fun of or laugh at him or her. Does this rule make sense to everyone? Great! No one needs to share an embarrassing moment if you don't want to. If you do choose to share, you may discover that many of us have had similar experiences. Now, would anyone be willing in this safe space to share a time when he or she felt embarrassed?"

If no child volunteers, the facilitator might begin the discussion by sharing one of his or her own experiences of feeling embarrassed. Doing this in a comfortable and authentic manner is a useful way to model mindful self-compassion while also encouraging others to speak. A little bit of humor can be helpful as well. For example, one facilitator described getting her first smartphone. Not knowing how to use a touch display, when the phone rang, she pushed on the "answer" button instead of swiping across the screen. When this didn't work, she called customer service to complain that her phone was broken because it wouldn't answer any phone calls. After describing what she was doing, the customer service person carefully explained how to swipe her finger across the screen to answer a phone call. She imagined that the customer service person was secretly laughing at her and felt stupid and embarrassed. Ideally you might share one of your own relatable experiences from childhood, adolescence, or even an experience of embarrassment you had during adulthood.

Then, invite the children again to share one of their embarrassing experiences, with an emphasis on examining a *small* embarrassment from which they have recovered. After one child shares, thank him or her for being courageous enough to share the embarrassing moment with the group. Remember to thank the rest of the group for being mindful listeners. Then you might invite the child to consider whether he or she would have felt embarrassed if he or she had been alone and no one had seen what happened? Most likely the answer will be "no," because embarrassment is usually an emotion that happens when we are in front of other people. If children are hesitant to share aloud, encourage them to just raise their hand if they can at least think of something embarrassing that happened to them.

"Today we're going think about a little time when we felt a little embarrassed, which has happened to all of us. I'm going to ask you to write about one of your small embarrassing moments in your mindfulness notebook. Afterwards, but only if you wish, we'll share some of these experiences with each other."

Then invite the children to close their eyes or gaze softly at the floor, and then remember clearly a time they were embarrassed. Maybe it was when they dropped a tray in the lunchroom, or walked down the street with their pants unzipped. Did they ever get toilet paper stuck on their shoe and have someone point it out to them? Or be called on in class and give the wrong answer to an easy question? Maybe they missed an easy catch during a game, or even scored on their own team! What other experiences could bring up feelings of embarrassment? Encourage the kids to pick a small experience that they can remember well.

"Visualize the experience first. What did the embarrassment feel like in your body, and where? What thoughts came up during the event? What were the thoughts about yourself and the thoughts about the people around you who saw you make this mistake? What did you think afterward? Then describe the experience in your journal—including as many details as possible. As you write, practice mindfully observing the entire event. Pretend that you are a reporter writing a story for another person to read. Write down all the details—who, what, when, where, why, and how."

Allow the kids about 10 minutes to write down their experiences, and then invite them to share what they wrote and how they felt as they were writing. As children share their responses, you can create a chart like the one in this example:

EXAMPLE CHART

Trigger event	Body sensations	Feelings	Unhelpful thoughts (may increase embarrassment)	Helpful thoughts (may decrease or help manage embarrassment)
Dropped my lunch tray in the cafeteria and everybody laughed.	Tears in eyes, body froze	Embarrassed, humiliated	This is the worst thing that's ever happened to me. Everyone is watching me and laughing.	This is a bummer, but no one will even remember it by next week.
Was called on in class and didn't know the answer.	Flushed face, heart racing	Self-conscious, felt stupid, bad about myself	This is awful. I can't believe I don't know the answer to this.	No one knows the answer to every question. I'll study harder so I can do better next time.
My little sister told everyone on the bus that I still sleep with my teddy bear.	Headache, fists clenched, teeth grinding	Embarrassed, ashamed, angry at my sister	Ughhh, now everyone will call me a baby or think I'm a dork.	I bet I'm not the only kid who sleeps with a stuffed animal that helps them feel safe. It's no big deal.

As children volunteer responses, write down the trigger event, the body sensations that they felt, the feelings they had in response, and the thoughts that went along with the emotions. You might observe that embarrassment often occurs in conjunction with other emotions such as guilt, shame, fear, or even anger. Children may voluntarily offer helpful or self-soothing thoughts in response to the embarrassing events. Thoughts that serve to heighten embarrassment are written in the "unhelpful thoughts" column and those that potentially reduce embarrassment in the "helpful thoughts" column. Encourage several children to share their responses. The children might consider what to say that might help a friend, or what might make things worse. You can ask the group each time if anyone else has had a similar experience. Watch for heads nodding in agreement, since it is common for others to have had similar experiences, and reflect on whether it helps to feel less alone when we are embarrassed.

Next, ask the group to explore the difference between the last two columns. If no child has described thoughts that reduce or manage embarrassment, that's perfectly fine. This would be a good time to help them identify a few helpful thoughts to put in the last column. If any child gets stuck picking helpful thoughts, invite the other children to brainstorm solutions, as described in this example.

FACILITATOR: Okay, so you dropped your backpack at the bus stop and everyone had to wait while you picked everything up, loaded it back into your pack, and got on the bus. What sensations did you notice in your body when this was happening?

CHILD A: My face got really red and I felt tight in my chest. I was scrambling around under the bus. The driver seemed kind of mad at me, or at least annoyed.

FACILITATOR: What were you feeling when this happened?

CHILD A: Embarrassed, ashamed, and frustrated because these kinds of things always happen to me.

FACILITATOR: What thoughts were going through your mind?

CHILD A: I was thinking that this always happens to me. And I knew that everyone was laughing at me and thinking what a klutz I am.

FACILITATOR: That's a very thorough description, and it helps all of us be more aware of what was going on inside you. I'll bet that others here have experienced things like this as well. So, let's write down *embarrassed, ashamed,* and *frustrated* in the feelings box. Then, I'll put "This always happen to me" and "What a klutz I am" in the unhelpful thoughts box. The next box is for thoughts that might help us feel a little less embarrassed when something like this happens. Helpful thoughts might not make the embarrassment go away completely, but they can help us be more mindful of the experience and help us respond next time in a way that is kinder and more helpful to ourselves.

CHILD A: I don't really know.

FACILITATOR: That's okay. Would anyone else like to help with a thought that might help [Child A] feel less embarrassed? Maybe a thought that makes whatever happens not seem like such a big deal?

CHILD B: He could tell himself that everyone drops things sometimes.

CHILD C: He could tell himself that although it probably seemed like it took a long time to pick everything up, it really only took a minute.

CHILD D: If people helped him, he could remind himself that most people are really nice, and his friends weren't mad at him.

FACILITATOR: These are all great ideas. How do some of these thoughts sound to you (*looking at Child A*)?

CHILD A: Good, I guess.

FACILITATOR: I think so too. Let's put those helpful thoughts right here in this last column.

The facilitator should distinguish between helpful and unhelpful thoughts, making clear that different thoughts affect our moods and emotions in different ways. It is also important to *avoid* conveying the idea that there are "good thoughts" and "bad thoughts." All thoughts are just thoughts. But some thoughts may be closer to the reality of a situation, and those are the thoughts might be more helpful. Our minds are very good at creating unrealistic mountains of catastrophe out of anthills. Brainstorm as many helpful thoughts for each event as possible. Reiterate two key points: first, that thoughts have the power to affect our emotions, and second, that all feelings change and embarrassment fades over time.

Additional Discussion Questions for Children/Teens

- "How is bringing mindful awareness to feelings of embarrassment different from the ways you typically experience embarrassment?"
- "Could mindfulness of your feelings of embarrassment change how you respond to a trigger event?"
- "Could mindful awareness of another person's embarrassment change how you speak or act toward them?"
- "Does practicing mindfulness of your own difficult emotions help you feel more compassionate toward others?"
- "Does practicing kindness to yourselves help create a mindful classroom or community? If so, how?"

Challenges and Tips

Children and teens are usually okay with sharing embarrassing moments, but some may need the reassurance of someone else going first. This provides an opportunity for the facilitator to model curiosity, openness, and nonjudgmental acceptance by disclosing one of his or her own embarrassing moments. You may want to consider what you might be willing to personally disclose in advance of this activity. Events that are common may resonate with more children (e.g., dropping or spilling something, tripping, being late, saying something silly). Smaller events associated with smaller embarrassments, even while practicing mindfulness, may also facilitate disclosure and discussion. I've often shared falling asleep in meditation class! If you choose to use humor, make sure that the laughter is *shared with*, not *directed at* any child.

Suggested Practice Activities

There is a wealth of possibilities for additional practices that can further expand the kids' mindful understanding of embarrassment. Here is an example of the variety:

- "One aspect of practicing mindfulness is related to how we treat others who might be having difficult experiences. We've talked about being mindful of choices to help ourselves cope with our own difficult feelings. We can also practice using mindful awareness to make choices that help others cope with their difficult feelings—for example, feelings of sadness, anxiety, anger, or embarrassment. Let's say that your friend drops her lunch tray in the school cafeteria. You could do some things that aren't particularly compassionate, like laugh at her, walk away from her, pretend like she's not your friend, or just stand there and watch as she struggles to clean up the food on the floor all by herself. Alternatively, you could choose to act in a mindful and compassionate way.

- "Brainstorm other, more compassionate choices. What else might you say or do to help your friend during this stressful event? List in your mindfulness journals some of the ways that you might help your friends manage their feelings of embarrassment. Here are some possibilities:
  - "Help your friend clean up the food.
  - "Smile at her and let her know that she's still your friend.
  - "Gently remind those who are laughing or teasing that it's not cool to do that because anyone could have an accident like this.
  - "Tell your friend that it's no big deal.
  - "Go get an adult to help clean up the food and get it out of the way.
  - "Remind her of a time that you did something just like it.
  - "Make a silly joke to help everyone laugh and relax.

- "Now let's try an imagery activity. Remember a situation during which you felt embarrassed. In your mind's eye, recreate the situation just as it was. Recall the body sensations and feelings that you experienced. Remember the thoughts that may have popped into your head. Remember the looks on people's faces or the things that they said while this event was happening. Once you have brought the thoughts, feelings, and body sensations into focus, take a few moments and just be with them. From the safety of this room and this moment, observe those thoughts, feelings, and body sensations. Then, let the image go and breathe in and out three times.

  "Now, imagine that the same thing happens to you again. However, this time you have mindfulness skills to help you. You feel the same body sensations you noticed; maybe your face gets red or your heart starts pounding. What could you do for yourself to calm those body sensations? Maybe you can begin to relax yourself by bringing attention to your breathing, your body, your feet on the floor or other points of contact. Then look at your thoughts. What are you telling yourself that may be making the feelings worse? What could you say instead that might be more helpful to yourself? Think of as many different choices as you can for this event.

- "The next time you experience feelings of embarrassment or shame, practice transforming them with the steps we have learned today:
  - "Recognize the emotions as they arise.
  - "Bring attention to your own thoughts, feelings, and body sensations. Become friends with your internal experiences.

- ○ "Accept whatever your experiences are in the moment—right now—exactly as they are.
- ○ "Remember that thoughts and feelings are not permanent.
- ○ "Tell yourself that thoughts are just thoughts and that feelings are not facts.
- ○ "Let the thoughts and feelings come and go. What is the 'life cycle' of an embarrassing feeling?"

Activity 52. Mindfulness of Envy

Time Requirement

Each of the four activities described below can be completed in about 15–20 minutes. Each activity can stand alone or be grouped, as time permits.

Themes

- Bringing mindful attention to feelings of envy cultivates the ability to be objective observers of strong emotions.
- Observing without reacting helps us better understand the thoughts and body sensations that are associated with feelings of envy.
- Some thoughts can reduce the intensity of painful emotions, whereas other thoughts will create, maintain, or exacerbate the discomfort.
- Desires are transient. Getting the things we want often does not result in the long-term happiness that we had anticipated.

Background

Envy is an emotion that arises from a thought or feeling that we don't have enough. More specifically, envy arises when we look at others or the world around us and conclude that things are not as they "should" be. Something is not "fair." Someone else has something that we feel should be ours. Our own thoughts generate feelings of envy: "I don't have what I want"; "In order for me to be happy, I must have that thing"; "I want what she has, not what I have"; "How I am isn't good enough"; "What I have right now is not enough or not good enough."

Because humans are social creatures, we look at others to determine how we are doing. Are we smart enough, tall enough, pretty enough, skinny enough, or athletic enough? Who has more than I do? Envy happens when we decide that to feel okay, we must first acquire the attribute, experience, or object we believe we want. We must be something more than we are. Have something more than we have. We might even act as if this belief is true. Envy can lead us to think less of another person or hold resentful feelings toward someone who does possess what we think we want. Is it possible to feel good enough, or feel like we have enough, just as things are?

The mindful alternative is to bring awareness to all these "shoulds." These are the things we tell ourselves that we must have or be; we must be something other than we are or the world around us must be other than it is. We practice getting to know these "shoulds" in order to accept who we are and how things are—just as they are. With mindful awareness, we simply look at our moment-by-moment experiences—just as they are—with interest, curiosity, and compassion. We practice accepting that these are actually our experiences.

We offer four activities that invite children to observe feelings of envy with mindfulness and self-compassion. The first offers children an opportunity simply to observe their own feelings of envy as "nonjudgmental and curious observers," without judgments or self-criticism. We all want things that we don't or can't have. We invite discussion of questions such as "What does envy feel like in your body?" or "What thoughts are associated with that feeling of envy?" The second and third activities bring in the idea that desires change over time, and that getting the things we think we want often does not bring the expected happiness. We begin to examine the nature of *wanting*. These activities seek to bring greater awareness to the thoughts that intensify our belief that we "must have" certain things in order to feel okay. We also explore how our feelings about the things we want change over time and the ways in which our thoughts and expectations change the experience of getting something we thought we wanted. The last activity integrates the idea of having choices in how we respond to feelings of envy—having unwanted or distressing feelings does not necessarily require us to act impulsively or on autopilot. By developing greater tolerance for strong emotions such as envy, sadness, and anger, children learn to slow down their emotional reactions and look for alternative choices in their speech and behaviors. As children bring greater awareness to their feelings and their behaviors, they learn that they have choices in how to respond to them.

Materials Needed

- Flip chart paper and markers.
- Mindfulness journals.

Vocabulary for Grades 4–8

Envious, desirous, resentful, covetous, long for, pine for, hanker for, wish for, hunger for, be obsessed with, crave.

Vocabulary for Grades K–3

Envy means that we want or think we need what someone else has.

First Mindfulness Activity

The facilitator begins by advising the group that today we will bring what we have been learning about mindfulness to feelings of envy. Sometimes, when someone else has something we want, or another person gets to do something that we wish we could do, feelings of envy come up. Today we are going to talk about how we can become more aware of those feelings in us, so they don't carry us away or cause us to act in ways we wish we hadn't. Has anyone ever felt envious of a sibling, classmate, or friend? We are going to start with a story about feeling envious. The story is told as a guided imagery. Invite the children to close their eyes and picture, as best they can, the story you are about to tell them. Ask them to picture the story clearly, as if they are living in it, making it seem real by seeing the story in their mind's eye as vividly as they can.

"You and your friends all want the brand new iPhone—with all its great new features [or insert any other smartphone, tablet, or other recent, age-appropriate, highly desired electronic device]. Thoughts about that iPhone are frequently on your mind. Everywhere you go, you see them. Every day you talk about getting one for your birthday, saving enough money to buy one, maybe even convincing your grandparents to buy you one. You've read about it, watched videos about it—you have even picked out which color you want. As the weeks go by, some of your friends get the phone. One day, you get home from school to find that you have received a present from your grandparents. You get very excited and hope that it's the iPhone that you want so much. You rip off the wrapping and open the box to discover that they gave you an old model of a no-name brand phone. That very night, your best friend calls. His voice sounds really happy and excited. He has just received a brand new, top-of-the-line iPhone and wants to come over and show it to you. You are feeling very envious and almost can't believe he got the exact iPhone that you wanted so badly. [long pause]

"What sensations are you feeling in your body? What are your thoughts? What are you telling yourself about this situation? You tell your friend that you have homework to do tonight, so he can't come over. The next day you go to school and you see your best friend with his shiny new iPhone. What are you feeling toward your friend now? How are you feeling about yourself? What thoughts are going through your mind? What sensations are you feeling in your body? What do you say to him? How do you act toward him? Take a few moments and, as best you can, observe the feelings in your body. Imagine taking a step back from yourself and simply watching what and where envy lives in your body, without needing to do anything to change it or make it go away. Looking closely at the envy and say to yourself, 'Hmm, I know that feeling. It's envy. Let me just look at that for a minute.' Just watching in an interested and curious way—without judging or trying to make the uncomfortable feelings go away. Seeing envy as it is, in your thoughts, in your emotions, and in your body sensations. [long pause] Now you are letting go of the story. Remembering that this is just a story and not real. Whenever you feel ready, open your eyes and bring your awareness back to the room."

Invite the children to share their experiences of this story, or with younger children, to draw or maybe doodle or write about the experience. What thoughts came up? Body sensations? How did he or she act, or want to act, toward this friend the next day? As children provide their answers, pay special attention to the thoughts associated with envy. You might elicit their reasons for wanting that iPhone. Is it to have the same thing that all their friends have? To fit in? To feel special or more important? To get the rush that goes along with getting something new? Because having it could make others feel envious? It is rarely (if ever) because the thing we want so badly is actually essential or necessary.

Prepare a chart like the following one as children offer their answers. Although children are told that envy is one of the feelings they experience, other feelings will likely emerge in this visualization as well. They may also describe feelings of anger, disappointment, frustration, or even depression along with envy.

EXAMPLE CHART

Trigger event	Feelings	Why I think I need this	Do I really need this?	Helpful thoughts (things I might tell myself to feel better about not getting what I wanted)
My friend gets the new iPhone and I get an old, no-name smartphone.	Envious, disappointed	I can't be happy unless I have everything that my friends have.	No.	I could be happier for my friend. It's great that he got one.
Same	Envious of my friend. Angry that I didn't get what I really wanted.	iPhones are cool and old, no-name phones are definitely not.	No.	It would be great to have one, but I can live without it. The phone my grandparents got me does most of the same things.
Same	Jealous, sad, frustrated	Everyone else has one. They'll think I'm a loser if I don't have one too.	No.	My friend lets me borrow his phone sometimes. I'm lucky to have a good friend like him.

As we discussed earlier, we can't always control what happens to us, but we can always choose how we respond to those events. We can choose to act in a way that helps us be more mindful of how we feel, or we can choose to get swept up in envy and make choices that may not be the best ones for ourselves or for the people around us:

"You might even act on your envy in a way that could have negative consequences. Can anyone think of some examples? For example, you might stop talking to the friend who received the iPhone, tell your grandparents you didn't like their gift, or even think about stealing or breaking your friend's new phone. How might doing any of those things work out for you?"

Second Mindfulness Activity

You might begin this activity by reminding children of the work they have done recognizing the choices that were available to them during the other activities, and that they have choices when it comes to envy as well. You might want to remind them of when such choices can be made:

"Choices arise in the moment before you say or do something driven by envy or any other strong emotion. In this moment, you can look at the different options you have and choose one that is most helpful for you and for the people around you. Sometimes the best choice is simply to practice being mindful of how you feel. Nothing else."

One of the ways we bring mindful compassion to our envy is to look at the thoughts that keep the envy alive (refer to the charted thoughts). Then help children consider other thoughts that might better manage these difficult feelings: "What are some thoughts that you might tell yourself that could help you make choices that will be better for everyone?" Add these to the last column of the chart. You can start by asking the child whose responses are already on the chart, but also invite the others to contribute their ideas.

Third Mindfulness Activity

"The next activity again explores the point that emotions change over time. How you are feeling now will most likely change over time. What are some things that you use to believe you really needed that you no longer think you need quite as much? Write down in your mindfulness journals an object (coat, necklace, bicycle), an experience (trip to Disney World, go to a concert), or something else (a pet) that you had really wanted a lot and that you received more than 6 months ago. Reflect on your thoughts and feelings before, during and after you got this thing. Some questions you might ask yourself are:

- "Was the actual experience the same as what you expected?
- "Was the anticipation of getting the item different from the actual experience?
- "Did your desire for the object change after you received it?
- "Did you feel any disappointment with the actual thing as compared to your belief about what it would be like?
- "Did your interest in the item change once you had it for a while?"

EXAMPLE CHART

What I wanted	How I felt *before* I got it	How I felt *when* I got it	How I felt 1 week later	How I felt 6 months later	How I feel *now*	Did my feelings change?
A puppy	Like I really, really have to have a puppy.	Excited. The best day of my life.	Really happy to have a puppy.	I love my dog, but he can be a lot of work.	I still love him, but I wish my mom would feed him.	Yes
A bicycle	I want that bike more than anything.	Surprised and excited when my dad gave it to me.	Still feel really good.	I still like it, but it's kind of scratched up now and one tire is flat.	Wish I had a newer bike.	Yes
Go to Disney World	This is the greatest place in the whole world.	I had fun, but it was hot and crowded. I got tired and wanted to go home early.	I had fun, but it wasn't as much fun as I thought it would be.	Okay, fine. It was cool to go.	Don't think about it much anymore.	Yes

Children can develop greater awareness of the thoughts, beliefs, and expectations that accompany the feeling of "gotta have it." The main idea to convey here is that, like thoughts and emotions, the feeling of "wanting" changes too. What we want now, we may not feel so strongly about in the future. And, once we do receive that thing we once wanted so badly, we may discover that we didn't actually want it as much as we thought we did. Cultivating this perspective on impermanence can bring greater awareness to how we feel about things we believe we "must have."

Fourth Mindfulness Activity

This is another guided imagery activity that focuses on bringing compassion to our feelings of envy. The inquiry following this activity can be conducted similarly to the ones described previously.

"Begin by thinking of a time in your life when you felt really envious of another person. It could be anything—like a new brother or sister being born, your best friend getting the starring role in the school play, or seeing a friend get something that you really want but can't afford or weren't allowed to have. It doesn't matter what the situation was as long as it brought up feelings of envy and you can remember the situation well.

"Once you have recalled this situation as clearly as you can, bring your attention to your body sensations, paying close attention to any thoughts that arise. Remembering back to how you reacted to those feelings. Thinking back to what you said and how you acted. Were you being kind to yourself? Considering what you have learned about mindful choices, would you make the same choices now? How might you respond differently today? What would you say? Would you be kinder to yourself or to the person of whom you envied? What are your mindful choices?

"Take three deep breaths. The next time you feel envy arise, sit, breathe, and bring your attention to the thoughts, feelings, and body sensations. Remind yourself that no feelings last forever. Give yourself a big pat on the back each time you practice mindful compassion for yourself or another person."

Additional Discussion Questions for Children/Teens

- "What makes us always want something, even though that something always seems to be changing?"
- "What does it mean to bring mindful awareness to our feelings of envy?"
- "How does this mindful awareness change the way we typically experience envy?"
- "How might mindful awareness increase our ability to better manage our envy?"
- "Could practicing self-compassion make managing envy or other difficult emotions a little bit easier?"

Challenges and Tips

Guided imageries that attempt to elicit strong or difficult emotions should be conducted with careful attention to how each child is responding. These activities are not intended to create overwhelming distress, but rather to bring up memories clearly enough to be able to explore them. Although this rarely happens, if you should notice a child becoming emotionally triggered or highly distressed, it's probably best to shorten or gently end the imagery.

Activity 53. Mindfulness of Gratitude

Time Requirement

10–20 minutes.

Themes

- Practicing gratitude makes us kinder people, more appreciative of our lives, and happier.
- Being mindful of the good things in our lives helps us feel more connected to the people around us and fosters new friendships while strengthening our existing relationships.

Background

Cultivating gratitude produces benefits both in terms of emotional well-being and in interpersonal relationships. Robert Emmons (2009) suggested that gratitude includes two key components: First is the affirmation that there are good things in the world—gifts or benefits that we have received, and second is the recognition that the source of this goodness is outside of ourselves. Gratitude strengthens relationships. Feeling gratitude does not mean that life is perfect. Nevertheless, it does encourage us to recognize the goodness that is in our lives.

Gratitude is experienced in the anterior cingulate cortex and medial prefrontal cortex, which are brain regions associated with pleasure and socializing, empathy, understanding other people's perspectives, and experiencing feelings of relief. These areas are also connected to parts of the brain that control our basic emotion regulation, stress relief, and pain reduction (Fox, Kaplan, Damasio, & Damasio, 2015). Therefore, cultivating gratitude not only brings psychological benefits, it may actually change the structure or functioning of our brains.

Materials Needed

Mindfulness journals.

Vocabulary for Grades 4–8

Appreciative, appreciation, acknowledge, recognize, value.

Vocabulary for Grades K–3

Thanks, thankful, grateful, glad, appreciate.

Mindfulness Activity

"Let's start by taking a mindful posture, sitting up straight and alert. If you are comfortable doing so, close your eyes. If you would rather keep your eyes open, that's okay too, just lower your eyes a little, and take a soft gaze.

"Gently bringing your attention to the sensations of the breath around your heart. You might wish to place your right hand on your heart and your left hand on your belly. Your hands are feeling how the breath and the heart are working together. You don't need to make your breath faster or slower—you only need to let it be whatever it is. There is no need to try to control the breath in any way—rest your attention while you let the breath breathe itself—just as you let your heart beat itself. You might think of it as breathing the way you do when you are asleep. Not really big deep breaths and not really short breaths, but the kind of breath you take when you aren't paying attention to it. We are letting our attention rest on the breath and the beat of the heart as they come together in the body. If one breath is long and another short, that's totally okay. With mindfulness, we practice just noticing what is already there. [long pause]

"Now of someone in your life for whom you are grateful. This might be a family member or a close friend. Maybe this person is a neighbor, or a teacher, or someone you don't know very well who has done you a kindness. Opening your heart and your mind's eye to all the things about this one person that you are grateful for. You might be seeing many small acts of kindness, or the hugs and other simple ways that this person shows love and caring for you. You might be remembering a very special gift you received from this person. Perhaps you remember something he or she said or did that touched your heart. Feeling your heart grow larger as you see this person's presence in your life as a gift that you will appreciate and cherish forever."

Additional Discussion Questions for Children/Teens

- "Where does gratitude live in your body?"
- "What does gratitude feel like in your body?"
- "What are some possible benefits of remembering things to be grateful for?"
- "How might practicing mindfulness of gratitude affect your everyday lives?"
- "Could cultivating gratitude change your relationships? If so, in what ways?"

Challenges and Tips

It is important to remember that mindful gratitude practices can potentially backfire in a number of ways. First, low self-esteem sometimes hides behind excessive gratitude. Some children are so careful to thank everyone else for anything good that happens that they ignore or minimize their own contributions and talents. Be mindful of when gratitude might be getting in the way of a child taking appropriate credit for his or her own successes. Second, trying too hard to identify things about which to be grateful can paradoxically leave a child feeling less grateful and happy than if he or she hadn't done it at all. The child might start focusing instead on all the things in his or her life that are not so good—things for which the child is not grateful at all. If any of the children are finding it hard to identify things to write about, don't push. Writing once a week will be more helpful than struggling to write something every day. Third, gratitude does help us focus on important things instead of getting caught up in all the little annoyances of everyday life. Nevertheless, some problems aren't little and may need some impetus from less pleasant emotions, such as fear or even justifiable anger, to motivate us to do something about them. Finally, the "near-enemy" of gratitude is a feeling of indebtedness. Gratitude leaves us feeling good about ourselves and others. Alternatively, feeling indebted to another person often brings up feelings of unworthiness or guilt, which can damage a relationship. If you suspect that any of these things are happening, try to redirect the child back to the positive components of gratitude.

"Write down five things for which you feel grateful. The written record is important—don't just do it in your head. The things you list might be something small, such as "the delicious hamburger I had for lunch today," or it might be something much bigger, such as "My mother was very sick for a long time, but now she is completely well." The goal of this activity is to remember people, events, experiences, or things for which you are grateful. Here are some tips to consider as you write*:

*Some of these tips were adapted from the Greater Good Science Center (*www.mindful.org/a-simple-weekly-mindfulness-practice-keep-a-gratitude-journal*).

- "Don't be trivial. Describe in detail a particular person or event for which you are grateful, instead of just making a list of many small things.
- "Be specific: 'I'm grateful that my brother let me borrow his bicycle on Saturday for my Girl Scout ride,' rather than, 'I'm grateful for my brother.'
- "Focus more on the people to whom you are grateful rather than on things that you might have received.
- "Focus on events and experiences you are grateful for, especially ones you might not have valued at the time.
- "Remember the minuses as well as the plusses. Consider what your life might be like without a particular person in it. Be grateful for his or her presence in your life. Thich Nhat Hanh suggests being grateful that you *don't* have a toothache right now.
- "All good things are gifts. If you see every good thing in your life as a gift, you won't take good things for granted.
- "Appreciate surprises. Remember events or small gifts that were unexpected or surprising."

Activity 54. Mindful Compassion

Time Requirement

5–10 minutes.

Theme

Practicing mindful compassion helps us focus the healing power of compassion toward ourselves and toward others in our lives.

Background

The need for social connection is a basic human desire. Research is making it increasingly clear that feeling connected to others confers both physical and mental health benefits (Hutcherson, Seppala, & Gross, 2008). In addition, practicing self-compassion increases our own psychological health and well-being (Neff, 2009; Neff & Germer, 2013). Sometimes called *loving-kindness* meditation, this activity is a simple practice of directing kind wishes toward ourselves and toward other people. Practicing mindful compassion can help us feel less isolated and more connected to ourselves and to those around us.

Materials Needed

None.

Vocabulary for Grades 4–8

Compassion, empathy, sympathy, concern, consideration, kind-heartedness, benevolence, thoughtfulness.

Vocabulary for Grades K–3

Kind, caring, loving, nice, gentle.

Mindfulness Activity

Forming the intention to put more compassion into the world is the first step in practicing mindful compassion. This is a guided visualization practice. After settling in and taking a few deep breaths, slowly lead the children through this five-step activity. The compassion phrases we use are, "May I/you be happy. May I/you be healthy and strong. May I/you be at peace." You may prefer your own variation of these wishes. The children can repeat after the facilitator either silently or out loud. Once they are familiar with the phrases, the chanting can be done in unison.

Step 1

"Start by directing these compassionate phrases to yourselves: 'May I be happy. May I be healthy and strong. May I be at peace.'"

Step 2

"Next, directing your compassion toward someone you love, for whom who you feel thankful, or toward someone who has helped you. Visualize this person clearly in your mind's eye as you say, 'May he or she be happy. May he or she be healthy and strong. May he or she be at peace.'"

Step 3

"Now visualizing someone that you feel neutral about—someone that you neither like nor dislike. Coming up with a neutral person can be harder than you might think—which helps us realize how quick we are to judge people in our lives in positive or negative ways. Maybe this person is another child that you see on the school bus every day but have never spoken to. Or the clerk at the corner market. Or a neighbor whom you see every morning walking his or her dog. Perhaps it's the school janitor or someone you only see from time to time. Visualize this person clearly in your mind's eye as you say, 'May he or she be happy. May he or she be healthy and strong. May he or she be at peace.'"

Step 4

"Oddly, this next person can sometimes be easier. Thinking about someone that you don't like or whom you are having a hard time with. This might even be someone who has not treated you very well. Children who are being teased by another child can feel quite empowered when they send compassion to the person who is making them miserable—but only if they feel comfortable doing so. Visualize this person clearly in your mind's eye as you say, 'May he or she be happy. May he or she be healthy and strong. May he or she be at peace.'"

Step 5

"Finally, directing your good wishes toward all living creatures in the world: all people, all animals, all beings everywhere. Opening your heart wide as you say, 'May all beings be happy. May all beings be healthy and strong. May all beings be at peace.'"

Variation for Younger Children

The mindful compassion statement may be simplified to, "May I be happy and healthy."

Suggested Practice Activities

Mindful compassion for others and for ourselves can be cultivated in brief interludes.

"Whenever you're feeling lonely or disconnected from other people, close your eyes and take three long inbreaths and three long outbreaths. Then bring the image of someone you really like into your mind. Imagine seeing him or her happy and smiling at you. Silently say to this person, 'May you be happy. May you be healthy and strong. May you be at peace.' Notice how your body, mind, and heart feel when you do this.

"Whenever you're feeling low, you can be compassionate to yourself by sending kind thoughts to yourself. Close your eyes and take three long inbreaths and three long outbreaths. Then silently say to yourself, 'May I be happy. May I be healthy and strong. May I be at peace.' Notice how your body, and mind, and heart feel when you do this."

Kids can create their own phrases that feel authentically kind and loving to them.

Caveat

Children should never feel pressured or even invited to send compassion to current or past abusers (physical, sexual, or emotional) or to those who have bullied them in the past or who may be currently doing so.

ACTIVITY 43 HANDOUT. Being Present

My name is: _____

I just checked in with myself. Right now I feel . . .

Today is (date)	Terrible	Awful	Bad	So-So	Good	Great	Fantastic
	1	2	3	4	5	6	7
	1	2	3	4	5	6	7
	1	2	3	4	5	6	7
	1	2	3	4	5	6	7
	1	2	3	4	5	6	7
	1	2	3	4	5	6	7
	1	2	3	4	5	6	7
	1	2	3	4	5	6	7
	1	2	3	4	5	6	7

(Author Unknown)

- Never pass up the opportunity to go for a joyride.

- Allow the experience of fresh air and the wind in your face to be pure ecstasy.

- When loved ones come home, always run to greet them.

- When it's in your best interest, practice obedience.

- Let others know when they have invaded your territory.

- Take naps and stretch before rising.

- Run, romp, and play daily.

- Eat with gusto and enthusiasm.

- Be loyal.

- Never pretend to be something you're not.

- If what you want lies buried, dig until you find it.

- When someone is having a bad day, be silent, sit close by, and nuzzle him or her gently.

- Avoid biting when a simple growl will do.

- On hot days, drink lots of water and lie under a shady tree.

- When you are happy, dance around and wag your entire body.

- No matter how often you're scolded, don't buy into the guilt thing and pout; run right back and make friends.

- Delight in the simple joys of a long walk.

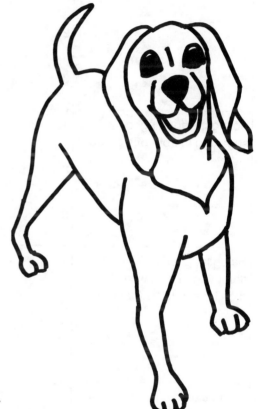

ACTIVITY 46 HANDOUT. Managing Worries and Anxieties

Stressful Event	Choices I Can Make or Things I Can Do
Taking a test that I haven't prepared very well for	1. 2. 3.
Meeting new people	1. 2. 3.
Acting, performing, or speaking in front of a group	1. 2. 3.
Being laughed at for something I said when I didn't mean to be funny	1. 2. 3.
Being called on in class and not knowing the answer	1. 2. 3.

(continued)

Stressful Event	Choices I Can Make or Things I Can Do
Going to a party where I don't know anyone	1. 2. 3.
Being called into the school office to speak with the school principal	1. 2. 3.
Hearing someone say something embarrassing about me to my friends	1. 2. 3.
Being bullied or harassed at school	1. 2. 3.
Being caught in a thunderstorm, hurricane, earthquake, or other natural disaster	1. 2. 3.

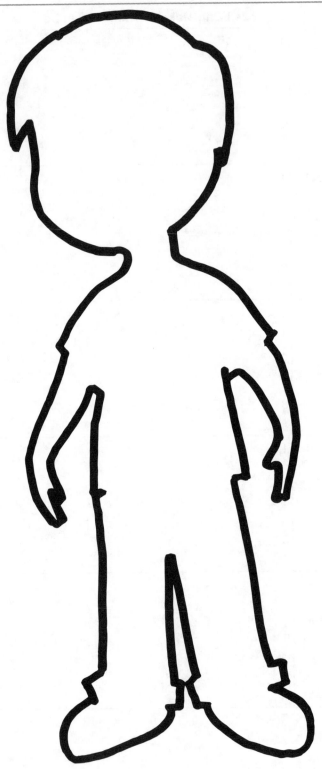

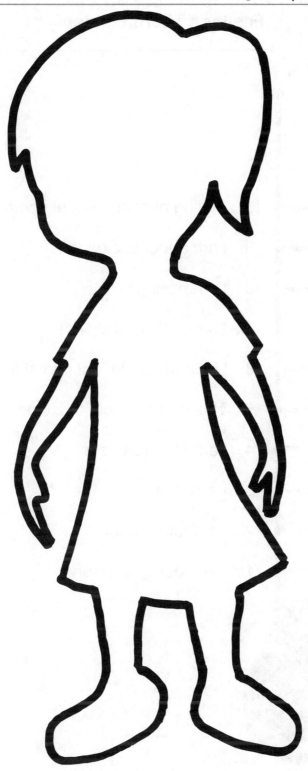

Feelings Thermometer

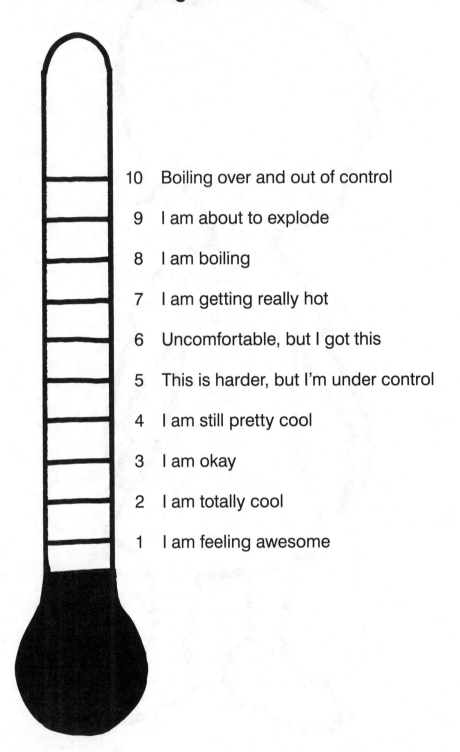

10 Boiling over and out of control

9 I am about to explode

8 I am boiling

7 I am getting really hot

6 Uncomfortable, but I got this

5 This is harder, but I'm under control

4 I am still pretty cool

3 I am okay

2 I am totally cool

1 I am feeling awesome

Thich Nhat Hanh (1991b)

The first step in dealing with feelings is to recognize each feeling as it arises. The agent that does this is mindfulness. In the case of fear, for example, you bring out your mindfulness, look at your fear, and recognize it as fear. You know that fear springs from yourself and that mindfulness also springs from yourself. They are both in you, not fighting, but one taking care of the other.

The second step is to become one with the feeling. It is best not to say, "Go away, Fear. I don't like you. You are not me." It is much more effective to say, "Hello, Fear. How are you today?" Then you can invite the two aspects of yourself, mindfulness and fear, to shake hands as friends and become one. Doing this may seem frightening, but because you know that you are more than just your fear, you need not be afraid. As long as mindfulness is there, it can chaperone your fear. The fundamental practice is to nourish your mindfulness with conscious breathing, to keep it there, alive and strong. Although your mindfulness may not be very powerful in the beginning, if you nourish it, it will become stronger. As long as mindfulness is present, you will not drown in your fear. In fact, you begin transforming it the very moment you give birth to awareness in yourself.

The third step is to calm the feeling. As mindfulness is taking good care of your fear, you begin to calm it down, "Breathing in, I calm the activities of body and mind." You calm your feeling just by being with it, like a mother tenderly holding her crying baby. Feeling his mother's tenderness, the baby will calm down and stop crying. The mother is your mindfulness, born from the depth of your consciousness, and it will tend the feeling of pain. A mother holding her baby is one with her baby. If the mother is thinking of other things, the baby will not calm down. The mother has to put aside other things and just hold her baby. So, don't avoid your feeling. Don't say, "You are not important. You are only a feeling." Come and be one with it. You can say, "Breathing out, I calm my fear."

The fourth step is to release the feeling, to let it go. Because of your calm, you feel at ease, even in the midst of fear, and you know that your fear will not grow into something that will overwhelm you. When you know that you are capable of taking care of your fear, it is already reduced to the minimum, becoming softer and not so unpleasant. Now you can smile at it and let it go, but please do not stop yet. Calming and releasing are just medicines for the symptoms. You now have an opportunity to go deeper and work on transforming the source of your fear.

The fifth step is to look deeply. You look deeply into your baby—your feeling of fear—to see what is wrong, even after the baby has already stopped crying, after the fear is gone. You cannot hold your baby all the time, and therefore you have to look into him to see the cause of what is wrong. By looking, you will see what will help you begin to transform the feeling. You will realize, for example, that his suffering has many causes, inside and outside of his body. If something is wrong around him, if you put that in order, bringing tenderness and care to the situation, he will feel better. Looking into your baby, you see the elements that are causing him to cry, and when you see them, you will know what to do and what not to do to transform the feeling and be free.

From Hanh (1991b, pp. 53–55). Reprinted with permission from Penguin Random House.

ACTIVITY 50 HANDOUT. Exploring My Own Trigger Events

With practice, bringing mindful awareness to a trigger event *while it is happening* can help us make wiser, kinder, and more compassionate choices. Practice with small triggers also helps us be better prepared to manage when the bigger ones come along.

Trigger event	What was I thinking?	What were my feelings?	What were my body sensations?	What can I do to be kind to myself now?	What happened afterward?
Example: Argued with my brother over what movie to watch	It's my turn to pick. It's not fair that he picks what he wants every time.	I was frustrated and annoyed.	Pressure feeling in my chest. Butterflies in my stomach. My face felt hot. I wanted to cry.	I took three deep breaths and thought about what to do.	I felt calmer and didn't yell the way I usually do. I told him it was my turn to pick the movie. We found one that we both wanted to see.

Concluding Activities

For many children, being in a mindfulness group can become a significant part of their lives. Kids in these groups often cultivate strong bonds with each other, frequently discovering an acceptance of themselves that brings comfort and self-assurance. So, they are often sad to see the group end. Something that they once counted on as an important part of their life is coming to an end. Getting closure requires letting go of what once was. Closure implies a complete acceptance of what has happened, an honoring of this time of transition away from what has finished, and a movement into something new. In other words, endings let us discover new possibilities. The Group 8 activities are aimed at helping kids to reflect on and articulate the insights they may have gained, generalize their understandings across the different parts of their lives, and share ways that they might continue cultivating mindfulness in their everyday lives. We also believe that rituals are powerful tools to help gain closure. Beyond talking and sharing, rituals affirm our shared intentions. So, we choose to close every group with a ritual of remembering—honoring the other group members and remembering to continue practicing mindfulness.

Activity 55. What Does Mindfulness Mean to Me Now? (Part II): Drawing

Time Requirement

15–20 minutes.

Themes

The children are invited to ask themselves the following questions:

- "After practicing mindfulness, what does mindfulness mean to me now?"
- "In what ways has practicing mindfulness changed some of the things I do?"
- "In what ways has practicing mindfulness changed how I think or feel?"

Background

This activity is intended to integrate and consolidate insights gained throughout the program and support the exploration of changes that may have occurred over the past weeks or months. Children have learned to cultivate mindful awareness using the breath, the body, and all of their senses. They may have learned that judging is not the same as describing, and they may have discovered that returning their attention to the present moment is always an option—at every moment of every day. Each moment offers us another opportunity to practice being present with our lives.

Over the past weeks or months of practicing mindfulness, the kids may have seen changes in themselves and in how they interact with others. The aim of this activity is to raise awareness of those changes and explore what discoveries they have made about living in the "here and now" of their lives.

Materials Needed

- Drawing paper.
- Colored pencils, markers, or crayons.
- The first drawing that each child completed during Part I of this activity (specifically, in Activity 2).

Mindfulness Activity

Just as with the first version of this activity, the children are invited to create their own drawings, using any colors, images, or words they choose. The drawing is meant simply to express what mindfulness now means to each person after having practiced it over the preceding weeks. You might wish to conduct a few minutes of mindfulness of the breath practice, and then invite each child to complete this sentence with colors, images, or words: "In my everyday life, mindfulness is. . . ."

Allow 10 or 15 minutes for drawing. Every few minutes, remind the children to stop for a moment, check in with their own thoughts and feelings, and then return attention to creating their drawings of mindfulness. The aim of this activity is simply for each child to express visually what mindfulness now means to them and how these practices might have influenced their lives. The first drawings that were done at the beginning of the group should be kept out of sight until these new drawings are completed. It can be helpful, once again, to emphasize that there is no "right" or "wrong" way to approach this drawing activity and that the quality of the drawing is unimportant.

Discussion

The discussion that follows the drawing activity takes place in two parts. First, invite the children to share their new drawings and describe what mindfulness means to them. They should now be more adept at describing the drawings and their experiences of drawing with mindful awareness and with fewer judgments. The child's awareness and mindful engagement in the activity is the focus, rather than the product of his or her efforts. Without requiring anyone to speak, invite each child to share what mindfulness means to him or her. Remember to include questions that elicit their thoughts and feelings as well as their nonjudgmental description of the drawing itself.

Following this discussion, return the drawings that were done at the beginning of the program during Activity 2 to the children and invite them to compare their two drawings and explore ways in which the meanings of mindfulness might have changed for them during the past weeks.

Suggested Practice Activities

Invite the children to reflect on any changes that may have emerged in the past few months of practicing mindfulness. Perhaps they feel a little less stressed out . . . or less irritable . . . or less fearful. They may be getting along better with their family members or friends. Perhaps they are relating a little differently to their own thoughts, no longer getting caught up in the stories quite as much. Perhaps they are not being hijacked by strong emotions as often. Invite them to write about the changes they have experienced in their mindfulness journals.

Activity 56. What Does Mindfulness Mean to Me Now? (Part III): Journaling

Time Requirement

Allow 15–20 minutes (or more) for discussion. Time permitting, the journaling activity can be done in the group or as a home practice activity.

Background

We have practiced bringing awareness to smells, tastes, music and sounds, and touch. We have looked closely at all our emotions, learning more about the ones that feel comfortable as well as those that feel uncomfortable. Perhaps we have learned to see what is around us with greater clarity—see when our own thoughts and emotions might be influencing what we experience. We have practiced grounding ourselves in the present moment using the breath and the body. Maybe we have integrated some of these body or breathing activities into our daily lives. We have practiced seeing that thoughts are just thoughts. We have learned how to be more compassionate and accepting of others and ourselves. We have seen how judging the world might interfere with seeing the choices we have available to us. Maybe we have learned different ways to respond to things that used to make us unhappy or uncomfortable. We have also explored what is different about living on autopilot versus bringing mindful awareness to our experiences.

We can watch thousands of thoughts arise and disappear every day. We have seen how thoughts, feelings, and body sensations are related. We recognize that our thoughts might not always be accurate about reality. We have learned the difference between describing and judging—and maybe even learned that judging rarely helps make our lives easier. We may be more aware of choices. We have learned how practicing mindfulness can create greater peace and happiness in our lives. We understand that challenges are inevitable in everyone's life. Living with awareness requires commitment, compassion, and ongoing practice. Having choices, we choose to face those challenges with awareness and compassion.

Materials Needed

Mindfulness journals.

Mindfulness Activity

Start by facilitating a group discussion of what the children have learned about mindfulness from being in this program. The meaning of mindfulness is different for every child. Some may be eager to share their experiences, and some may choose not to do so. Remember to continue modeling mindfulness of personal choices. Some questions you might ask are:

- "Have your ideas about mindful awareness changed since you started in this program? If so, in what ways?"
- "What have you learned from participating in this program?"
- "What was the most difficult part for you?"
- "Which activities did you find most useful?"
- "Would you like to continue developing mindful awareness in your everyday life?"
- "In what ways might you practice mindfulness in the future?"
- "What could you do that will help you remember to practice?"
- "What would you like most to remember about being in this group?"

After they have shared their experiences of the program, guide the children in an exploration of how they might continue to bring mindful awareness to their daily lives and how bringing mindfulness into their everyday lives might be helpful. Invite them to share with the group what mindfulness means to them personally and explore their commitment to continuing to practice mindfulness. You might use Socratic inquiry to make explicit the wisdom that thoughts and emotions are not facts. Invite the children to reflect on the activities they practiced in the group and how they might use those mindfulness skills to improve their lives. Discuss the transition from guided group activities to a self-directed daily practice. You might normalize the reality that nearly everyone has difficulty remembering to practice every day, and brainstorm ways to help all the kids remember to continue integrating mindfulness into their days.

Additional Discussion Questions for Children/Teens

- "How might you continue to bring greater awareness to your lives and meet your experiences with more clarity and self-compassion?"
- "In what ways might you practice mindful awareness, even in little ways, every day?"
- "In what specific areas of your life might cultivating mindfulness be helpful to you?"
- "When strong thoughts come up, how might you help yourselves remember that thoughts are just thoughts?"

- "When strong emotions come up, what could you do to help yourselves remember that emotions are just emotions?"
- "What might you do for yourselves to remember that thoughts are not always accurate?"
- "Could this help you deal with strong emotions when they arise?"
- "Does knowing that your thoughts influence your emotions, change how you experience events around you and change how you speak or act? In what ways?"
- "How can you cultivate mindful awareness and compassion in your daily lives?"
- "What have you learned from practicing mindful awareness in your everyday lives?"
- "What might you do to continue to build on what you have learned?"
- "What are some tangible benefits of continuing to practice mindfulness?"

Suggested Practice Activity

Invite the children to allocate a specific time in the next few days for quiet reflection and writing in their mindfulness journals. They may start by completing the sentence, "To me, mindfulness means. . . ."

Activity 57. Appreciation of the Group

Time Requirement

25 minutes.

Themes

- Appreciating ourselves and our peers.
- Practicing compassion and kindness.

Materials Needed

Colorful paper and markers or writing implements.

Mindfulness Activity

At this point we introduce a group activity to create a shared experience of gratitude:

"Sometimes it is hard to see our own best qualities, or we are surprised to hear about them from others. We've just spent a few weeks [or longer] together in this group, really getting to know each other, and we will be offering each other kind compliments now at the end of our time together. Everyone, please take a piece of paper and write your name at the bottom of the paper. [Facilitators can join in this activity as well.]

   "Now hand the paper to the person sitting to your left. Look at the name at the bottom of the paper you received, and write a compliment to this person at the top of the paper. A good compliment is personal and specific, maybe even an example from something you saw that person do. We will take 1 minute and just write down a sentence or two. You could also make a little drawing or a doodle for that person. Then fold over what you wrote, so it can't be seen, make a silent kind wish for that person, and pass the paper on to the left again each time I ring the bell [at about 1-minute intervals]."

The kids keep passing and folding until each paper has gone around the whole group. The students can read their letters together or save them until later. Close the activity with a brief loving-kindness practice.

"Close your eyes and take three long inbreaths and three long outbreaths. Then bring up an image of the group. Allow yourself to make a kind wish for yourself. Take a few breaths and then make a kind wish for the facilitator or facilitators of the group, then a kind wish for the whole group, and lastly, a kind wish for everyone in the world."

Activity 58. Here-and-Now Stones

Time Requirement

5–10 minutes.

Themes

* Anchoring awareness in an external object.
* Contemplating our place in the universe.
* Having a tangible reminder of the mindfulness class for informal practice after the group ends.

Background

Practicing mindfulness is not too difficult, but remembering to practice can be the real challenge. It can help to have a "touchstone" by which to remember. This activity was adapted from mindfulness-based cognitive therapy for children (MBCT-C; Semple & Lee, 2011) and the mindful self-compassion program (MSC; Bluth, 2017; Neff, 2011).

Materials Needed

Simple stones or pebbles that can be collected during mindful walking, a child's daily life, or purchased and passed out to the group.

Mindfulness Activity

The group is seated comfortably in rows or a circle. Each child selects (maybe with eyes closed in the interest of time and fairness) a stone, or gets out his or her own stone and holds it in the palm of his or her hand.

"Let's begin by just exploring this stone with our senses and thoughts. First bringing awareness to the sensations—noticing the weight, temperature, and textures against your hand and fingers. Noticing also the colors and shapes. Noticing what makes your stone unique, as well as the qualities that let you know that it's a stone. Perhaps even smelling the stone. Becoming aware also of the fact that this stone is millions or even billions of years old, and yet here we are—holding it in our hands. Allow yourself to connect with the stone. Letting it be a reminder of your mindfulness practice—a reminder to breathe—a reminder to become aware of your thoughts and your emotions. And as you slip your stone into your pocket, remember that any time you notice or touch the stone, you can come back to the present moment."

Suggested Practice Activity

"Carry the stone with you as a reminder that mindfulness can be practiced in every moment, with each new breath. Or keep it somewhere meaningful where you will see it and remember to practice bringing mindfulness into each day of your lives."

PART III
Pathways to Mindfulness

Introduction to the Pathways

Welcome to Part III, which is the "pathways" section of the *Mindfulness Matters* program. Here we explore the structure and rationale of each of five suggested pathways to mindfulness that address the most common cognitive, emotional, and behavioral issues faced by the kids with whom you work or plan to work. Rather than focusing on specific diagnoses or psychopathology, the pathways are designed to speak to five broad problem areas:

- Stress and anxiety
- Depression
- Attention problems
- Problems of emotion regulation and impulse control
- Trauma, abuse, and neglect

Each pathway follows a broadly similar structure. We begin with some background information that defines the scope of the issue and the overall demographics of the children who are affected. Then we describe the specific issues and problems faced by these kids. Each pathway includes a table that lists the most common symptoms, how each symptom looks from the child's perspective (subjective description), and how it might manifest to the adult observer (objective description). We intend these tables be to be practical, helpful, and user-friendly for teachers, parents, and other nonclinicians, as well as for mental health providers. We offer descriptive details as to what these symptoms might look like behaviorally, both in and out of a classroom or session with a child, and also how symptoms tend to manifest at different ages. Where relevant, we note any developmental issues (cognitive, emotional, physiological, and behavioral) that may arise. We also describe some of the unique challenges and opportunities that may arise on each pathway with each group, along with tips for engaging the kids. Before describing the suggested pathway, we offer a few cautions, contraindications, or potential complications that might arise.

From there the pathway itself is laid out for you, including goals and reasons why each activity was suggested. We also mention particular areas or issues on which to focus, which we feel might be helpful for that group, and that we encourage you to emphasize. Each pathway is divided into five sections:

- Introductory Activities
- Core Activities
- Intermediate Development Activities
- Advanced Deepening Activities
- Maintenance, Generalization, and Concluding Activities

We close Part III with an overview table, Summary of Activities within the Pathways (on pp. 239–240), which lists all the activities described in Part II mapped onto each pathway.

The pathways are intended to provide background information and general guidance for applying mindfulness approaches to specific problem areas. The state of mindfulness research with kids and teens has not yet advanced to studying the effects of specific activities on different problems. Our knowledge of the empirical research literature, our many years of clinical experience, and our own mindfulness practices have informed our construction of these pathways. As we mentioned in Part I, we do not intend this book to be a traditional treatment manual or class curriculum to follow blindly, but rather a "choose your own adventure" book that allows you—the expert on your own students or clients—to select a flexible path that meets the unique needs of your group.

Pathway through Stress and Anxiety

The following pages offer an introductory pathway that can be used without any adaptations, for most populations of stressed or anxious children and teens. With record rates of stress in young Americans (Merikangas et al., 2010); stress rising worldwide (Baxter, Scott, Vos, & Whiteford, 2012); and a strong link between stress, adverse childhood events, and subsequent mental health problems, behavioral concerns, and even medical issues later in life, this pathway is effectively meant to be a preventive public health intervention for a broad, fairly general population of children and adolescents. Anxiety disorders are also relatively common in children and adolescents, with data from the National Comorbidity Survey showing lifetime prevalence rates of about 25% for any anxiety disorder among teens ages 13–18 (Merikangas et al., 2010).

We offer this pathway for most groups that have no other major learning, behavioral, medical, or mental health concerns beyond stress or generalized anxiety. As always, we do recommend that teachers always remain attentive to the possibility of mental health issues, and work as needed in consultation with an experienced mental health professional.

Symptoms of Stress and Anxiety

Symptoms of stress and anxiety are increasingly common in our children, and may show up in children's own comments (the *subjective* column in Table III.1) or in an adult's observation of behavior (the *objective* column). When assessing stress and anxiety, a balance of these subjective and objective reports is most informative—integrating information from the child with your own observations and with those of parents, caregivers, teachers, or other adults in the child's life.

Symptoms may be behavioral, such as avoidance of anxiety- or stress-inducing people, interactions, places, and things. Avoidance behaviors might include irritable or "on edge" behaviors, alcohol or drug use, self-harming behaviors, disordered eating, excessive use of technology as an escape, creating quasi-crisis situations that may get a child out of an uncomfortable situation (e.g., engaging in disruptive behavior to avoid upcoming schoolwork or an unpleasant interaction), or seeking constant approval or reassurance.

TABLE III.1. Symptoms, Subjective Descriptions, and Adult Observations

Anxiety symptoms	Child description (subjective)	Adult observation (objective)
Cognitive		
Feeling restless, keyed-up, or edgy	• My thoughts won't slow down. • I can't get my mind to stop. • I'm always on edge. • I can't stop thinking.	• Excess nervous energy • Can't "settle down" • Talking too much or too fast • Catastrophic ruminations (e.g., "Daddy is 15 minutes late—he must have gotten in a car accident!")
Difficulty concentrating or paying attention	• I can't focus on schoolwork, or even TV or video games. • My mind just goes blank. • I can't think straight. • I forget everything I learned. • Brainfart.	• Schoolwork suffering • Academic work not getting done or grades falling • Unable to focus on other tasks like chores or even play activities • Quality of work poor • Appears forgetful
Emotional		
Worried, fearful, or scared; feelings of dread	• Something is wrong. • Something bad will happen.	• Clinging, tearful when facing separation from parent or caregiver • Temper tantrums • Avoids going places • Avoids being near other children or adults
Irritability or anger	• Everyone is annoying. • I have a "short fuse." • Everything annoys me more than it used to.	• Snapping at people • Less patience • Easily frustrated
Physiological		
Easily fatigued	• I'm really tired. • Things tire me out. • That takes too much energy.	• Worn out easily • Less energy for school, social life, or other activities • Avoids sports or other strenuous physical activities
Psychomotor agitation or muscle tension	• I feel like my heart is beating really loud [hard, fast]. • My hands are sweaty. • I feel jittery [jumpy, fidgety]. • I have butterflies in my stomach.	• Appears jittery, hand tremor might be observable • Nervous tapping of fingers or toes, whistling, or other repetitive behavior • Doesn't stop moving around
Somatic distress	• My neck [head, jaw, back] hurts. • My stomach is upset.	• Mysterious aches and pains • GI distress • Frequent trips to the bathroom • Frequent headaches
Sleep disturbances	• I can't fall asleep. • I can't stay asleep. • I can't wake up. • I wake up really early. • I sleep a lot but am still tired. • Worrying is keeping me up or waking me up.	• Difficulty falling asleep • Difficulty staying asleep • Difficulty waking up • Waking up early but not feeling rested • Sleeping but still fatigued
Appetite disturbances	• I'm hungry all the time. • Eating relaxes me. • I'm never hungry anymore. • I don't feel like eating anything.	• Eating too little or too much • Constant snacking • Weight loss or gain

Symptoms may also be physical, or appear to be, in the forms of sleep difficulties, gastro-intestinal distress, headaches, muscle tension and mysterious aches and pains (largely in jaw, neck, and back), or a weakened immune system that manifests as frequent colds or infections. Psychological and cognitive symptoms are more subjective, but might be observed as difficulty focusing on schoolwork, forgetting daily tasks, or looking worried or scared. Children need to meet only one of the symptoms listed in Table III.1 to receive a diagnosis of generalized anxiety disorder (GAD).

How Stress and Anxiety Manifest at Different Ages

Different age groups, cultural factors, and co-occurring mental health issues may cause symptoms to manifest in different ways or different settings. Like many diagnoses, stress and anxiety in children are likely to show up in their behaviors. In adolescents, these behaviors might include substance abuse, self-harm, or other risky behaviors to avoid feelings of anxiety. In younger kids these behaviors may include acting out aggressively, tantrums, silliness, and other disruptive behavior to avoid or override the feelings of anxiety. Younger children are also more likely to report and exhibit physiological distress (stomachaches and headaches, etc.) than they are to describe cognitive symptoms of worry. Children of all ages, but especially preadolescents, may engage in "magical thinking" and obsessive–compulsive disorder (OCD)-like rituals to manage their anxiety. There is evidence to suggest that children of different cultural groups may have more or fewer somaticized complaints than others that accompany their anxiety and stress (Crijnen, Achenbach, & Verhulst, 1999).

There is, of course, a range of relatively common anxiety disorders in children, from the more cognitive GAD to the more physiological panic disorder. Many childhood anxiety disorders commonly co-occur and overlap with GAD and with each other (Baxter et al., 2012; Merikangas et al., 2010). These include social anxiety disorder and subclinical anxiety triggered by social interactions. Panic attacks commonly precede agoraphobia, which can result in significant fear and avoidance of situations that provoke panic or feelings of being trapped, including school. Separation anxiety is a fear of separating from caregivers or leaving home, which also impacts social and school functioning. OCD includes symptoms of uncontrollable thoughts or obsessions, as well as uncontrollable ritualized and repeated behaviors or compulsions. Phobias comprise another anxiety disorder that includes irrational fears or aversions. Any of these co-occurring anxiety disorders can complicate the child's engagement in the group, even to the extent of just getting him or her in the door.

Although we do not explicitly address these particular disorders, we expect this pathway to lower baseline anxiety, which should then decrease the severity of the anxiety symptoms. Children and teens with more severe anxiety will likely respond best to a mindfulness group if they also have regular psychotherapy or sometimes an anxiolytic medication.

Adults may unwittingly reinforce avoidance behaviors that accompany anxiety by overly accommodating kids and protecting them from appropriate exposure to anxiety triggers. If you are concerned about a child being overly anxious, consult with a clinician who can help you assess the need for professional support. However, by themselves, mindfulness and physiological relaxation practices are ultimately therapeutic because these skills can reduce or manage the stress or panic response by using the principle of *exposure with response prevention* when a child or teen is triggered by an anxiety-producing situation. Mindfulness helps the child stay present with whatever is happening—long enough to make a better assessment and choose a more skillful response to the trigger. Trauma and posttraumatic stress disorders [PTSD] are addressed in the Pathway through Trauma, Abuse, and Neglect, pp. 231–238.

Some of these anxiety disorders may respond better to certain practices. For example, even mild social phobia presents a challenge if teaching in a group setting, which involves group discussions. Separation anxiety may present a challenge to these children to attend meetings without their caregivers or to focus on learning mindfulness skills even when present. OCD and perfectionistic tendencies may also present challenges regarding "doing mindfulness correctly," and so forth. GAD will likely respond well to both physiological and cognitive practices such as mindful breath counting, whereas more physiologically oriented anxiety disorders such as panic disorder may respond more effectively to slow breathing, relaxation, and movement-based practices.

Teaching Tips

Almost all children and teens experience stress, whether they recognize it as stress or not. Given kids' greater awareness of physical than emotional experience, it can be useful to start by talking with them about the ways we experience stress in the body. Shortness of breath, feeling constricted in the chest, butterflies in the stomach, sweaty or shaking hands, heart racing, and other experiences are readily recognized and described in physical terms for kids. The subjective descriptions in Table III.1 can be a useful starting place for a conversation about how we experience stress and anxiety.

One of the advantages of teaching mindfulness to anxious and stressed kids is that the benefits are often immediate and readily apparent in the both body and mind. From tension in the chest and shallow breathing, a few deep, mindful breaths can shift the child's physiology and subjective experience almost immediately. As with depression, ample research indicates that light to moderate exercise can prove useful in reducing stress and anxiety (Jayakody, Gunadasa, & Hosker, 2014), so we have integrated plenty of mindful walking and stretching activities into this pathway.

In the cognitive domain, kids may also be able to describe feeling more clear and calm in their minds after even a brief practice, especially as they approach adolescence. This immediacy may help motivate kids initially, but can also present a challenge when other kids feel that it isn't "working" for them as well as they would like it to. Managing expectations is an important component of the initial sessions. Given that the initial benefits feel like they "wear off" over time, discussing the cultivation of patience and an ongoing practice is essential.

Developing a metacognitive approach to "thinking errors" (e.g., black-and-white thinking and catastrophizing) that make up the cognitive basis of anxiety can be eased with mindfulness. By more clearly examining these types of thoughts after calming the nervous system, we can more mindfully examine and weigh those thoughts as distorted or not accurate in relation to reality. As with depression, the goal is not to change the thoughts, as in traditional cognitive therapies, but to help children change their relationship and emotional reactions to negative, anxious, or overwhelming thoughts, and ultimately, to identify with them less. Thoughts become "just" events in the mind. Not facts—not "real."

Cautions and Contraindications

Breath practices can sometimes present a challenge among anxious populations. Perfectionistic kids may worry that they are "breathing wrong" and become more anxious; hence extra guidance and patience may be warranted. For kids with past experience of panic or breathing problems such as asthma, a focus on the breath can paradoxically trigger more anxiety. Kids with a history of physical trauma may find that too much focus on deeper body sensations may present a challenge, and thus a lighter focus on the body, an emphasis on the outside rather than inside of the body (e.g., feet on the floor), or on external anchors such as sounds, may be easier for them. Walking and stretching activities can also help if stillness practices feel too challenging. As always, each pathway offers a range of choices to leave kids with at least a few practical skills that they can take away and use in their own lives. If kids are still struggling, some tips from the Pathway through Trauma, Abuse, and Neglect may prove helpful.

Activities for a Pathway through Stress and Anxiety

The ultimate goals of the anxiety and stress pathway are threefold: first, to reduce the children's physiological overarousal; second, to bring greater cognitive awareness to anxious and stressful situations; and third, to master a few activities that the child can use independently in situations that trigger high stress or anxiety.

Introductory Activities

As with all the pathways, we begin with an introduction to mindfulness and how it relates to anxiety and stress. The introductory activities we recommend include a ***What Does Mindfulness Mean to Me? (Part I)*** drawing activity, which also offers us a baseline of understanding. From there we recommend ***Taking a Mindful Posture, Taking a Mindful SEAT,*** and ***A Cup of Mindfulness*** with queries about anxiety. Then select one of the simple breathing practices such as ***Mindfulness of the Breath*** or ***Mindful Breath Counting,*** which builds focus; ***Belly Breathing*** and ***Taking Three Mindful Breaths,*** which are helpful for sleep and panic, and/or ***Mindful Humming,*** which is useful for lowering physiological stress. ***Mindful Silliness*** can also be a fun and engaging activity for kids and "break the ice" if they are feeling a bit shy or self-conscious at first, and ***Mindful Humming*** is also a fun, informal activity that can help kids relax.

Core Activities

Once the basic introductory practices and explanations of anxiety and stress have been established, we turn toward the beginner movement- and body-oriented practices. For anxiety that is experienced in the body, we suggest beginning with ***Mindful Walking, Mindful Movements*** (yoga postures), and ***Mindful Flower Stretch.*** Movement-based body awareness is often a much more tolerable place to begin with anxious and stressed-out kids. Body awareness practices based in stillness can make focus a challenge, and are also, well, less fun and engaging than movement—although the ***Mindful Smiling While Waking Up*** and the ***Mindful***

Mountain Visualization activities can help kids internalize feelings of equanimity and are excellent introductions to the longer stillness practices. We recommend *Mindfulness of Discomfort* to help kids begin to explore the impermanence of sensations and emotions, become aware of mind–body connections, and explore their own coping styles.

Intermediate Development Activities

Once the kids have grown comfortable with these beginner practices both in and out of the group time, we suggest moving toward the intermediate body-based stillness practices such as *Mindful Eating (Parts I and II)*, the shorter and longer *Body Scan*, the *Mindful HALT* activity, as well as *Mindfulness While Lying Down* variations with a look toward locating stress and anxiety in the body. *Mindful Body Relaxation* is a progressive muscle relaxation activity that can help kids let go of stress and anxiety-related tension, and is particularly helpful for sleep challenges. *Mindfulness of My Feet* can be a helpful short practice when anxiety is triggered.

Advanced Deepening Activities

Once children have successfully learned and practiced at least a few of the intermediate body practices—at least enough so that they use one or two on their own—we turn toward more advanced sensory and cognitive awareness practices. Beginning with sensory practices and learning to get curious about and tolerate these, they can move toward emotional awareness. We suggest beginning with *Listening to Silence, Mindful Seeing (Parts I and II), Finding Five New Things,* and *Mindful Smells (Parts I and II),* with an emphasis on the sensations and thoughts that accompany excitement, anticipation, and uncertainty, which overlap with anxiety. From there, we suggest moving toward *Mindfulness of Judgments,* then the practices that include mindfulness of range of feelings and emotions, with an emphasis on *Mindfulness of Worry and Anxiety (Parts I and II),* and *Mindfulness of Embarrassment* in an effort to locate emotions in the body. Children who struggle with stress or anxiety in a way that results in anger might explore the activities related to *Mindfulness of Frustration and Anger (Parts I and II),* or other topical practices. Kids whose anxieties are related to sadness or envy might practice those activities. *Mindfulness of Gratitude* and *Mindful Compassion* can also be explored toward the end.

Maintenance, Generalization, and Concluding Activities

In closing, we encourage a discussion that includes what has changed—specifically, what skills can be carried forward into stressful and anxiety-producing situations. We recommend *What Does Mindfulness Mean to Me Now? (Part II Drawing and Part III Journaling)* and closing with *Appreciation of the Group* and the *Here-and-Now Stones.*

Pathway through Depression

This pathway offers a suggested route for children and adolescents who are experiencing mild or moderate depression. This can be one of the more challenging groups to motivate and engage, particularly outside of the group time. As always, we recommend prescreening potential participants for motivation, commitment, and safety concerns, as well as working in consultation with an experienced psychotherapist. Before beginning, please also review the specific cautions and contraindications that we discuss below.

Depression and other mood disorders are relatively common in children and adolescents, with a lifetime prevalence rate for adolescents of 14.3% (Merikangas et al., 2010). There is a marked difference between genders, with girls experiencing depression at nearly twice the rate of boys. Children and teens who identify as lesbian, gay, bisexual, transgender, or queer (LGBTQ) are also at elevated risk. The rates of persistent depressive disorder (PDD; formerly *dysthymic disorder and chronic depression*), which is a milder but long-lasting or chronic form of depression, is about equal between boys and girls. Bipolar disorders (BPs) are notable for their marked mood swings between hypomania or mania and depression. Although BP is less common than unipolar depression, it is also seen in children and teens, with a lifetime prevalence rate for teens of 2.5% (Merikangas et al., 2010).

Early treatment of mood disorders can reduce academic, legal, or conduct problems (Buka, Monuteauz, & Earls, 2002) as well as future problems such as loneliness and problematic relationships in adulthood (Allen, Chango, Szwedo, & Schad, 2014). Although the long-term mindfulness research has yet to be conducted, offering this pathway to at-risk kids and teens may help prevent more significant problems down the road. At the least, we believe that this pathway can offer some useful self-care skills. Although we hope this pathway might be helpful to those with pediatric bipolar disorders, we recommend consulting with a mental health professional before adapting these practices for kids who are experiencing severe mood swings.

Symptoms of Depressive Disorders

Depressive symptoms may manifest in a variety of ways. As with the anxiety and stress pathway, we have created a table that includes a child or teen's subjective comments as well as objective adult or peer observations. We have further divided the table into four clusters of symptoms: cognitive, emotional, physiological, and social–behavioral. When assessing for depression, PDD, or BP, a balance of these subjective and objective reports will likely be most helpful and useful. Information from your own observations, as well as available observations from other adults in the child's life, should all be considered. We also recommend that caregivers have a pediatrician examine the child to rule out the presence of physical conditions such as hypothyroidism or anemia that can mimic symptoms of depression.

A depressive episode includes a significant change in mood with five of the symptoms in Table III.2 lasting more than 2 weeks. One of the symptoms must be either depressed mood or loss of interest and pleasure. With children and teens, however, the mood is often *irritable* rather than depressed. For children and adolescents, a PDD diagnosis requires depressed or irritable mood plus two or more symptoms, which last for more than 1 year.

Cognitive symptoms are more readily identified in adolescents than in children. There may be marked pessimism and negativity that are overly generalized and overly personalized. You may notice significant worries or preoccupations with death or other "dark" subjects. If they can articulate it, kids and teens may express feeling excessively guilty, ashamed, or remorseful. Emotionally, the child's mood can be sad, anxious, irritable, or a mix of all three. You might notice that most symptoms in Table III.2 fall into the physiological category. One common symptom that can result in a significant functional impairment is poor attention/concentration. This symptom manifests in the child as an inability to focus or stay on task; the child has the appearance of being unmotivated, easily distracted, or "not working up to potential." Attentional problems can significantly hinder academic and social performance and are discussed in more detail in the Pathway through Attention Problems. Other physiological symptoms include unspecified aches and pains, low energy, not sleeping well or significant oversleeping, appetite changes, and psychomotor changes. These may be observed by caregivers or teachers, or may also be evident in the child or teen's own complaints. Behaviorally, depression in children may manifest as low motivation, feeling ill or feigning illness, clinginess, school refusal, and disinterest or boredom with activities or people that the child had previously enjoyed. Bear in mind, however, that a loss of interest in activities that were previously interesting may also reflect developmental changes or be influenced by peers, especially as kids approach adolescence.

How Depression Manifests at Different Ages

Younger children tend to express depression through sulkiness, irritability, crankiness and restlessness, and may have low self-esteem, social difficulties, and pessimistic attitudes. School performance may suffer, partly through lack of motivation or resulting from the cognitive and attentional impairments that often accompany depression. Older children and teens may "act out" their depression though alcohol or substance abuse, self-harming behaviors, disordered eating, and other risky behaviors in an attempt to manage their moods and uncomfortable feelings of emptiness. As with anxiety and stress, there is some evidence to suggest that different cultural groups may have more or fewer somatic complaints than others (Chentsova-Dutton, Ryder, & Tsai, 2014).

TABLE III.2. Symptoms of Depressive Disorders, Child Descriptions, and Adult Observations

Depressive symptoms	Child description (subjective)	Adult observation (objective)
Cognitive		
Excessive guilt, shame, self-blame, or remorse	• I'm a bad person for [doing or not doing] things • I shouldn't have said/done that • I've never done anything right in my life	• Out-of-proportion guilt and shame • Low self-esteem and self-worth
Negativity about oneself, others, the world	• I'm not enough [good, worthy, deserving, smart, pretty] • I have low self-esteem • I'm unlovable • I'm just a bad kid • Everyone hates me • Everything sucks	• Acting in ways that suggest feelings of low self-worth, such as self-deprecating comments, compromising, and giving up too quickly • Cynical, untrusting, and negative outlook about others. often manifesting in disengagement and isolation • Cynicism about the world and future; giving up easily
Hopelessness and pessimism about the future	• No one will ever love me • I will never be a success at anything • Nothing is going to work out • I have nothing to look forward to • The future looks bleak • Nothing good will ever happen to me	• Expressing pointlessness or negativity about the future • Acting in ways that suggest things will not get better or are not worth trying to improve • Not planning for the future and not future-oriented
Thoughts of death or dying; suicidal wishes or ideation; making suicide plans	• I wish I were dead • I want to die • I have nothing to live for • I'd be better off dead	• Frequently preoccupied with issues of death or dying • Talking about death and dying • Talking about suicide (active or passive) • Making overt plans for suicide by giving away possessions, saying good-bye to people, pets, places, etc.
Emotional		
Sad, empty, depressed, down, blue	• I feel [sad, bad, down, empty, hollow, numb]	• Appears sad and lethargic • Crying over seemingly minor things
Worried, anxious, nervous	• I'm [worried, anxious, scared, tense] • I'm too nervous to [undertake an activity]	• Excessive worries and contingency planning • Appears nervous, fidgety
Irritability, restlessness	• Everything is annoying • Everything is lame	• Irritable mood • Irritated by minor inconveniences

(continued)

TABLE III.2. *(continued)*

Depressive symptoms	Child description (subjective)	Adult observation (objective)
Physical		
Impaired attention and concentration	• I can't remember anything • I can't study anymore • What did you say?	• Unable to stay on task with activities • Appears not to be listening or following conversations • Frequently says "What?" or asks for things to be repeated • Is easily distracted by irrelevant or minor sounds, sights, movements, etc. • Complains about not being able to pay attention • Quality of schoolwork declines
Aches, pains, cramps, and digestive problems that don't respond to the usual treatment	• Tummyaches • Butterflies in stomach • Neck and back pain	• Complaints of soreness • Appetite changes • Frequent trips to the bathroom • Mysterious medical complaints and discomforts
Feeling exhausted or having much less energy	• I'm always tired • I don't have the energy to do it • I don't feel like it • Wow, that wore me out • I just want to stay in bed or on the couch all day	• Small tasks appear to require more effort • Still tired despite sleep • Low energy and easily worn out by typical activities • Lethargic • Reluctance to do even mildly strenuous activities
Insomnia, disrupted sleeping, or sleeping too much; significantly more or less sleep than developmental needs or academic and social demands	• I'm too sleepy to think • I can't fall asleep • I can't wake up • I keep waking up all night • I'm sleeping a ton but still exhausted all the time	• Difficulty falling asleep • Difficulty waking up (oversleeping beyond typical adolescent sleep changes) • Difficulty staying asleep • Note that a lack of sleep *and* lack of tiredness is one indication of a manic or hypomanic episode
Loss of appetite or increased appetite *Over- or undereating with more than a 5% weight gain or loss that is unintentional*	• I'm hungry all the time • I never feel like eating • All food is gross to me these days	• Overeating • Constant eating for emotional comfort • Over- or undereating • Skipping meals • Increased pickiness in choice of foods • Significant weight gain or loss
Psychomotor changes	• I feel slow • I feel like I'm moving underwater • I'm feeling so [jumpy, fidgety, jittery]	• Noticeably more sluggish, slow and clumsy in movement and speech • Appears agitate; is fidgety, pacing; repetitive tapping of fingers or feet • Speech rapid, louder than usual, or pressured • Appears to feel "uncomfortable in [his or her] own skin"

(continued)

Depressive symptoms	Child description (subjective)	Adult observation (objective)
TABLE III.2. *(continued)*		
Social–behavioral		
Loss of interest, enjoyment, or engagement in normally pleasurable activities beyond what is developmentally appropriate; social withdrawal	• I don't enjoy anything any more • I don't want to do anything • Everything is boring • I won't enjoy doing that • I'm bored • No one wants to be around me	• Not enjoying or engaging in school, hobbies, social life, and other activities • Avoids seeing friends • Stays in room all day • Skips school • Talk of, or efforts to, run away from home
Use of alcohol, marijuana, or other substances to "self-medicate" the depression	• I'm not sad when I drink • It's only the [substance] that keeps me going • It's the [alcohol, substance] that makes me feel better	• Increasing use of alcohol or substances is more common in males than in females • Steals money, alcohol, or substances from parents
Suicidal or parasuicidal attempts	• Self-harm behaviors [cutting, burning oneself] • Overdosing on alcohol and/or drugs	• Any suicidal gesture or suicide attempt is serious • Immediately refer the child or teen to a professional for evaluation

Teaching Tips

The challenges of teaching depressed children and teens mindfulness are mostly related to motivation, especially encouraging them to take action on their own behalf outside of the group. Getting some kids who are depressed to do much of anything is often a challenge. In fact, loss of interest, pleasure, and motivation is diagnostic of depressive disorders. What caregivers, teachers, facilitators, or even peers may see as resistance or boredom may be symptoms of depression. Lack of motivation, a cynical, dismissive or irritable "attitude" in teens and tweens, or not following through on assigned homework exercises outside of group are common. For that reason, we also suggest calling it home *practice* rather than home*work*.

Depressed children and teens may experience greater difficulties initiating and regulating their attention and concentrating on tasks than their nondepressed peers. Depressed kids also may report that they become more aware of only negative thoughts when they sit down and focus attention on their thoughts. It is easy for mindful awareness to spiral down into unhelpful depressive ruminations. For that reason, learning to disconnect (decenter) from the stream of thoughts and "not believe everything you think" is particularly important for those kids—especially when negative thoughts or difficult emotions become the focus of attention. Movement-based activities and the external anchors provided by sensory-based activities also seem to help manage ruminative thinking.

Along with the challenges, depression also presents unique opportunities for a mindfulness group. Much of the way mindfulness may "work" in treating depression is by shifting the pessimistic outlook—in Aaron Beck's terms, the "cognitive triad" of negativity toward oneself, the world, and the future (Beck, Rush, Shaw, & Emery, 1979)—in a more realistic direction about the difficult experiences all of us inevitably have at times with people, events, and situations in our lives. Paradoxically, however, the aim of mindfulness practice is not to change thoughts (as in the traditional cognitive therapies), but rather to change the child's relationship to his or her negative thoughts (Segal, Williams, & Teasdale, 2002, 2013), and then learn to respond to them with new awareness that promotes less problematic thought patterns and behaviors.

Although returning one's focus to the anchor of attention over and over again may feel frustrating, it also offers opportunities to practice self-compassion by not judging oneself negatively—a practice that can be applied outside of formal practice activities. This often reduces negative thoughts and shame about oneself. The affective flatness that sometimes accompanies depression can improve with activities that bring nuanced awareness to moment-by-moment experiences. To spark an exploration of emotions beyond the experience of them as simply "flat" and "numb," the depression pathway emphasizes awareness of even the most subtle of physical and emotional experiences, helping the child to become aware of the slightest flicker of emotion—however subtle it may seem.

In consideration of the ample research on behavioral activation (Dimidjian et al., 2006) and physical activity (Ströhle, 2009) as helpful in managing depressed moods, the depression pathway also encourages mindful movement activities. In other research with adults, mindfulness appears to boost motivation for exercise and make it more enjoyable (Ruffault, Bernier, Juge, & Fournier, 2016; Tsafou, De Ridder, van Ee, & Lacroix, 2016). In addition, mindfulness-based interventions with adults are associated with greater medication compliance (Gregg, Callaghan, Hayes, & Glenn-Lawson, 2007), which suggests that mindfulness might also help kids who are taking antidepressants or other medications.

Cautions and Contraindications

As with the other pathways, there are a few notes of caution to consider when working with depressed kids. One primary concern is introducing activities that are initially too challenging, which can impact motivation in an already difficult-to-motivate group. For that reason, we encourage you and the group to start smaller and slower than with the stress and anxiety pathway. Keep activities short and build on small successes with plenty of motivational encouragement and authentic validation of each child's progress along the way. There is no problem with slowing down the pathway and doing more and shorter activities, particularly if kids appear to be frustrated, bored, or simply unable to focus. If kids express feelings of incompetence or hopelessness, you might wish to strongly emphasize the elements of non-judgment and self-compassion in the practices more than the elements of attention, awareness, and present-moment focus.

Another concern, primarily seen in kids with depressive episodes that include more somatic symptoms, is lack of energy, fatigue, and even falling asleep, as well as kids reporting "more negative thoughts than before I started mindfulness." Both of these concerns are addressed by steering away from activities that are too relaxing and "opening." You may want to avoid activities that include long periods with closed eyes, or have prolonged durations, or require stillness of the body. Depression may occur alongside trauma and may even share some symptoms. Fortunately, the practices that we recommend for depression, which focus on external anchors and movement, also overlap with some of the recommended activities for working with trauma.

Suicide Risk Management

The most serious concern when working with depressed youth involves the possibility of suicidal thoughts. Even many clinicians are uncomfortable working with suicidal kids or adults, but we have been trained in how to handle this when it comes up. If you are a teacher or other nonclinician, however, we strongly recommend consulting closely with a trained therapist who has experience with the population of kids you work with, or who knows the specific child and his or her treatment history. The information that follows is meant to help you become a more informed facilitator and is not intended to provide clinical training in risk management.

Suicide is the second leading cause of death among young people in the United States (Centers for Disease Control and Prevention, 2015). Although the rate of suicide is higher in boys than girls, the latter have higher rates of suicidal ideation and attempted suicide (Cash & Bridge, 2009). Children and adolescents with severe depression or mood disorders have the devastating potential to end their own lives. Risk factors include a history of suicide in the family, exposure to sexual or physical abuse, marked impulsivity, alcohol or substance use, bullying or victimization, and/or access to lethal means (Cash & Bridge, 2009). When working with kids who may be severely depressed or otherwise at risk of attempting suicide, we strongly advise consulting with a mental health professional and being attentive to the presence of the following significant warning signs:

- Talking about suicide or about death or dying more generally.
- Searching on the Internet for ways to commit suicide.
- Making a specific suicide plan.
- Acquiring, hiding, or hoarding the necessary provisions (e.g., weapons, poisons, pills).
- Expressing significant shame, guilt, self-blame, or hopelessness.
- Saying that he or she feels like a burden to others and that loved ones would be better off if he or she were dead.
- Saying goodbye to family members, pets, friends, or places.
- Giving away important possessions.
- Escalating alcohol or substance use.
- History of risky or impulsive behaviors.
- Previous self-harming behaviors or suicide attempts.
- Sudden improvement in mood, energy, or expressions of peace or relief.

Activities for a Pathway through Depression

There are a few ways mindfulness may "work" with depression. One is addressing the cognitive symptoms by offering a greater awareness of negative thoughts and skills to disempower thoughts as being "just" thoughts. On the physiological level, greater somatic awareness can help kids identify the body sensations they most associate with depression, and understand the relationship between those sensations and the thoughts that trigger or exacerbate their depression. Mindfulness may also ease symptoms related to sleep problems (Blake et al., 2016) and over- or undereating (Godsey, 2013), increase optimism (Schonert-Reichl & Lawlor,

2010), and increase tolerance and management of pain and somatic symptoms (Jastrowski Mano et al., 2013; Petter, Chambers, & Chorney, 2013). The following is one suggested pathway through depression, which we developed based on the limited existing research, our own clinical experience, and the theoretical considerations discussed previously.

Introductory Activities

As with all the pathways, we begin with an introduction to mindfulness, with an additional focus on how it relates to depression and the negative outlook that can keep depression going. The introductory activities we recommend open with an *Introduction to Mindfulness,* followed by the *What Does Mindfulness Mean to Me?* (Part I: Drawing) activity, which also offers us a baseline of understanding. From there we recommend *Taking a Mindful Posture* and/or *A Cup of Mindfulness,* and then one of the simple breathing practices such as *Mindfulness of the Breath* or *Mindful Breath Counting,* which builds focus. *Belly Breathing* and *Taking Three Mindful Breaths* may help with sleep and managing stress.

Mindful Silliness or *Matching Movement Moments* can serve as fun and engaging activities for kids and "break the ice" if they are feeling a bit shy or self-conscious at first. These also introduce some bodily awareness in a fun way. Kids can then learn about *Taking a Mindful SEAT* early on. Another engaging and fun introductory activity is to bring mindfulness into eating, with *Mindful Eating (Part I).* This can be followed with a discussion about noticing more pleasant things in life, as well as life's subtleties, from tastes to thoughts and emotions. The *Mindful Smiling While Waking Up* and *Mindfulness of Gratitude* are engaging, mood-boosting home-based activities. *Mindfulness of Discomfort* can help kids begin to explore the impermanence of sensations and emotions, become aware of mind–body connections, and explore their own coping style.

Core Activities

Once the basic introductory practices and education about depression and depressive symptoms are established, we turn toward the beginning body-oriented practices, particularly those that are activating and movement-oriented. We suggest beginning with *Mindful Walking,* including the slow variation; *Mindful Movements* (yoga postures); and the *Mindful Flower Stretch.* We also recommend these as home practices. Movement-based body awareness may help depressed kids stay engaged more than body awareness practices that involve stillness, which can make it challenging to focus or stay awake, and may also be, well, less fun and engaging than movement activities.

Intermediate Development Activities

Once the group has experienced success and demonstrated some independence with the beginning activities, both in and out of the group time, we suggest moving toward the intermediate still body-based practices. To keep it fun, we suggest the *Mindful Eating (Part II)* as a way to bring more awareness to the subtleties of experience and enjoyment of everyday activities, and to help regulate eating if under- or overeating is present. A short *Body Scan* or *Mindful Body Relaxation* (with its progressive muscle relaxation) might be easier for kids to focus on than longer activities, and can also help with sleep difficulties and managing accompanying stress. The *Mindful Mountain Visualization* is an activity that can teach kids equanimity in the face of life's stressors and setbacks. The *Mindful HALT* activity helps kids remember to check in with some of their more basic needs and physiological symptoms. However, some of these eyes-closed activities might be modified to eyes open if acute post-traumatic distress is a concern.

Advanced Deepening Activities

Once children or teens (1) have successfully learned and practiced at least a few of the intermediate body practices, (2) feel comfortable with the practices, and (3) understand how their thoughts may relate to their depression, we can turn toward more advanced sensory and cognitive awareness practices. Beginning with sensory practices, learning to develop curiosity about and tolerance of sensations moves kids toward a deeper emotional awareness. We suggest beginning with *Listening to Silence, Mindful Seeing (Part I), Finding Five New Things,* and *Mindfulness of Smells (Parts I and II),* with an emphasis on bringing awareness to the sensations, thoughts, and urges to action that accompany these sensory experiences.

From there, we suggest moving into the activities that foster mindfulness of emotions, with a particular focus on locating emotions in the body and connecting the bodily experiences to depression. One of the pervasive qualities of depression is a flattening of emotional experience, so deeply exploring the nuances of emotions can bring greater awareness to the full range of human emotions. Practicing the longer *Body Scan* can bring more awareness to body sensations and energy, helping kids to recognize emotions when they begin as sensations in the body and to tolerate and manage their somatic symptoms.

We suggest beginning the emotions sequence by exploring *Mindfulness of Pleasant Events* followed by *Mindfulness of Unpleasant Events,* with attention to what thoughts and behaviors might manifest during these practices. Children who struggle with forms of depression that lead to strong negative emotions (or vice versa: those who struggle with strong negative emotions that lead to depression) might more deeply explore the activities related to *Mindfulness of Sadness and Loss (Parts I and II)* or *Mindfulness of Embarrassment,* then *Mindfulness of Worry and Anxiety (Parts I and II)* and mindfulness of any other "negative" or unpleasant emotions that may be relevant to the children in your group. *Mindfulness of Gratitude* or *Mindful Compassion* may be a helpful introduction to more "positive" feelings and effect some cognitive shifts as well. Kids who are irritable or triggered by envy might practice *Mindfulness of Frustration and Anger (Parts I and II)* or *Mindfulness of Envy.* We then recommend bringing in *Mindfulness of Happiness (Part I),* because kids learn well with marked contrasts, then explore more unpleasant emotions, before ending with *Mindfulness of Happiness (Part II).* Moreover, beginning with the "happy" emotions may lead kids to feel frustrated or get down on themselves because they aren't experiencing happy feelings. Teaching emotions by alternating contrasting valences may therefore be easier and less frustrating.

Maintenance, Generalization, and Concluding Activities

In closing, we encourage a discussion that includes explorations of (1) what has changed, (2) the skills and insights that can be brought to managing depression, and (3) situations that might trigger another depressed mood. ***Mindfulness of Judgments*** can help kids maintain awareness of their thoughts and attitudes going forward after the group has terminated. We also recommend including ***What Does Mindfulness Mean to Me Now? (Part II Drawing*** and/ or ***Part III Journaling)*** and the ***Here-and-Now Stones*** that give kids a concrete and tangible transitional object and reminder that they can always bring mindful awareness into each moment, as well as reinforcing equanimity. The final activity, ***Appreciation of the Group,*** leaves kids with positive feedback from their peers, which they can take with them. We suggest really taking time with this activity for kids who struggle with depression, so that they can "drink in" the appreciations they receive from other children in the group. You may want to include an activity in which they write appreciations for themselves as well.

Pathway through Attention Problems

My experience is what I agree to attend to.
—WILLIAM JAMES (1890)

Clear and effective thinking depends on the ability to focus one's attention while managing disruptive thoughts, intrusive feelings, and external distractions. Although all kids, especially younger ones, tend to have short attention spans and be more easily distracted than adults, some kids and teens have much more trouble focusing, sustaining attention, and staying on task than others. Attentional problems are common and can have a strong, negative impact on health and well-being, social functioning, academic performance, and happiness.

Attention is a complex phenomenon. Long ago, the great American psychologist William James wrote:

> Everyone knows what attention is. It is the taking possession by the mind, in clear and vivid form, of one out of what seem several simultaneously possible objects or trains of thought. Focalization, concentration, of consciousness are of its essence. It implies withdrawal from some things in order to deal effectively with others, and is a condition which has a real opposite in the confused, dazed, scatter-brained state which in French is called distraction. (1890, pp. 403–404)

More recently, researchers have divided the study of attention into three components: alerting, orienting, and executive functioning (Petersen & Posner, 2012; Posner & Petersen, 1990). *Alerting* is what occurs when something catches our attention. For example, you might hear a sound and turn to see what it is. *Orienting* is how we put that alert signal into context. So, we might look outside to see what's happening in the schoolyard, see no one there, and then keep looking to discover what the source of the sound might be. *Executive functioning* involves, in part, using the "planning" part of our brain to reach a goal, by seeing the steps to take, and understanding what is needed to complete the task. Essentially, *alerting* is achieving and maintaining a state of high sensitivity to a stimuli; *orienting* refers to the selection of sensory information; and executive functioning is involved in processing ambiguous, incongruent, or conflicting stimuli, and then deciding how to respond to them (Yin et al., 2012).

In his investigations of attention, James (1890) suggested that the ability to intentionally bring back a wandering attention was "the very root of judgment, character and will." But after discussing the importance of volitional control of attention, he then wrote, "it would be easier to describe this ideal than to give practical directions for bringing it about" (p. 424). Yet, despite James's pessimism, mindfulness training is essentially attentional training. One definition of mindfulness is "paying attention to things as they actually are in any given moment, however they are, rather than as we want them to be" (Williams et al., 2007, p. 47). Note that in this definition, mindfulness is simply a special kind of attention. Mindful attention is intentional, focused directly on present experience, nonjudgmental, and accepting of oneself and others. A number of research studies with children and adolescents have already shown mindfulness training to be beneficial in managing attentional problems in this population (Droutman, 2015; Huguet, Ruiz, Haro, & Alda, 2017; Semple, Lee, Rosa, & Miller, 2010; Singh & Singh, 2014; Tarrasch, 2018), and there are some indications that mindfulness training may improve academic performance as well (Bakosh, Snow, Tobias, Houlihan, & Barbosa-Leiker, 2016; Bennett & Dorjee, 2016).

Problems of Attention

Although many people immediately think of attention-deficit/hyperactivity disorder (ADHD) when childhood attentional problems are discussed, there are a number of other problem areas that are also marked by disruptions of attention. We don't know for sure how many children are misdiagnosed with ADHD every year, but one study estimated the number could be nearly 1 million (Elder, 2010). So, after discussing ADHD, we briefly describe some of the attentional problems associated with learning disabilities; stress and anxiety; OCD; trauma, neglect, and abuse; and the use of alcohol or drugs. Sleep deficits and depression are also associated with attentional problems.

Attention-Deficit/Hyperactivity Disorder

Considered a heritable brain disorder, ADHD is one of the most common behavioral disorders of childhood, and is associated with academic underachievement, poor social functioning, and suicidality (Kessler et al., 2014). The Centers for Disease Control and Prevention found that in 2016, an estimated 6.1 million U.S. children ages 2–17 years (9.4%) had received an ADHD diagnosis by a professional at some point, with approximately 5.4 million children currently having ADHD (Danielson et al., 2018). One in 12 kids in this country has been diagnosed with ADHD! Nearly two out of three of these kids and teens (63.8%) had also been diagnosed with at least one other psychological or behavioral disorder. Behavior or conduct problems were the most common comorbidity, followed by anxiety disorders, depression, autism spectrum disorder, and Tourette syndrome. Boys are almost three times more likely than are girls to be diagnosed with ADHD. About 3.3 million children were receiving medications, while about 2.5 million had received some form of behavioral health treatment. Young children and boys were more likely to receive a behavioral health treatment than teens and girls (Danielson et al., 2018).

One common misconception is that having ADHD means having a short attention span. A better way to look at it is that those with ADHD have a dysregulated attention system, or underdeveloped executive functioning. Three ADHD behavioral patterns are described in the *Diagnostic and Statistical Manual of Mental Disorders, Fifth Edition* (DSM-5; American Psychiatric Association, 2013), which are based on the dominant symptoms for the previous 6 months. These three behavioral patterns are predominantly hyperactive/impulsive, predominantly inattentive, and combined type. Behaviors associated with these are shown in Table III.3.

In addition to hyperactivity, impulsivity, and/or inattention, kids with ADHD often gravitate to what feels exciting or pleasurable, and are unenthusiastic about doing things they have decided are "boring." They also may have difficulty shifting attention from one thing to another. On the other hand, when they are doing something they enjoy or find intrinsically rewarding, they can "hyperfocus" on it, continuing the activity for hours after other kids would move on to other things. You might see this behavior when the child is playing video games, watching television, or surfing the Internet for hours on end. Combine this hyperfocus with poor social, organizational, and time management skills, and the teen may end up playing video games alone for an entire weekend. Channel it appropriately into productive activities, however, and hyperfocus may become a superpower for ADHD kids. Other consistently reported strengths associated with ADHD include a high level of energy and drive, creativity, agreeableness, empathy, and willingness to assist others (Mahdi et al., 2017).

TABLE III.3. Behaviors Commonly Associated with Attention-Deficit/ Hyperactivity Disorder

Signs of hyperactivity

- Is overly active
- Frequently fidgets or squirms in his or her seat
- May tap fingers, feet, pencil, fork, etc., or make other repetitive movements
- Finds it difficult to sit quietly in class, read, watch TV, or participate quietly in other activities
- May run around, jump, or climb up on things when it's not appropriate

Signs of impulsivity

- Talks loudly, rapidly, and/or excessively
- Often interrupts others before they finish speaking
- Finds it hard to wait in line or wait his or her turn when playing with other children
- Jumps from one task to another, frequently leaving each task unfinished
- Can act intrusively (e.g., barging into a sibling's bedroom without knocking)

Signs of inattention

- Sometimes appears not to be listening when someone is speaking to her or him
- Has difficulty keeping attention on one task or activity at a time
- Forgets or skips details when doing assignments or when following instructions
- Is easily distracted, so often makes seemingly careless or thoughtless mistakes
- Forgets responsibilities and doesn't follow through with promises
- Fails to finish homework without close supervision, guidance, and structure
- Habitually misplaces or loses possessions

Note. List based on DSM-5 diagnostic criteria for ADHD (American Psychiatric Association, 2013).

Learning Disabilities

When a child seems to be giving her attention to everything except the book she is supposed to be reading, one reason might be that she has a learning disability. A teen with undiagnosed dyslexia might be upset that he can't seem to do what the other kids do—and also be ashamed and concerned about covering up that fact. Learning disabilities (LDs) are neurologically based information-processing problems that interfere with a child or teen's ability to learn basic skills such as reading, writing, or math. LDs may also interfere with executive functions such as organization and planning, goal setting, decision making, short- and long-term memory, and attention. It is important to understand that LDs can also affect the lives of kids and teens beyond the classroom—in particular by impacting their relationships with friends and family. Mindfulness has been shown to improve the lives of some children with LDs by reducing stress, anxiety, and social problems (Beauchemin, Hutchins, & Patterson, 2008); improving self-monitoring skills (Haydicky, Wiener, Badali, Milligan, & Ducharme, 2012); improving sustained and selective attention, and reducing impulsivity (Tarrasch, 2018); and strengthening reading skills (Tarrasch, Berman, & Friedmann, 2016).

Stress and Anxiety

Stress makes it more difficult for pretty much anyone to pay attention to new information or to memorize new facts. A kid who seems to be inattentive in school might actually be mired in chronic worries about which teachers or parents are not aware. Anxiety interferes with concentration by shifting the focus of attention toward the specific worry or fear (Ehrenreich & Gross, 2002). Since we don't have a limitless capacity for attention, redirecting attention to one thing means that other things will be disregarded. For example, a kid with separation anxiety might be so preoccupied about something bad happening to his mom while he is at school that he can't pay attention to the class lesson. Some kids with social anxieties are so worried about making a mistake or saying something embarrassing that they spend all their time internally rehearsing what they might say—so internally focused that they don't even hear what is being said to them in that moment. When a teen takes an unusually long time to finish her homework assignment, sometimes it's not because of inattention, but rather that she has perfectionistic fears that her work won't be good enough.

Obsessive–Compulsive Disorder

Children with OCD are often obsessed with ritualized, compulsive behaviors that are carried out to prevent "something bad" from happening. Instead of paying attention to what is happening in the present moment, a child with OCD might be compulsively tapping her fingers or counting in her head. Or he may be busy lining his books up just so on his desk—over and over again. A teen with an obsession about germs might go to the bathroom dozens of time every day to wash his hands—while missing out on important class time. For kids and teens with OCD, the mind can be consumed with irrelevant tasks and information, and therefore have less attention to give to more task-relevant information (Muller & Roberts, 2005).

Trauma, Neglect, and Abuse

Children can also appear to be suffering from inattention when they have experienced trauma, neglect, or abuse (Semple & Madni, 2014). A child who witnesses chronic domestic violence in the home, for example, is likely to be preoccupied by his home environment and have difficulty paying attention in class. One symptom of trauma is a persistent sense of insecurity that results in a hypervigilant scanning of the environment. When that happens, the child or teen is not paying attention to what may be more relevant information or things happening in that moment. *Traumatic dissociation* is a lack of connection in the person's thoughts, memories, and sense of self-identity with what is happening in the present moment. When traumatic thoughts, memories, images, emotions, or body sensations become too intense to bear, dissociation is a common way of managing the unbearable fears. Essentially, the mind simply "checks out" for an indeterminate amount of time.

Alcohol and Substance Use

Beginning in adolescence, a key area of concern is increased risk of tobacco, alcohol, and cannabis use. Teens with ADHD and conduct disorders are more likely than others to develop nicotine, alcohol, or substance use disorders (Lee, Humphreys, Flory, Liu, & Glass, 2011). It's overly simplistic to assume that ADHD results in alcohol and substance use, in part because conduct disorder, which is highly comorbid with ADHD, is also an important factor (Tuithof, ten Have, van den Brink, Vollebergh, & de Graaf, 2012). Alcohol has both short- and long-term effects on the brain, such as confused or abnormal thinking, loss of inhibition, increased impulsivity, and poor decision making (Dougherty, Marsh, Moeller, Chokshi, & Rosen, 2000). Heavy or chronic drinkers may also experience impaired attention and memory loss. Given that the brains of teenagers are in a highly plastic neurodevelopmental period, it's not surprising that binge drinking by teens is associated with long-term attention and memory problems (Cservenka & Brumback, 2017).

   In recent years, marijuana has become more readily available and socially acceptable. In one meta-analysis, children with ADHD were nearly three times more likely to have reported using marijuana than those without ADHD (Lee et al., 2011). Given that, like alcohol, cannabis is also a central nervous system depressant with calming and relaxing effects, it also makes sense that marijuana is the preferred "self-medication" of hyperactive adolescents (Patel et al., 2018). Unfortunately, its disadvantages may outweigh the benefits. Findings from a longitudinal study indicated that adolescents who started smoking between 14 and 22 years old, despite stopping by age 22, had significantly more cognitive problems, health problems, and lower academic achievement and functioning at age 27 than their nonusing peers (Brook, Stimmel, Zhang, & Brook, 2008). Table III.4 describes the most common symptoms of attention problems in the domains of executive functioning, emotions, and physical and behavioral expressions along with child (subjective) and adult (objective) examples.

How Attention Problems Manifest at Different Ages

Younger children, in particular, have difficulty delaying gratification—they generally want everything right now. This behavior is exacerbated if they also have attention problems. They

TABLE III.4. Symptoms of Attention Problems, Child Descriptions, and Adult Observations

Problems of attention	Child description (subjective)	Adult observation (objective)
Executive functioning		
Distractibility means having difficulties maintaining focus as intended because attention is easily pulled away by internal or external extraneous stimuli.	• I can't focus—it's too noisy in here • What did you say? • I forgot what we were talking about. • Hey look at that over there!	• Appears not to be listening or following conversations • Frequently asks "What?" or asks for things to be repeated • Has difficulty staying on task with activities that are less interesting • Can't stay focused on work if there is any noise or visual stimuli • Can't complete tasks that have multiple elements • Changes conversation topic frequently • Is easily distracted by irrelevant or minor sounds, sights, movements, etc. • Quality of schoolwork declines • Skips school
Concentration is impaired when the ability to direct and maintain attention in a sustained way is poor.	• I can't pay attention • I can't learn anything • I don't remember • Reading is boring	• Complains about not being able to pay attention • Constantly forgets things • Makes careless mistakes • Takes an unusually long time to complete schoolwork • Frequently complains about being bored
Inattention refers to the inability to select relevant information to pay attention to, while ignoring information that is less relevant.	• I don't know [who is winning, what the score is] • I can never focus on just one thing • I often forget where I'm going	• Doesn't seem to be listening to the person talking • Can't remember what was just said • Has difficulty sorting out important information from what is not as important • Has difficulty connecting new information with information already known • Appears to be daydreaming
Hyperfocus is a difficulty shifting attention from one activity to another.	• I can [watch television, play video games, surf the Internet] for hours.	• Is able to sustain attention to selected high-interest, high-stimulation activities • Takes longer to shift attention to other tasks • Focus of attention is so strong that he or she appears to be oblivious to the world around him or her.
Emotional		
Worried, anxious, nervous	• I'm [worried, anxious, scared, tense] that I will fail • I'm scared to [undertake an activity]	• Worries excessively • Incessant contingency planning • Appears afraid to start new activities or to challenge him- or herself
Sad mood, low self-esteem, and negativity	• I'm not smart enough • I'm dumber than other kids • Something is wrong with me • I'm just a bad kid	• Adults may hear self-disparaging comments or comparisons • May lose or give away possessions • Is socially withdrawn or disengaged

(continued)

TABLE III.4. *(continued)*

Problems of attention	Child description (subjective)	Adult observation (objective)
Physical and behavioral		
Hyperactivity and restlessness	• Everyone else moves too slowly • I always have a lot of energy • I can't sit still • I feel so [jumpy, fidgety, jittery]	• Appears agitated, nervous, or fidgety • Paces, repetitively taps fingers or feet • Shows irritation when forced to sit still • Appears to be uncomfortable in [his or her] own skin
Impulsivity	• I can't control myself. • I don't know why I just did that! • I really need to do that right now.	• Has difficulty planning and organizing activities • Acts without thinking about the consequences
Use of alcohol or marijuana to "self-medicate" hyperactivity or sad mood	• Alcohol makes me feel [calmer, happier, better] • It's only the [substance] that keeps me going	• Appears intoxicated, hungover, or other symptoms of substance use • Money, alcohol, or prescription drugs go missing from the home • Marked change in functioning (e.g., grades decline, drops out of activities previously enjoyed) Note: Use of alcohol and marijuana is more common in males than in females.

also tend to be impatient and have trouble keeping strong emotions in check, resulting in angry outbursts or temper tantrums. These kids have difficulty waiting their turn, and they never seem to finish anything, becoming easily distracted or getting bored with a task before it's completed. They may move around a lot—constantly fidgeting, squirming, running, jumping, and climbing. They can't seem to sit still or play quietly. They can be overly talkative and will guess at answers instead of taking time to work through a problem. These are the kids who often interrupt others—for example, blurting out answers in class without waiting to be called on, or even without waiting to hear the entire question. They also have trouble staying organized, planning ahead, and finishing projects. So, they frequently lose or misplace their homework, books, toys, or other items.

In older kids and teens, organizational difficulties are pervasive. These teens may constantly be late for everything and have trouble keeping track of time. They are easily distracted, so sometimes "flake out" on important promises (e.g., forgetting to pick up a younger sibling at school). They forget or misplace things constantly. They have difficulty staying focused, so find it hard to complete long-term assignments. They may look like they're confused or daydreaming, and don't seem to be listening when spoken to. Impatience leads them to interrupt other people or make unexpected, rude, or inappropriate comments. They struggle to follow directions, and appear slower and less accurate at processing information than other teens. Because they are easily bored and impulsive, they can act recklessly without considering the consequences.

Teaching Tips

Kids with attentional problems can be supported by establishing short, simple rules and consistent routines in the group. They may need more modeling and supervision, which you can provide by pairing them with motivated peer buddies who model expected behaviors and help them remember to do home practice assignments. This pairing also benefits the more mature child by giving him or her opportunities to be responsible and empathic at the same time. Reducing potential distractions goes a long way toward creating an environment for all the kids and is conducive to learning and practicing mindfulness. For teens, in particular, this is likely to mean not allowing cellphones to be on in the group. And last, be mindful that nearly all kids respond much better to rewards than to punishment. Positive attention can be a great motivator. Rather than banning an overly active child from the group or sending him or her to a time-out, you might assign the teen to be your helper to pass out supplies, act as the timekeeper, ring the bells, etc.

Cautions and Contraindications

When working with children and teens who have attentional problems, it's important to remember that they do not necessarily have a motivational problem. They are not purposely being disruptive, nor are they intentionally ignoring you. Conducting a group of kids with attentional problems (and often co-occurring conduct problems) can feel like hard work. Expect that kids will show up late . . . or be texting during mindfulness activities . . . or listening to music on their headphones while practicing mindful walking. If there are a number of hyperactive kids in your group, we strongly recommend having a co-facilitator present to help meet their individual needs for attention, while the other facilitator continues the group activities. It's also useful to emphasize physical movement activities more than the still or seated ones. These kids may also have more difficulty with the longer practices, such as the body scan. However, we do not recommend skipping these altogether, but rather inviting the kids to extend the practice as long as they feel able—plus 1 minute longer. With a healthy dose of patience, teaching mindfulness skills (which directly address attention and impulsivity problems) may be the best gift you can give the attention-disordered child.

Activities for a Pathway through Attention Problems

The first goal of this pathway is to teach practical attention regulation skills that can be used every day. In the postactivity discussions, we recommend eliciting ideas about how the skills learned in the group might be applied in daily life, and then encouraging the kids to try implementing those ideas right away. The second goal of this pathway is to help kids and teens with attention problems gain more self-acceptance and comfort in their own skin. We can facilitate this by speaking openly about the problems associated with dysregulated attention and how it might be affecting their lives. Ignoring or minimizing the problems is not helpful. The last goal is to expand awareness of their emotional and behavioral choices. Having attentional dysregulation is not a choice. Learning how to respond to the difficulties this produces with emotional equanimity, mindful awareness, and skillfulness is what we aim to teach.

Introductory Activities

Adults are always telling children to pay attention, but never actually explain how to do it. Kids with attention problems likely hear this command more frequently than others and respond either by tuning out or getting frustrated. This response pattern makes taking your time to introduce mindfulness with patience and respectful awareness especially important. As with all the pathways, we recommend starting with the ***Introduction to Mindfulness.*** Following that with ***A Cup of Mindfulness*** is a useful activity because it is short and engaging, and offers the experiential understanding that mindfulness can be increased. ***What Does Mindfulness Mean to Me? (Part I)*** can be used to focus attention on ways in which mindfulness might help manage everyday problems and increase motivation to practice. Teaching patience can be challenging with kids who have attention problems, so discovering meaningful reasons to practice is important. ***Matching Movement Moments*** can be a good way for kids to get comfortable with each other, and is also useful to lower the energy level in the room by gradually slowing down the movements—like a wind-up toy running down.

Core Activities

Taking Three Mindful Breaths is a practical activity that can and should be practiced at many moments throughout the day. Particularly when strong impulses arise, this activity is helpful in creating a brief space to consider what choices may be available in that moment. When strong emotions are present, practicing ***Mindful Breath Counting*** is a skillful way to avoid reacting thoughtlessly. ***Mindful Movements*** (yoga postures) can be practiced at home to provide a brief break when studying or doing chores, while maintaining a nondistracting attentional focus. Emphasize body awareness as a useful grounding skill. Although it is a still-body activity, ***Three Minutes in My Body*** is short and focused enough to keep children and teens engaged, as is the ***Mindfulness of My Feet*** activity. ***Taking a Mindful SEAT*** helps cultivate self-awareness, which is a necessary skill before teaching self-management strategies.

Intermediate Development Activities

The ***Mindfulness of Thoughts*** and ***Mindfulness of Judgments*** activities are intended to promote decentering from thoughts and increase awareness of the influence of judgments on experiences. These are useful understandings for kids who may not be in the habit of looking at their own thoughts as "just thoughts." ***Mindfulness of Discomfort*** can be a stimulating activity to challenge teens with impulse-control problems to extend their own capacity to experience discomfort without needing to act on it. ***Finding Five New Things*** and ***Mindfulness in Everyday Life*** help increase present-focused awareness of ordinary daily activities, as does ***Mindful Eating (Part II), Mindful Listening and Speaking,*** and ***Mindful Touching. Mindful Seeing (Parts I and II)*** support the cultivation of new perspectives. All of the sensory-based activities also reinforce the concept that mindfulness is meant to be integrated into one's life—not just practiced in a group room or on a cushion at home. We encourage the creative exploration of related home practices following each of these activities, which are then shared with the group at the next session.

Advanced Deepening Activities

Mindfulness of Urges: Urge Surfing can be practiced regularly so that it becomes another useful daily management skill. The *Body Scan* may one of the most challenging activities for this group, so we recommend not teaching this until late in your program (or sometimes not at all). This can be replaced with shorter body activities such as *Mindfulness While Lying Down* or a shortened version of *Mindful Body Relaxation.* The *Mindful Mountain Visualization* is an intermediate-length activity that can move teens toward longer practices. Moving into the mindfulness of emotions sequence, we suggest providing positive experiences by starting with *Mindfulness of Happiness (Part I),* followed by *Mindfulness of Happiness (Part II),* which bring awareness to the impermanence of emotions. Spending extra time on the *Mindfulness of Frustration and Anger (Parts I and II)* activities highlights the influence of thoughts on behaviors and the importance of making choices that are not influenced by strong emotions. *Mindfulness of Embarrassment* begins the process of cultivating mindful self-compassion. Each of the other emotion-focused activities can be introduced as needed and as time permits.

Maintenance, Generalization, and Concluding Activities

Kids with attentional problems frequently have problematic relationships that create a good deal of distress in their lives. *Mindfulness of Gratitude* and *Mindful Compassion* support the cultivation of self-compassion and empathy for others. These group practices also strengthen each child's sense of social connectedness. As the group approaches its conclusion, we encourage facilitating discussions focused on identifying the skills and insights that can be usefully brought into everyday life. *What Does Mindfulness Mean to Me Now? (Part II): Drawing* and *What Does Mindfulness Mean to Me Now? (Part III): Journaling* can motivate kids to continue practicing mindfulness by raising awareness of its personal benefits. You may also wish to go back to the beginning and repeat some of the basic activities, such as *Taking Three Mindful Breaths, Listening to Silence,* and *Taking a Mindful SEAT* that can be useful when the child or teen becomes stressed out or frustrated. As we began, we close by emphasizing choices—not in what happens—but rather in how the kids choose to respond to what happens. Practicing *Mindfulness of Judgments* can help kids maintain awareness of thoughts as "just thoughts," remember that they always have choices, and commit to not letting unrealistic thoughts or intense emotions drive how those choices are made. The *Here-and-Now Stones* are gifts that we give each member of the group. These provide a solid reminder of what they have learned, and a prompt to continue practicing. The activity *Appreciation of the Group* particularly helps kids with low self-esteem recognize the ways that they contributed to the group. Hearing appreciative feedback from the other group members is a gift of compassion that each child gives to one another.

Pathway through Problems
of Emotion Regulation
and Impulse Control

This pathway offers a suggested sequence of activities for children and adolescents who are struggling with regulating their emotions or behaviors, or exhibiting worrisome speech or behaviors that place them or others at significant physical or legal risk. These include kids with problematic personality traits, perhaps diagnosed initially as having oppositional defiant disorder (ODD), which often overlaps with substance use disorders. Although personality disorders are not diagnosed before adulthood, many professionals who work with these often challenging populations are familiar with the traits and symptoms we describe in the following pages. Kids don't always fall neatly into one diagnostic category and can certainly offer challenges to teachers and mental health professionals.

For the most part, the kids best supported by this pathway are teens or tweens. Adolescence tends to be a period of increased emotional reactivity and psychopathology (Costello, Mustillo, Angold, Erkanli, & Keeler, 2003), and younger children are still developing the neurocognitive competencies necessary to self-regulate their emotions and behaviors (Ahmed, Bittencourt-Hewitt, & Sebastian, 2015). The teens with severe emotional and behavioral difficulties are often seen in substantially separated special educational settings, therapeutic schools, residential treatment facilities, the juvenile justice system, or other forensic or mandated settings.

Emotion Regulation and Impulse-Control Disorders

Disruptive and aggressive disorders that are marked by difficulties with emotion regulation and poor impulse-control skills include ODD, intermittent explosive disorder (IED), and conduct disorder (CD). ODD is characterized by angry or irritable mood and behaviors, with aggressive and often violent interpersonal behavior falling under categories of angry/irritable, argumentative/defiant, and vindictive (DSM-5; American Psychiatric Association, 2013). IED is characterized by recurrent difficulties with anger management. Frequent angry outbursts of verbal and physical aggressions are far out of proportion to the triggering situation. IED is associated with interpersonal childhood trauma and neglect (Nickerson, Aderka, Bryant, & Hofmann, 2012), tends to emerge in late childhood or early adolescence, and is more common in boys than girls (Kessler et al., 2006). The diagnosis of CD captures similar but more severe behaviors, and more emotional dysregulation than ODD. CD includes many worrisome traits of the adult antisocial personality disorder (ASPD). These include physical and sexual aggression toward people or animals, theft or destruction of property, deceitfulness, and serious violation of rules and social norms. Boys tend to act out with aggression, lack of discipline, and criminal behaviors, whereas girls are more likely to exhibit deceit, substance abuse, prostitution, truancy, and running away (Matthys & Lochman, 2017).

Here, a word of caution about diagnosis is warranted. There is a great deal of symptom overlap and co-occurring ODD, IED, and CD. In addition, PTSD, ADHD, substance use disorders (SUDs), and attachment disorders are commonly diagnosed instead of (or in addition to) the disruptive, impulse-control, or conduct disorders (Kessler et al., 2006). These may sometimes look similar and the distinctions can be challenging to detect. Many of these teens exhibit a confusing grab bag of symptoms, and go through a number of these diagnoses over the course of their adolescent development. The most common symptoms associated with this cluster of diagnoses along with child (subjective) descriptions and adult (objective) observations are listed in Table III.5. The symptoms are grouped into four domains (identity and cognition, emotional, behavioral, and interpersonal and social).

Personality disorders (PDs) are characterized by inflexible and persistent patterns of thinking and behaviors that interfere with functioning in emotional experiences, interpersonal relationships, and managing impulses across a range of situations. People with PDs have trouble dealing with everyday stressors and problems. Although not generally diagnosed until at least age 18, traits associated with these disorders begin to emerge in adolescence, notably antisocial PD, borderline PD, histrionic PD, and narcissistic PD (DSM-5; American Psychiatric Association, 2013).

ASPD describes a pattern of disregard for others since at least age 15, including at least three socially unacceptable behaviors such as failing to conform to rules and laws, deceit, impulsivity, aggression, disregard for safety of self and others, pervasive irresponsibility, and a lack of remorse. ASPD is more typically seen in males, and is often preceeded by symptoms of CD.

Borderline personality disorder (BPD) is characterized by a pattern of instability in relationships, emotions, and self-image. It includes five or more of the following: frantic efforts to avoid real or imagined abandonment, unstable relationships, unstable sense of self, impulsivity, suicidal threats or gestures, reactive mood, chronic feelings of emptiness, anger problems, and transient paranoia or dissociation. BPD traits are largely seen in females, and may include self-harming or mutilating behaviors such as cutting, scratching, or burning.

Histrionic personality disorder (HPD) is also largely seen in females, and is marked by a pervasive pattern of dramatic, attention-seeking behavior with five of the following symptoms: discomfort with not being the center of attention, rapidly shifting and shallow emotions, excessive attention to appearance, vague and impressionistic speech style, exaggerated and dramatic expression of emotion, easily influenced by others, and misinterpreting the depth of interpersonal relationships.

Narcissistic personality disorder (NPD) is characterized by a sense of grandiosity and a need for admiration, along with a lack of empathy for others. The prevalence of NPD skews

TABLE III.5. Problems of Emotion Regulation and Impulse Control, Child Descriptions, and Adult Observations

Emotion dysregulation and impulse-control symptoms	Child descriptions (subjective)	Adult observations (objective)
Identity and cognition		
Lack of trust that disrupts interpersonal functioning	• I don't trust anyone • I hate everyone • There's always "drama" in my life • They are out to get me • I'll get them back!	• Black-and-white perceptions of others • Misjudgments about who may be trustworthy or untrustworthy • Chaotic and unstable interpersonal relationships with peers and adults (particularly with adults in positions of authority) • May have enemies and rivals as well as allies, as if he or she were on a reality contest show
Identity concerns that are beyond typical or developmentally appropriate adolescent identity concerns	• I'm a [bad, evil, worthless] person • I don't know who I am	• Frequently talks about existential issues
Deliberately deceptive to attain material or emotional desires	• I deserve this, so it's okay to [lie, cheat, steal]	• Lies for status, emotional needs, or material gain • Manipulates others for his or her own self-aggrandizement
Grandiose sense of self-importance and future status beyond what is typical or developmentally appropriate for adolescence	• Don't you know who I am? • If I ran this place, . . . • I'm kind of like a reality star • No one is as smart as me • I'm going to be a professional athlete • I'm going to be a billionaire	• Unrealistic view of present and future status
Consistently needing to be the center of attention; demands special attention Demanding sense of entitlement	• I should get special treatment • Did you hear about/see my [achievement, recognition, success, fame] • Do you know that I know [famous or important person]	• Acting or presenting self as a celebrity, reality TV star, or person of high status who is deserving of recognition and adulation • Dramatic behaviors, provocative interpersonal style • Extreme or inappropriate fashion style • Excessive name dropping
Consistent sense of entitlement beyond what is developmentally typical	• My parents would take me right out of here if they really knew about this place • You are completely terrible compared to my old [school, teacher, therapist, etc.]	• Makes unreasonable demands on adult caregivers • Expects "special treatment" • Acts as if he or she were a reality show star

(continued)

TABLE III.5. *(continued)*

Emotion dysregulation and impulse-control symptoms	Child descriptions (subjective)	Adult observations (objective)
Emotional		
Low motivation, interest, or engagement outside of highly stimulating activities	• I'm too tired • I don't have the energy to do it • This is really boring • I just want to be playing [video games, sports] • I just want to [get high, cut myself, act out] • Everything is lame • Leave me alone	• Low motivation and resistance to accommodate even small or simple tasks or requests • Reluctant to do even mildly strenuous activities • Engages in unusually risky and high-stimulation behaviors related to sex, substances, or physical safety
Hopelessness, pessimism	• Nothing is ever going to work out for me • I'm doomed • Everything sucks • The future looks bleak • Nothing good ever happens to me • Nothing/no one can help me	• Expresses consistent negative attitude about self, world, others, and future • Nihilistic attitudes, beliefs and behaviors
Feeling empty or numb	• I don't care • I feel [empty, dead, hollow, numb] • I don't know who I am	• Appears dull, listless, or apathetic • Moves or speaks slowly or not at all
Depression or anxiety	• I'm always [sad, down, depressed, miserable, unhappy, blue] • I'm [nervous, anxious, worried, scared, afraid]	• Appears sad and/or anxious • Excessive crying or sadness over seemingly minor triggers • Excessive focal or overly generalized anxieties and fears
Angry or aggressive feelings	• Everyone is out to get me • I'll show them • You'll be sorry • I hate you	• Extreme anger and aggression in response to real or perceived slights • Emotional or physical aggression toward people, animals, property
Irritability or restlessness	• Everything is annoying • I hate [you, everybody, what's happening or not happening]	• Irritable mood • Easily loses temper, "touchy" argumentative, resentful, vindictive
Emotional reactivity	• Comments like these that are out of proportion to the situation: • This *is* a big deal! • I can't believe you would treat me this way!	• Sudden swings in mood and emotions • Inappropriate emotional reactions to triggers

(continued)

TABLE III.5. *(continued)*

Emotion dysregulation and impulse-control symptoms	Child descriptions (subjective)	Adult observations (objective)
Behavioral		
Deliberately cruel or vindictive to others emotionally or physically	• Let's beat them up • Let's play this [mean, cruel, nasty] trick on them • I'm going to make them sorry • I'll make that chump pay for [something I wanted or planned to do]	• Physically cruel or aggressive toward people or animals • Emotionally cruel to others; relational bullying • Spreading false rumors • Intentionally "sets up" other kids for failure • Blaming or framing others when caught doing something wrong
Deliberately destructive or criminal activity [setting fires, vandalism, shoplifting or other thefts]	• Let's mess this up just for fun • Let's steal it • Let's break in here	• Vandalism • Stealing • Trespassing, especially in ways that violate the space of others
Interpersonal and social		
Difficulty with social norms	• This group sucks • The rules don't apply to me • I'm too good for all this • I'm too sick and messed up to be helped	• Acting out with silliness, anger, aggression, attention seeking, interpersonal chaos or other disruptions to group dynamics • Deliberately annoying and provoking peers and adults • Disregard for social rules and norms, including laws
Blames others; takes little or no responsibility for behavior or emotions; shows little or no guilt or remorse	• It's not my fault • They made me do it • I don't care • It doesn't bother me • I'm not sorry, they deserved it • It's their fault, I don't feel bad for them • I'd do it again in a minute	• Takes little or no responsibility for mistakes or getting into trouble • No guilt or remorse expressed or evident when caught
Impulsivity and carelessness	• I'm just going to do this [then does it without regard for consequences] • I don't care about [another person, property damage]	• High-risk sexual behavior that is developmentally inappropriate • High-risk alcohol or substance use (e.g., binge drinking, driving drunk) • Self-harm behaviors (e.g., cutting, scratching, or burning his- or herself) • Risky or harmful behaviors (e.g., academic suspension, failing grades) • Impulsivity and lack of planning or regard for consequences • Indifferent or abusive in relationships
Recurrent suicidal or self-harming behaviors or threats used to manipulate others	• I want to kill myself • Here's how I would kill myself • I'll hurt/kill myself if you don't do/say what I want	• Threating to self-harm or commit suicide • Talking about death and suicide • Past history of plans or nonlethal attempts at suicide

toward men and must include five of the following symptoms: a grandiose sense of importance, fantasies of unlimited success and power, belief in their own specialness, needing
excessive admiration, excessive entitlement, takes advantage of others, lacking empathy, arrogant, and preoccupied with envy.

Another issue that comes up frequently with individuals with personality disorders is
co-occurring SUDs. Symptoms of SUDs include taking more of a substance or for longer than
intended; is unable to cut down despite wanting to; spends a lot of time and money obtaining
substances; experiences significant interference with school, work, and relationships; and
continues to use despite problems, dangers, or consequences (DSM-5; American Psychiatric
Association, 2013). Some substances, including nicotine, alcohol, sedatives, amphetamines
(uppers), and opioid painkillers, are addictive and result in growing tolerance and withdrawal
symptoms when the substance is stopped. Be aware that many of the qualities of chronic
substance users and those who are in early recovery can look a lot like emotion regulation,
conduct, or impulse-control problems: for example, deception, theft, manipulative behaviors,
impulsivity, erratic anger outbursts, and sudden mood swings.

How Emotion Regulation and Impulse-Control Problems Manifest at Different Ages

Although the symptoms and behaviors of emotion regulation and impulse-control problems are largely associated with teens and sometimes tweens, worrisome signs may develop
earlier in childhood and latency-age children. These include frequent tantrums, excessive
argumentativeness and defiance, deliberate attempts to annoy or upset others, developmentally inappropriate blaming of others, lack of responsibility, lack of remorse, and high
reactivity.

Teaching Tips

Kids with behavioral and emotion regulation issues are among the most challenging to engage,
and keep consistently engaged, while maintaining group cohesion and order. Safety of the
kids and others may also be more of a concern than with other groups, although we expect
that you will know your kids best—both as individuals and within the group's interpersonal
dynamics. Managing a group of teens with emotion or behavior regulation problems can be
daunting in terms of group or classroom dynamics and management of acting-out behaviors
that emerge more frequently in groups. As always, we recommend prescreening potential
participants for motivation and commitment when possible. We also recommend screening
for any safety concerns to assure the well-being of all participants in the group. If feasible, it
can be helpful to have a co-therapist or teaching aide in the room to help manage disruptive
behaviors. We strongly suggest having an experienced psychotherapist available for consultation. Concomitant parent and child mindfulness training also offers a promising approach
to working with kids who have more severe externalizing problems (Bögels, Hoogstad, van
Dun, de Schutter, & Restifo, 2008).

As with depression, resistance to participating may look like psychiatric symptoms, and symptoms may look like resistance. Behaviorally challenging kids who fall into this category are far less likely to follow through on mindfulness homework, or even fully participate when the group or class gets together. They may engage in disruptive behaviors and comments that appear to deliberately sabotage the teacher or undermine other kids. Irritability, disengagement, and cynicism may be more passive forms of resistance seen in the adolescent years. Particularly acute kids may disrupt group dynamics. We recommend carefully considering seating arrangements, such as the use of rows rather than circles, to prevent participants from distracting each other, and separating kids you know will struggle to focus if seated near each other. Some challenging kids may also simply be unable to regulate themselves to sit still for a long time, and offering them a job may be helpful (e.g., timekeeper, bell ringer) to keep them in the group but in a different role. In extreme cases, a child or teen may need to leave the group for a few minutes to settle him- or herself down. Having a supervised space nearby is ideal but often not practical. With younger children, having a designated "quiet space" in one corner of the room can be helpful.

Research suggests that mindfulness-based interventions may help with self-management of emotions and behaviors (Droutman, 2015; Teper, Segal, & Inzlicht, 2013). Problematic symptoms and behaviors may be reduced due to apparent brain changes in regions associated with emotion regulation and impulse control, thereby boosting positive emotions (Lutz et al., 2014; Tang, Tang, & Posner, 2016), as well as reducing the emotional pain associated with interpersonal rejection and perceived rejection that may drive problem behaviors (Peters, Eisenlohr-Moul, & Smart, 2016).

Mindfulness also appears to help teens more effectively regulate their behavioral impulsivity as it relates to reacting to strong emotions (Franco, Amutio, López-González, Oriol, & Martínez-Taboada 2016). In turn, this increased regulation may reduce aggression, drug use, self-harm, and other risky behaviors. Mindfulness may also boost empathy and compassion, reducing hyperactivity and interpersonal aggression (Viglas & Perlman, 2018), perhaps by helping kids take the perspective of others and become more concerned about the negative impact of their behaviors on others.

Much of the mindfulness-based intervention research on individuals who have difficulty regulating their emotions and behaviors has been conducted using dialectical behavior therapy for adolescents (DBT-A; Miller, 1999), which uses shorter mindfulness exercises than used with adults, along with other skills. Consequently, we have emphasized shorter activities in this emotion regulation pathway. Many in this population tend to be sensation seeking, so we suggest activities that involve movement such as mindful walking or mindful sensory activities. Sensations can be increased during mindful eating activities by using hot or spicy foods or bold flavors, such as strong mints, while emphasizing impulse control during all of the activities.

Cautions and Contraindications

As with each of the other pathways, there are a few things to be on the lookout for when working with these complex children and teens. With unresolved, often undiagnosed trauma more prevalent in this group, we recommend a few specific tips. Closed-eyed breathing may be too triggering for some. Closing the eyes in a group can feel unsafe, particularly if there is a lack of trust between the kids. One alternative is to invite them to rest their eyes on the floor or desk in front of them, which can help minimize internal and external distractions. Deeper and longer body-based practices like body scans may also lead to acting out with either silliness and distraction or aggression. Compassion and self-compassion practices may also lead to what Germer and Neff (2013) have described as "backdraft," which is a firefighting term to describe what happens when opening a door in a burning building—oxygen rushes in and the flames increase. Compassion practices should be closely monitored to ensure that they don't "open the door" to emotional overload or trauma reactions, such as dissociation. "When we bring the light of loving-kindness and compassion to our experience, we discover our hidden wounds and fears. Then we bring kindness to ourselves and the wounds begin to lose their sharp edge. The process may be understood as compassionate exposure therapy" (Germer & Neff, 2013, p. 863).

Another concern involves an increased awareness of thoughts of self-harm and suicide, or, alternately, increased aggression toward others. As clinicians, these risks always present a challenge, but we have been trained in how to handle these behaviors when they arise. If you are a teacher or other nonclinically trained facilitator, we strongly recommend working closely with a therapist or behavior specialist who is experienced with this population, knows the kids, and is familiar with their individual issues.

One more wild-card variable that can be more of an issue in the teen population, especially in mixed-gender groups, are the unique group dynamics that emerge in every group. These are as important for a facilitator to monitor as are the individual reactions and responses to each activity. Intragroup conflict, competition, or rivalries; power struggles; sexual posturing; and bullying, victimizing, and scapegoating are a few dynamics of which to be aware. We strongly recommend having co-facilitators or other staff present who are familiar with the dynamics of the group.

We would also like to note that many of the characteristics of PDs often look like the worst stereotypes of adolescence. This is a major reason why PDs are not diagnosed until adulthood. These "symptoms" include rapidly shifting moods and identities, impulsivity, lack of planning, lack of empathy for others, and a flair for the dramatic. But PDs are not what drives the behaviors of the average struggling teen, but instead represent the pathological extremes of those behaviors.

Activities for a Pathway through Problems of Emotion Regulation and Impulse Control

This pathway has three main aims. The first is to reduce the cognitive and physiological arousal that can distort perceptions or interpretation of events, influence judgments, or drive impulsive behaviors and exaggerated reactivity to events. The second goal is to bring greater emotional awareness to triggering situations, and in getting to know and accept the full range of human emotions, cultivate empathy and compassion for others and self. The third aim is to master a few mindfulness skills that the child or teenager can use independently in potentially triggering situations.

Introductory Activities

As with all the pathways, we begin with an introduction to mindfulness and how it relates to recognizing and managing strong impulses and emotions. We suggest linking these two for the kids: a strong emotion can lead to a strong impulse, which can lead to serious consequences. The introductory activities we recommend include a *What Does Mindfulness Mean to Me? (Part I)* drawing activity. Starting with this activity also provides a baseline with which to assess kids' engagement and understanding. The settling and grounding effects of *Taking a Mindful Posture* may be enhanced by the children placing the palm of one hand flat on the ground or desk. From there we recommend *Taking a Mindful SEAT,* which helps kids recognize and begin to work with the connections between sensations, emotions, thoughts, and actions that might land them in more difficulty. Introductory breath training can include *Mindfulness of the Breath* and *Mindful Breath Counting,* which build focus and cognitive regulation; and *Belly Breathing* and *Taking Three Mindful Breaths,* which can offer calmness through grounding and reducing physiological activation. However, we do recommend you begin these activities and visualizations with the eyes open. The *Mindful Mountain Visualization* offers a taste of equanimity, although we recommend starting with a shorter version to give kids a positive experience. A longer or "eyes closed" version might not be indicated, depending on your group dynamics. *Mindfulness of My Feet* gives kids a chance to experience simple grounding that can disrupt an overwhelming emotion or urge. The initial goals are to introduce the kids to mindfulness and give them immediate positive experiences on which to build.

Core Activities

Once kids have engaged with the basic introductory practices, see the benefits for themselves, and are able to trust the group dynamic and the facilitator, we turn toward body-oriented core practices. Movement may be easier for this population than still practices. At the same time, many kids might be self-conscious about making any moves while others are watching, depending on group dynamics.

Mindful Walking is a good place to start, though slow walking may raise self-consciousness, whereas *Mindful Movements* (yoga postures) might be easier for these kids, especially as they can just do these stretches in whatever they are wearing. A *Mindful Body Relaxation* (progressive muscle relaxation), which is more active and immediate in its effects than a simple body scan, can also engage kids, and can be done with eyes open, if needed, or encouraged as a practice that can be done at home. At this point *Mindful Eating (Parts I and II)* is likely to be fun and engage this particular group, especially if more stimulating foods like chocolate, strong mints, or cinnamon candy are provided. Kids might also learn to listen to their bodies—to tune into their emotional and physical needs more—using the *Mindful HALT,* which will be easier and may feel less threatening than a protracted body scan.

Intermediate Development Activities

Once the kids have grown comfortable with the core practices, we suggest moving toward the *Body Scan* and *Mindfulness While Lying Down* variations, with a look toward locating the origins of emotion in the body. ***Listening to Silence*** and ***Mindful Hearing*** are worth exploring and discussing as practice deepens and lengthens during this phase. We also suggest exploring shorter practices such as ***Finding Five New Things, Mindfulness in Everyday Life, Mindful Touching,*** and ***Mindfulness of Smells (Parts I and II).*** Given the nature of this group, at this point we recommend ***Mindfulness of Urges: Urge Surging.*** If the kids and group dynamics work, we recommend ***Mindful Silliness, Matching Movement Moments,*** and ***Mindfulness of Gratitude.***

Advanced Deepening Activities

As the kids master the intermediate practices and engage more fully with the group and facilitator, we nudge them toward greater emotional awareness. ***Mindful Listening and Speaking*** practice may teach impulsive kids to slow down long enough to hear what the other person is saying. We may want to review and keep up with ***Taking a Mindful SEAT, The Mindful Stop,*** and other check-in practices for insight into urges and impulses, before turning toward mindfulness of emotions. This includes ***Mindfulness of Judgments, Happiness, Worry,*** and ***Frustration*** before turning to ***Mindfulness of Sadness, Embarrassment, Envy,*** and other more vulnerable emotions.

Maintenance, Generalization, and Concluding Activities

As the group closes, we encourage a discussion that includes what has changed, and which skills can be carried forward into potentially triggering situations. We recommend closing with developmentally appropriate ***What Does Mindfulness Mean to Me Now? (Part II: Drawing for younger children*** or ***Part III: Journaling for teens), Appreciation of the Group,*** and the ***Here-and-Now Stones.***

Pathway through Trauma, Abuse, and Neglect

Childhood Trauma

Unfortunately, childhood often is not the idyllic experience portrayed in poetry and song. Every day in the United States, children are exposed to violence—in their homes, schools, and communities. The second National Survey of Children's Exposure to Violence (NatSCEV II; 2011) found that 54.5% of children and adolescents (birth–17 years old) have experienced some form of physical assault: 24.6% were victims of physical intimidation (i.e., physical bullying); 51.8% were victims of relational aggression (i.e., emotional bullying); and 10.3% were victims of assault with a weapon (Finkelhor, Turner, Shattuck, & Hamby, 2013). More than two-thirds of all children will be exposed to one or more potentially traumatic events before the age of 16 (Copeland, Keeler, Angold, & Costello, 2007).

Early childhood trauma affects both brain structure and functioning of the brain (Grasso, Greene, & Ford, 2013), and the rapidly developing brains of young children are especially vulnerable to trauma. Trauma appears to impact the size of some cortical areas (Dickie, Brunet, Akerib, & Armony, 2013; Tomoda, Navalta, Polcari, Sadato, & Teicher, 2009; Tomoda, Polcari, Anderson, & Teicher, 2012). The frontal cortex is responsible for many executive functions, including attention, perceptual awareness, and self-awareness; thinking, learning, and memory; and the child's ability to self-regulate his or her emotions and behaviors.

Traumatic events can have profound and lasting impacts. A child's sense of safety may be shattered by frightening images, loud noises, violent movements, pain sensations, and other stimuli associated with unpredictable and/or frightening events. Children commonly blame themselves or their caregivers for not preventing a scary event or for not being able to change its outcome. Not having an accurate understanding of cause-and-effect relationships, some children may believe that their own thoughts have the power to make bad things happen. A sense of helplessness and lack of control further exacerbates the traumatic impact. Younger children are less able to anticipate danger or to know ways to keep themselves safe, and therefore are particularly vulnerable to experiencing posttraumatic distress. Children are less able than adults to express in words what they are feeling. However, their behaviors can give us important clues about how they are being affected.

Adverse Childhood Experiences

Children are completely dependent on parents or other adult caregivers for their physical and emotional protection and survival. When a caregiver is abusive or neglectful, the child is certain to be strongly affected—cognitively, emotionally, behaviorally, and developmentally. Without the support of a trusted parent or caregiver to help them learn to regulate intense emotions, the child is likely to experience overwhelming distress and be unable to effectively communicate his or her needs or explain what he or she is feeling. Adult caregivers can exacerbate the distress by not recognizing the symptoms and uncharacteristic behaviors as trauma-related responses, and they may not know how to respond appropriately.

Although adverse childhood experiences (ACEs) sometimes occur independently, they more often occur in combination and frequently have serious consequences that last into adolescence and adulthood. These include increased health risks related to smoking, alcoholism, and drug abuse; sexually transmitted diseases; depression and suicide attempts; physical inactivity and severe obesity; and are related to the emergence of adult diseases that include ischemic heart disease, cancer, chronic lung disease, skeletal fractures, and liver disease (Felitti et al., 1998). ACEs generally fall into three broad categories:

- *Abuse:* psychological abuse, physical abuse, and sexual abuse.
- *Neglect:* physical neglect and emotional neglect.
- *Household dysfunction:* mental illness, alcohol or substance abuse, domestic violence, incarcerated relative, and divorce.

The national statistics on child maltreatment are simply horrendous. According to the Children's Bureau (U.S. Department of Health and Human Services, 2017), in 2015:

- 3,358,000 children in the United States were referred for a child protective services investigation.
- 683,000 children were found to be victims of child abuse or neglect.
- Of those children, 75.3% were neglected; 17.2% were physically abused; and 8.4% were sexually abused.
- A nationally estimated 1,670 children died of abuse and neglect.

Overview of Stress Disorders

DSM-5, the most recent edition of the *Diagnostic and Statistical Manual of Mental Disorders* (American Psychiatric Association, 2013), made significant changes to the spectrum of stress disorders, including differentiating them from the anxiety disorders and removing a criterion that required the individual's response to involve "fear, helplessness, or horror." A new dissociative subtype was added, and separate diagnostic criteria for preschool children (6 years or younger) are now included.

All of the stress disorders that we discuss in the following material require exposure to a traumatic or stressful event. This may involve experiencing or witnessing the event in person;

indirect exposure, such as learning that a parent or caregiver was exposed to a trauma; or secondary exposure, as experienced by emergency first responders and medical personnel. Other symptoms are specific to each disorder. Trauma-related signs and symptoms manifest in four domains: cognitive, emotional, physiological, and behavioral.

Symptoms of PTSD include persistent reexperiencing of components of the trauma, avoidance of trauma-related stimuli, negative thoughts or feelings that began or worsened after the trauma, and physiological arousal or hyperreactivity. The symptoms must last for more than 1 month. *Acute stress disorder* (ASD) symptoms are similar to PTSD, but there are no mandatory symptoms from any cluster and a greater emphasis on dissociative experiences. Symptoms must last for more than 2 days and less than 1 month. Many different events can trigger symptoms of *adjustment disorder* (AD). You may see defiant or impulsive behaviors, nervousness or physical tension. The child may cry, feel sad or hopeless, and withdraw from other people. These symptoms follow a stressor, are more severe than would be expected, and are not part of normal bereavement following the death of a loved one. *Reactive attachment disorder* (RAD) is marked by emotionally withdrawn and inhibited behaviors, whereas *disinhibited social engagement disorder* (DSES) is characterized by indiscriminate and disinhibited social behaviors. Both are associated with extreme childhood abuse or neglect, social deprivation, multiple changes of caregivers, and being reared in unusual settings. *Other specified trauma or stressor-related disorders* can include adjustment-like disorders with a delayed onset or with a duration of more than 6 months without a prolonged stressor being present, subthreshold PTSD, grief that is complicated by depression or another mental disorder, ataque de nervios, and other culture-bound symptoms. *Persistent complex bereavement disorder* (PCBD) is also included in this category. PCBD lasts more than 12 months after the death of a loved one and results in significant distress or functional impairment. The bereavement reaction must be out of proportion or inconsistent with cultural, religious, or age-appropriate norms.

As shown in Table III.6, traumatic stress symptoms are broadly clustered as symptoms of reexperiencing, avoidance, dissociative experiences, and physiological arousal.

How Trauma Symptoms Manifest at Different Ages

Younger children tend to express somatic symptoms and show behaviors more than they verbally express their worries or fears. These include complaints of headaches, stomachaches, or other unidentified pains, along with concentration, sleep, or appetite problems. Children are less likely to show dissociative experiences than do teens and adults. Behaviorally, they may be clingy and fear being separated from their caregiver, cry or throw temper tantrums, or act out to avoid triggering situations or being near adults who remind them of the trauma. Young children frequently show signs of PTSD in their play. For example, they may repeatedly reenact parts of the trauma through drawing or in play with dolls or other toys. A child might want to play shooting games after he or she witnesses a school shooting, for example. These games may have a compulsive quality about them and do not reduce the worries or distress. Elementary school-age children may not experience visual flashbacks or amnesia for aspects of the trauma. However, they do experience what's known as "time skew," which

TABLE III.6. Traumatic Stress Symptoms, Child Descriptions, and Adult Observations

Traumatic stress symptoms	Child descriptions (subjective)	Adult observations (objective)
Reexperiencing • *Recurrent intrusive images or thoughts* • *Nightmares or recurrent dreams* • *Flashbacks (a sense of reliving the event)* • *Distress when reminded of the event*	• Scary stuff keeps coming into my mind over and over. • I can't stop thinking about it. • I'm afraid to go to sleep. • It just keeps happening.	• Frequent talking about the event in a ruminative or obsessive way. • Sometimes acts as if the trauma is happening again. • Screaming or excessive crying.
Avoidance • *Event-related people, places, activities* • *Thinking or talking about event*	• I don't want to talk about it. • I don't want to go there. • I don't like doing that any more. • I don't want X to take care of me. • I don't want to go to X's house.	• May show fear of adults associated with the trauma, abuse, or neglect. • Excessively clingy, especially when anticipating separation from a caregiver. • Refuses to talk about the event. • Refuses to go back to the location or activity where event occurred. • Appears sad or withdrawn.
Dissociative experiences • *Emotional numbing, detachment, or absence of emotional responsiveness* • *Reduced awareness of his or her surroundings* • *Derealization* • *Depersonalization* • *Dissociative amnesia (can't remember some parts of the traumatic event)*	• I feel dead inside. • I don't care about anything. • I forget where I am. • I feel funny, not like myself. • I feel spacey. • The world feels weird sometimes.	• Unusually quiet. • Socially withdrawn. • Little expression in face or voice. • Appears to have no emotions. • Loses track during conversations. • Eyes and face may go blank during a dissociative episode. • May show little awareness of people or events around them.
Physiological arousal • *Difficulty sleeping* • *Irritability* • *Poor concentration* • *Hypervigilance* • *Exaggerated startle response* • *Motor restlessness or agitation*	• I can't go to sleep. • I wake up in the middle of the night and can't get back to sleep. • I'm tired all the time. • I'm mad at everyone. • Everything bothers me. • I can't think straight. • My mind just goes blank. • I forget everything I learned. • I feel jumpy, jittery, edgy. • I can't sit still. • I have butterflies in my stomach.	• Acts jumpy, startles easily. • Hands trembling. • Repetitive movements (e.g., tapping fingers, motor tics). • Temper tantrums. • Regressive behaviors that are age inappropriate (e.g., thumb sucking in a 12-year-old). • Exhibits aggressive behaviors. • Frequent requests for reassurance. • Appears nervous or irritable. • Memory problems, forgetful. • Quality of schoolwork declines. • Poor appetite, low weight, or gastrointestinal problems. • Somatic complaints (e.g., frequent headaches, stomachaches, unspecified aches or pains).

is an inaccurate or "off" sequencing of the trauma-related events when recalling the experience.

Older children and teens who have experienced multiple traumas can be easily triggered, which may precipitate brief dissociative episodes. They may display sadness, irritability, or anxiety and have difficulties focusing or learning in school. It's not uncommon that they become untrusting of others and less confident in themselves, which may result in social withdrawal. Teens are more likely than younger children to show impulsive or aggressive behaviors. They may act out in ways that are risky or carry the potential for self-harm (e.g., cutting or other self-mutilating behaviors, unsafe sex or otherwise risky sexual behavior, alcohol or substance abuse) or in socially unacceptable or destructive ways (e.g., lying, stealing, or vandalizing property).

Nearly everyone experiences some short-term distress following exposure to a traumatic event. Cognitive and emotional resources, ethnicity and cultural factors, previous trauma exposure, and preexisting child or family problems all contribute to how this distress will manifest. It's important to recognize that these short-term responses are not necessarily problematic. Some behavioral changes may be adaptive attempts to cope with the difficult experience. Many symptoms will resolve by themselves within a few days or weeks. Long-lasting posttraumatic distress, however, increases the risk of subsequently experiencing a host of other problems, including major depression or chronic anxieties (Hodges et al., 2013), alcohol or substance abuse (Dube et al., 2006), and academic problems (Holt, Finkelhor, & Kantor, 2007).

Teaching Tips

Whereas some children are less affected by experiencing a traumatic event, others can experience posttraumatic symptoms that significantly interfere with their well-being and development. Particularly in light of the high incidence of trauma, abuse, and neglect in children, it's important to be aware of some potential pitfalls.

- Don't assume that all kids respond to trauma in the same way. As professionals are fond of saying, when you've met one child with a trauma history, you've met one child with a trauma history.
- Don't be too quick to pathologize early distress or behavioral reactions.
- Don't assume that all trauma-exposed children will experience long-term consequences or need treatment. In time, the majority will recover.
- Don't create conditions in which trauma-exposed children have few choices or feel that they have no control.
- Don't force children to share their stories (but remember to listen respectfully if they choose to do so).
- Don't require any child to close his or her eyes during group mindfulness practices. For many children, but particularly for those who have been traumatized, closing eyes with others present can feel unsafe and frightening.
- Remain aware of your legal and ethical obligations as a mandated reporter.

Cautions and Contraindications

With anxiety or depression, the signs are generally clear. With trauma, however, the signs often go unrecognized. Trauma symptoms can look like other problems, such as boredom, frustration, conduct problems, or having difficulty concentrating, following directions, or getting along with other children. These behaviors are often attributed to anxiety, behavioral problems, and attention disorders, rather than being recognized as symptoms of trauma, abuse, or neglect. Physiological hyperarousal and hypersensitivity to bodily sensations are common reactions to trauma, as are difficulties with regulating strong emotions. Increased levels of alertness, jumpiness, scanning the environment for danger, difficulty sleeping, and rapid breathing are indicators of hyperarousal. Children who have a high level of sensitivity to physical stimuli (e.g., sounds, sights, touch, or smell) may feel overwhelmed or exhausted, and show exaggerated physical reactions such as being easily startled or easily provoked to tears.

Emotional and behavioral reactivity are often seen following physical or sexual abuse, but also emerges in response to other stressful events such as bullying, family discord, physical injury, or other medical emergencies. The hyperarousal along with associated memories are sometimes managed by blocking out both body awareness and emotions—essentially the child chooses to live in his or her head, rather than in his or her body. With severely traumatized children, focusing attention on body sensations may trigger emotional upsets, flashbacks, or dissociative episodes. Maintaining a sense of safety and self-control are important. Mindfulness can provide a stable platform that allows children to reconnect with their body sensations at their own pace—in ways that feel safe. Movement activities such as walking, stretching, or yoga postures may be more tolerable than internally focused activities such as the body scan. Whether you're teaching in a classroom or conducting a therapy group, always remain attuned to expressions of distress, particularly when conducting any of the body practices. There are also some indications that individual therapy may be more effective for severely traumatized children (Tucker & Oei, 2007).

Mental health professionals may be needed to provide therapy and support for severely abused or traumatized children. Most teachers do not have this specialized training. Since teachers spend many hours each week with their students, however, they have an important role in which they get to know the students in other ways that include identifying and referring these children for assessment.

Activities for a Pathway through Trauma, Abuse, and Neglect

Introductory Activities

We recommend starting any mindfulness program by introducing the concept of mindfulness both verbally and with at least one or two introductory activities. If you are working for a longer duration with a group (e.g., as a classroom teacher with the same children for an entire year), it's perfectly okay to work your way through all of the activities in this book. *A Cup of Mindfulness* is an externally focused introductory activity that nearly all children enjoy. *Mindful Silliness* is a good icebreaker activity that involves externally focused movements, so is unlikely to trigger traumatic memories. ***Listening to Silence*** is a very short calming activity that can be repeated throughout a school day or across group sessions. Although ***Taking a Mindful SEAT*** is a calming and grounding activity for most children, it might be a little more challenging for severely traumatized children. The settling effects of ***Taking a Mindful Posture*** can be enhanced by the child's placing the palm of one hand flat on the ground. The initial goals are to introduce children to the concept of mindfulness and guide them in exploring the experience of cultivating mindfulness.

Core Activities

Core practices teach basic skills that can easily be incorporated into everyday life. Breathing practice is the heart of mindfulness. We encourage you to include all five of the breathing activities described in Part II and to practice at least one of them with the kids in every session. If a child is feeling emotionally overwhelmed, ***Belly Breathing*** and ***Mindful Breath Counting*** can be excellent grounding and centering practices. The latter is also useful for shifting attention away from thoughts that may be escalating the child's distress. ***Mindful Silliness*** and ***Matching Movement Moments*** can be fun introductions to body practices. We recommend teaching ***Mindful Walking*** and ***Mindfulness of My Feet*** early in the program, as these can be useful grounding skills to quickly lessen emotional distress. The ***Mindful Mountain Visualization*** may be helpful in down-regulating intense emotions. ***Mindful Flower Stretch*** and ***Mindful Movements*** (yoga postures) can be helpful in reducing physical tension. Extended stillness-based body practices such as the ***Body Scan*** may be more challenging or even triggering for some kids, and so should be introduced later as a more advanced practice, although a very brief nonmoving body practice like the ***Three Minutes in My Body*** may be helpful in grounding an emotionally overwhelmed child whose trauma is not highly body-focused.

Intermediate Development Activities

After the group is comfortable with the basic breath and body activities, we work to develop specific skills that can be used in daily life. ***The Mindful STOP*** and ***Mindfulness of Urges: Urge Surfing*** can be taught, then practiced in real time as skills for managing impulsive, emotionally driven behaviors. ***Mindful Touching*** and ***Mindful Humming*** are useful grounding practices when emotions feel like they are spiraling out of control. ***Mindfulness of Thoughts*** and ***Mindfulness of Judgments*** help kids develop insights into how frequently their own emotions and behaviors are driven by thoughts and judgments—and learn from experience that these are "just thoughts," not facts. The kids learn that what they think may not be true, and that these thoughts are rarely a good guide on which to base skillful choices.

Advanced Deepening Activities

Emotion-focused practices that may be useful to help traumatized kids manage uncomfortable emotions include Parts I and II for ***Mindfulness of Worry and Anxiety, Mindfulness of Sadness and Loss,*** and ***Mindfulness of Frustration and Anger. Mindful Compassion*** may be the most important, as these kids are often far too hard on themselves. However, it's important to be aware that initially, mindful self-compassion practices might elicit "back-draft" in which long repressed emotions come rushing to the surface (Germer & Neff, 2014). When troubled children or teens give themselves permission to stop judging themselves and be just as they are, there can sometimes be a release of years of pent-up anger, longing, sadness, grief, and despair. *Mindfulness of Pleasant Events* can help to refocus attention from traumatic memories to the pleasant events that are present in this moment.

Maintenance, Generalization, and Concluding Activities

During the last few sessions, we encourage making time for a group discussion that includes sharing what has been learned, what might have changed, and how mindfulness skills can be used to manage traumatic stress. One important component in this discussion is to explore ways that can help sustain a regular mindfulness practice. James Pennebaker has studied the psychological effects of writing about trauma and found that, although initially emotional distress may increase, the act of writing appears to speed up the healing process (Pennebaker, 1997, 2000). With this research in mind, the activity *What Does Mindfulness Mean to Me Now? (Part III): Journaling* can be expanded to include writing about ways in which mindfulness could be helpful in managing emotional distress. Cultivating self-compassion and empathy for others can be an important component of healing following trauma, so *Appreciation of the Group* is a recommended activity. We suggest always concluding your group with the *Here-and-Now Stones* activity.

Summary of Activities within the Pathways

Activity	Group	Stress and Anxiety	Depression	Attention Problems	Emotion Regulation and Impulse Control	Trauma, Abuse and Neglect
1. Introduction to Mindfulness	Introduction	•	•	•	•	•
2. What Does Mindfulness Mean to Me? (Part I) [Drawing]	Introduction	•	•	•	•	
3. A Cup of Mindfulness	Introduction	•	•	•		•
4. Listening to Silence	Introduction	•	•	•		•
5. Taking a Mindful Posture	Introduction	•	•		•	•
6. Taking a Mindful SEAT	Introduction	•	•	•	•	•
7. Mindfulness of the Breath [with Handout]	Breath	•	•	•	•	•
8. Taking Three Mindful Breaths	Breath	•	•	•	•	
9. Mindful Smiling While Waking Up [with Handout]	Breath	•	•			
10. Belly Breathing	Breath				•	•
11. Mindful Breath Counting	Breath		•	•	•	•
12. Mindful Silliness	Body		•		•	•
13. Mindful Flower Stretch	Body		•			•
14. Three Minutes in My Body	Body			•		
15. Mindful Walking	Body		•		•	•
16. Mindful Movements [Yoga Postures]	Body		•	•		
17. Matching Movement Moments [Paired Activity]	Body		•	•	•	
18. Mindfulness While Lying Down	Body	•			•	
19. Mindful Mountain Visualization	Body			•	•	
20. Mindfulness of My Feet	Body	•		•	•	•
21. Body Scan	Body	•	•	•	•	
22. The Mindful HALT	Body	•			•	
23. Mindful Body Relaxation [Progressive Muscle Relaxation]	Body	•		•	•	
24. Mindfulness in Everyday Life	Awareness			•	•	
25. Finding Five New Things [with Handout]	Awareness	•	•	•	•	
26. Mindfulness of Pleasant Events [with Handout]	Awareness		•			•
27. Mindfulness of Unpleasant Events	Awareness		•			
28. Mindfulness of Discomfort	Awareness	•	•	•		
29. Mindfulness of Urges: Urge Surfing	Awareness			•	•	•

(continued)

Activity	Group	Stress and Anxiety	Depression	Attention Problems	Emotion Regulation and Impulse Control	Trauma, Abuse and Neglect
30. The Mindful STOP	Awareness				•	•
31. Mindful Listening and Speaking	Awareness			•	•	
32. Mindful Eating (Part I)	Sensory	•	•		•	
33. Mindful Eating (Part II)	Sensory	•	•	•	•	
34. Mindful Seeing (Part I)	Sensory	•	•	•		
35. Mindful Seeing (Part II)	Sensory	•			•	
36. Mindful Touching	Sensory			•	•	•
37. Mindful Humming	Sensory	•				•
38. Mindful Hearing	Sensory				•	
39. Mindfulness of Smells (Part I)	Sensory	•	•		•	
40. Mindfulness of Smells (Part II)	Sensory	•	•		•	
41. Mindfulness of Thoughts	Thoughts			•		•
42. Mindfulness of Judgments	Thoughts	•	•	•	•	•
43. Mindfulness of Happiness (Part I)	Emotions		•	•	•	
44. Mindfulness of Happiness (Part II)	Emotions		•	•		
45. Mindfulness of Worry and Anxiety (Part I) [with Handout]	Emotions	•	•		•	•
46. Mindfulness of Worry and Anxiety (Part II)	Emotions	•	•		•	•
47. Mindfulness of Sadness and Loss (Part I)	Emotions		•		•	•
48. Mindfulness of Sadness and Loss (Part II)	Emotions		•		•	•
49. Mindfulness of Frustration and Anger (Part I) [with Handout]	Emotions			•	•	•
50. Mindfulness of Frustration and Anger (Part II)	Emotions			•	•	•
51. Mindfulness of Embarrassment	Emotions	•	•	•	•	
52. Mindfulness of Envy	Emotions				•	
53. Mindfulness of Gratitude	Emotions	•	•	•		
54. Mindful Compassion	Emotions	•	•	•		•
55. What Does Mindfulness Mean to Me Now? (Part II) [Drawing]	Closing	•	•	•		
56. What Does Mindfulness Mean to Me Now? (Part III) [Journaling]	Closing	•	•	•	•	•
57. Appreciation of the Group	Closing	•	•	•	•	•
58. Here-and-Now Stones	Closing	•	•	•	•	•

PART IV

Research Support
for Mindfulness with Kids

O ver the past decade, research on mindfulness-based interventions with children and teens, like the research on mindfulness in general, has grown exponentially. Still, our understanding of what works, who it works for, and how it works remains far from complete. Although there have been over 12,000 professional journal articles published on this topic since 2000, less than 20% of these describe research studies and only a small percentage of those studies evaluated the effectiveness of mindfulness interventions with children and adolescents. Funding for mindfulness studies with youth lags far behind the funding support that has been provided for adult studies (see Figure IV.1). Furthermore, many of the studies reported have serious methodological problems that limit what we can really infer about their findings. These limitations include small sample sizes, the absence of a control group or lack of randomization to groups, nonstandardized facilitator training, few consistent and manualized protocols, inadequate measures of fidelity or adherence to the treatment protocol, measures of mindfulness that lack reliability or validity, inappropriate data analyses, no long-term follow-up, and conclusions that go well beyond the scope of the research design or data collected (Davidson & Kaszniak, 2015; Semple & Burke, 2019). Other challenges include the logistical and ethical difficulties of conducting research with minors, who rarely have consistent schedules and for whom obtaining informed consent/assent is extremely complicated. Nonetheless, our knowledge of how mindfulness programs might be effective for youth at different ages, across different settings, and in addressing differing problems is expanding.

Mindfulness, Executive Function, and Attention

Few doubt that student mental and physical health and academic performance are related, and most of us agree that rising expectations of K–12 students are placing heavy demands on their attention and other executive functions. Executive function (EF) is a neuropsychological concept that refers to high-level cognitive processes. EFs make it possible to mentally play with ideas; to take the time to think before acting; to plan and initiate activities; to begin tasks

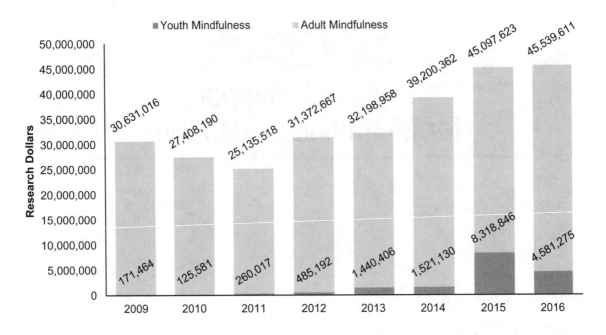

FIGURE IV.1. National Institutes of Health funding for youth mindfulness research and adult mindfulness research from 2009 through 2016.

and follow through with them; to meet new or unanticipated challenges; to manage impulses as they relate to speaking or behavior; to resist temptations; and to stay focused on the task at hand. EFs also include working memory and cognitive flexibility, which means thinking creatively or "outside the box," seeing things from different perspectives, and flexibly adapting to changed circumstances. These are all functions that are essential when functioning on autopilot or relying on intuition or instinct is ill-advised (Diamond, 2013). Children aren't born with EF skills, however; they are born with the potential to learn and develop them. The development of EF begins at birth and continues through adolescence and into early adulthood.

Attention is both an essential component of EF and essential to the development of EF. The skills of focusing attention, sustaining attention, and redirecting attention are necessary for learning to occur—including the learning of EFs. With impairments of attention, learning occurs more slowly or not at all (Mirsky, 1996; Rueda et al., 2004). The United States has a high prevalence of childhood mood and anxiety disorders (as high as 20% by some estimates), and these common disorders are known to impair attention (Roeser, Skinner, Beers, & Jennings, 2012). Environmental stressors also impair attention. For example, the heavy emphasis on standardized testing in schools has further increased levels of student and teacher stress, which also impairs attention. Our kids and teens are under record levels of stress, whether it's related to academic pressures or to stress associated with poverty, bigotry, and other ACEs. Attention is the doorway to our lives. Where and how we direct our attention governs our daily experiences, our relationships, and the quality of our lives. As the poet William Blake wrote, giving attention to the experiences that make up our lives is "to see a world in a grain of sand and heaven in a wild flower." We frequently hear parents and teachers telling children to "pay attention." Unfortunately, however, children are rarely taught *how* to pay attention. At its most basic, mindfulness training is the training of attention. Before a child can make conscious, skillful choices, he or she must first be aware that choices are available. This awareness requires present-focused attention to both internal and external events.

Several studies have shown that mindfulness can reduce problems associated with ADHD. One team of researchers evaluated an adapted MBCT intervention for adolescents ages 13–18 years with ADHD and their parents (Haydicky, Shecter, Wiener, & Ducharme, 2015). Eighteen adolescents and 17 parents attended parallel group sessions for 8 weeks. The participants reported on adolescent ADHD symptoms, internalizing and externalizing problems, functional impairment, family functioning, parenting stress, and mindfulness. Following the intervention, parents reported significant reductions in their adolescents' inattention, conduct problems, and peer relations problems. Parents also reported experiencing reductions in parenting stress and increases in mindful parenting. Interestingly, although the teen participants did not endorse any improvements immediately following the intervention, they did report reductions in internalizing problems 6 weeks after the program ended.

The effectiveness of an adapted 8-week mindfulness-based stress reduction (MBSR) program for teens ages 11–15 years with ADHD was evaluated in conjunction with mindful parenting training for their parents (van de Weijer-Bergsma, Formsma, Bruin, & Bögels, 2012). This study used computerized tests of attention and self-report questionnaires to measure changes immediately after, 8 weeks after, and 16 weeks after the program. After the mindfulness training, the teens' attention and behavior problems decreased, and their EF improved. Improvements in their performance on the computerized attention tests were found after the training. Interestingly, the effects of mindfulness training became stronger at the 8-week follow-up, but then waned at 16-week follow-up, which suggests that mindfulness practices need to be implemented consistently to maintain long-term effectiveness.

Another study examined the effectiveness of a shorter mindfulness intervention for reducing impulsivity in teens who were in treatment for ADHD (Rynczak, 2012). Twelve kids ages 12–15 were assigned either to the mindfulness group or to "treatment as usual." Following the intervention, significant increases in attentiveness and decreases in impulsivity were found for the mindfulness group participants.

Studies of mindfulness training for children and teens have also shown reductions in general attentional problems (Lee, Semple, Rosa, & Miller, 2008; Semple et al., 2010); improvements in attention and decision making (Droutman, 2015); improvements in alertness, attention, concentration, and focus (Singh & Singh, 2014); and improved classroom behaviors, which included paying attention, self-control, participation in activities, and caring/respect for others (Black & Fernando, 2014).

Mindfulness and Metacognitive Awareness

A central component of effectiveness in cognitive therapies is believed to be the development of *metacognitive knowledge,* which refers to an acquired knowledge of one's own cognitive processes and an understanding of how to regulate those processes (Wells, 2008). With metacognitive knowledge, thoughts can be explored, challenged, and altered (Teasdale, 1999). Alternatively, mindfulness-based therapies are believed to promote *metacognitive awareness* (or decentering), which describes the ability to experience thoughts as transient events in the mind (Teasdale, 1999; Teasdale et al., 2002). Mindfulness training does not teach skills to examine or challenge the accuracy of thoughts, but rather aims to change how an individual relates to his or her own thoughts (Segal et al., 2002, 2013).

Essentially, cognitive therapy focuses on the contents of the thoughts, with a goal of changing unhelpful patterns of thinking. In contrast, mindfulness training focuses on the process of thinking, with the goal of enhancing the awareness of thoughts as events in the mind, without self-judgment and criticism. With mindful awareness, thoughts, emotions, and body sensations are perceived as transient phenomena to observe rather than to judge, and as internal events to be identified rather than changed. Greater awareness of the patterns of connections between thoughts, emotional states, and body sensations tends to interrupt these habituated patterns, and that interruption increases an individual's ability to respond to internal and external events with conscious awareness, rather than with habituated emotional reactivity.

Because decentering is believed to be a central mechanism of change in mindfulness training programs, it is important to ascertain if children are capable of metacognitive awareness at all, and if so, at what age this ability develops. Satlof-Bedrick and Johnson (2015) explored children's awareness of the flow of their breathing; their awareness of the natural flow of consciousness and thoughts in the mind; and the ability of children to self-monitor the thoughts, emotions, and body sensations that is cultivated with mindfulness practices. This study evaluated 68 children ages 4, 6, or 8 years old and found significant age-related differences and a developmental progression of abilities. By the age of 6, children demonstrated understanding of awareness of breathing only by artificially altering their breath. At age 8, children were able to consistently monitor their own natural breathing. Age 6 appeared to be the pivotal age in terms of the ability to monitor natural breathing. No significant differences in awareness of thoughts were found across the three age groups. No children were adept at demonstrating awareness of their own thoughts; however, the ones who first learned a breath awareness task subsequently performed better on the thought awareness task than those who didn't. This finding is consistent with traditional mindfulness practices, which suggest that cultivating awareness of the breath promotes awareness of other internal processes, such as awareness of thoughts and emotions (Grossman, 2010). It also suggests that cultivation of metacognitive awareness may begin in children as young as 8 years old.

Training in breath awareness with young children may be improved using sensory-based grounding techniques (Semple, Reid, & Miller, 2005). However, Satlof-Bedrick and Johnson (2015) noted that attention to externally oriented tasks might disrupt internal awareness of thoughts, whereas attention to internally oriented tasks (e.g., attention to the breath) might facilitate development of metacognitive awareness.

Mindfulness and Social–Emotional Development

One major concern within the current learning environment is that the social–emotional development of children is often neglected. Another is recognizing that the process of learning, understanding, and reasoning about ideas discussed in a classroom is not always quantifiable. An old platitude about research is that scientists often measure what is easy to measure rather than what is important to measure. Perhaps educators do this too. As we look toward educating the whole child, McNeil (1986) noted that "measurable outcomes may be the least significant results of learning" (p. 18). Research data strongly support positive relationships between attention, EFs, emotional self-regulation, and academic outcomes (Buckner, Mezzacappa, & Beardslee, 2009; Greenberg et al., 2003; Tang, Yang, Leve, & Harold, 2012). In particular, a child's ability to self-regulate his or her own responses to stress is a powerful predictor of future life outcomes (Moffitt et al., 2011). Moffitt and her colleagues followed a cohort of 1,000 children from birth to age 32 and found that childhood self-control predicted later physical health, substance dependence, personal finances, and criminal offending outcomes. Schoolwide mindfulness programs aimed at improving attention, EF, and social–emotional resiliency seem to be decreasing social–emotional and behavioral problems (Semple & Burke, 2011).

Mindfulness in Schools

A recent meta-analysis of 24 school-based studies with nearly 4,000 students concluded that mindfulness interventions in school settings showed small to medium effect sizes, but that their effectiveness differed according to the age of the students receiving the intervention, the type of intervention delivered, and the individual who facilitated the intervention (Carsley, Khoury, & Heath, 2017). Older teens appeared to benefit somewhat more than younger children did. Adolescent development is a time in which the brain is malleable, so mindfulness training may be particularly effective during these years. Interventions that included a combination of varied mindfulness activities with yoga-based mindfulness activities seemed to be more effective than basic mindfulness practices alone. This may be because a program that includes a variety of activities is more engaging than single-activity programs. In an unexpected twist, Carsley and her colleagues found greater effects when trained classroom teachers delivered the program than when the program was delivered by an outside facilitator. Although teachers may have less familiarity or experience with a given mindfulness program, they know their students better than an outside facilitator and therefore may be better suited to adapt the program to be more responsive to the specific needs of their students. Keep this in mind as you consider partnering with facilitators within or outside of the school setting.

One study found that, compared to a control program on social responsibility, children randomized to a mindfulness program showed greater improvements in cognitive control and stress physiology; reported greater empathy, perspective taking, emotional control, and optimism; had greater reductions in depressive symptoms; and were rated by peers as being more prosocial (Mendelson et al., 2010). Other studies have reported significant reductions in depression and anxiety (Esmailian, Tahmasian, Dehghani, & Mootabi, 2013; Liehr & Diaz, 2010; Raes, Griffith, Van der Gucht, & Williams, 2014).

The evidence for the effectiveness of mindfulness in improving academic performance has been mixed (Bakosh, Tobias Mortlock, Querstret, & Morison, 2018; Semple, Droutman, & Reid, 2017). A recent review (Maynard, Solis, Miller, & Brendel, 2017) found indications that mindfulness-based interventions do improve cognitive and social–emotional outcomes for children, but found little support for consistent improvement in academic achievement.

In addition, although many studies have reported an assortment of beneficial effects, none has yet followed children longitudinally to determine the sustainability of these benefits over time. Nevertheless, *potential* long-term benefits of teaching children mindfulness include:

- Development of resiliency and stress management skills (van de Weijer-Bergsma, Langenberg, Brandsma, Oort, & Bögels, 2014). We know that chronic stress impairs EF and predicts worse life outcomes (Reising et al., 2018).
- Improvements in attention and concentration. A child's ability to concentrate was the strongest predictor of success at age 32 (Moffitt et al., 2011).
- More adaptive social–emotional development, which includes cognitive flexibility and delay of gratification, which positively influenced later educational achievements, employment, crime rates, alcohol or substance abuse, and mental health outcomes (Meiklejohn et al., 2012; Moffitt et al., 2011; Semple & Burke, 2019; Semple et al., 2017).

Mindfulness for Teachers

A review of studies of mindfulness interventions for teachers found broad support that mindfulness can reduce teacher stress and burnout as well as depression and anxiety symptoms (Hwang, Bartlett, Greben, & Hand, 2017). The potential of mindfulness-based interventions to enhance teachers' psychological health and well-being seems evident. Other studies have reported benefits for teachers who complete mindfulness training that include:

- Lower levels of stress and burnout (Flook, Goldberg, Pinger, Bonus, & Davidson, 2013; Gold et al., 2010; Jennings, 2015; Roeser et al., 2013).
- Performance enhancements and greater job efficiency (Jennings, Frank, Snowberg, Coccia, & Greenberg, 2013).
- More emotionally supportive and better-organized classrooms. Mindfulness and efficacy were positively associated with perspective taking and sensitivity to discipline, particularly with students who were perceived as being challenging to manage (Jennings, 2015).

Caveats

Although most studies have reported promising results, a few have found little or no effects. In one study, for example, one group of sixth-grade students was randomized to an Asian studies class and practiced daily mindful breathing, while a control group of students was randomized to an African studies class to make a sarcophagus. Although positive mental health outcomes were found for both groups, the only advantage found for the mindfulness group was that those students were less likely to develop suicidal ideation or thoughts of self-harm than students in the control class (Britton et al., 2014). The ".b" program (pronounced dot-be) is an eight-lesson school-based mindfulness curriculum for 11- to 18-year-olds. Although .b is a well-researched program, one randomized controlled study of young adolescents found no beneficial effects on anxiety, depression, weight or shape concerns, or overall well-being (Johnson, Burke, Brinkman, & Wade, 2016). These authors suggested that more time might have been needed to engage these students. Other suggestions included using a different room to change the classroom dynamics, conducting smaller groups, and holding twice-weekly sessions to facilitate greater interaction and reinforcement of ideas. We suggest keeping all of these in mind for potential tweaks as you consider challenges you may be facing with regard to progress in your group.

Conclusion

What can we conclude from the wide variety of studies that have been conducted? First, and perhaps most importantly, we know that more rigorous research is required. Needed are larger sample sizes, active control groups, and more objective and meaningful clinical outcomes (e.g., symptom reduction and improvements in functioning) or school-related outcomes (e.g., attendance, behavioral referrals, suspensions, academic performance). We need more longitudinal follow-ups to ascertain the sustainability of effects over time. We also have little understanding at this point of how much mindfulness is "enough" to be an effective dose. We don't really know the quality, quantity, or duration of facilitator training that is needed to be effective; what the active components are of different interventions; or how interventions need to be adapted to best help children at varying stages of intellectual or emotional development. We don't know much about how children from differing cultural backgrounds, or those with histories of trauma or other special needs, will respond to standardized programs—or what might need to be changed in the training programs to better respond to children with special needs such as autism spectrum disorder (Semple, 2019). A recent review of 10 school-based mindfulness programs in the United States discussed the wide variability across programs and encouraged researchers, educators, and mindfulness practitioners to work collaboratively to conduct rigorous program evaluations (Semple et al., 2017).

We now have a great deal of research that supports the effectiveness of mindfulness-based interventions for adults in reducing stress and improving psychological well-being (Goyal et al., 2014; Sedlmeier et al., 2012); as a treatment for psychiatric disorders (Chiesa & Serretti, 2011; Hilton et al., 2016; Hofmann, Sawyer, Witt, & Oh, 2010); and in health care (Carlson et al., 2009; Gotink et al., 2015; Ruffault et al., 2017). We have less research to support the effectiveness of mindfulness interventions for kids and teens, and the research we do have is less robust. The interest in mindfulness programs with children and adolescents is very strong—much stronger than the current research support. Better research for these programs will increase their legitimacy and guide our efforts to create effective interventions—for which problems, with whom, at what age, and in which setting. Despite the lack of standardization in approach, specific techniques, facilitator training, or mode of intervention, the empirical support that we have now appears very promising.

References

Ahmed, S. P., Bittencourt-Hewitt, A., & Sebastian, C. L. (2015). Neurocognitive bases of emotion regulation development in adolescence. *Developmental Cognitive Neuroscience, 15*, 11–25.

Allen, J. P., Chango, J., Szwedo, D., & Schad, M. (2014). Long-term sequelae of sub-clinical depressive symptoms in early adolescence. *Development and Psychopathology, 26*, 171–180.

American Psychiatric Association. (2013). *Diagnostic and statistical manual of mental disorders* (5th ed.). Arlington, VA: Author.

Baer, R. A., Walsh, E., Lykins, E. L. B., & Didonna, F. (2009). Assessment of mindfulness. In F. Didonna (Ed.), *Clinical handbook of mindfulness* (pp. 153–168). New York: Springer Science+Business Media.

Bakosh, L. S., Snow, R. M., Tobias, J. M., Houlihan, J. L., & Barbosa-Leiker, C. (2016). Maximizing mindful learning: Mindful awareness intervention improves elementary school students' quarterly grades. *Mindfulness, 7*(1), 59–67.

Bakosh, L. S., Tobias Mortlock, J. M., Querstret, D., & Morison, L. (2018). Audio-guided mindfulness training in schools and its effect on academic attainment: Contributing to theory and practice. *Learning and Instruction, 58*, 34–41.

Baxter, A. J., Scott, K. M., Vos, T., & Whiteford, H. A. (2012). Global prevalence of anxiety disorders: A systematic review and meta-regression. *Psychological Medicine, 43*, 897–910.

Beauchemin, J., Hutchins, T. L., & Patterson, F. (2008). Mindfulness meditation may lessen anxiety, promote social skills, and improve academic performance among adolescents with learning disabilities. *Complementary Health Practice Review, 13*, 34–45.

Beck, A., T., Rush, A. J., Shaw, B. F., & Emery, G. (1979). *Cognitive therapy of depression.* New York: Guilford Press.

Bennett, K., & Dorjee, D. (2016). The impact of a mindfulness-based stress reduction course (MBSR) on well-being and academic attainment of sixth-form students. *Mindfulness, 7*(1), 105–114.

Black, D. S., & Fernando, R. (2014). Mindfulness training and classroom behavior among lower-income and ethnic minority elementary school children. *Journal of Child and Family Studies, 23*, 1242–1246.

Blake, M., Waloszek, J. M., Schwartz, O., Raniti, M., Simmons, J. G., Blake, L., . . . Allen, N. B. (2016). The SENSE study: Post intervention effects of a randomized controlled trial of a cognitive-behavioral and mindfulness-based group sleep improvement intervention among at-risk adolescents. *Journal of Consulting and Clinical Psychology, 84*(12), 1039–1051.

Bluth, K. (2017). *The self-compassion workbook for teens: Mindfulness and compassion skills to overcome self-criticism and embrace who you are.* Oakland, CA: New Harbinger.

Bögels, S. M., Hoogstad, B., van Dun, L., de Schutter, S., & Restifo, K. (2008). Mindfulness training for adolescents with externalizing disorders and their parents. *Behavioural and Cognitive Psychotherapy, 36*, 193–209.

Briere, J., & Semple, R. J. (2013). *Brief treatment for acutely burned patients (BTBP).* Unpublished treatment manual, University of Southern California, Los Angeles, CA.

Briñol, P., Petty, R. E., & Wagner, B. (2009). Body posture effects on self-evaluation: A self-validation approach. *European Journal of Social Psychology, 39*, 1053–1064.

Britton, W. B., Lepp, N. E., Niles, H. F., Rocha, T., Fisher, N. E., & Gold, J. S. (2014). A randomized controlled pilot trial of classroom-based mindfulness meditation compared to an active control condition in sixth-grade children. *Journal of School Psychology, 52*(3), 263–278.

Brach, T. (2004). *Radical acceptance: Embracing your life with the heart of a Buddha.* New York: Bantam Books.

Brook, J. S., Stimmel, M. A., Zhang, C., & Brook, D. W. (2008). The association between earlier marijuana use and subsequent academic achievement and health problems: A longitudinal study. *American Journal on Addictions, 17*(2), 155–160.

Buckner, J. C., Mezzacappa, E., & Beardslee, W. R. (2009). Self-regulation and its relations to adaptive functioning in low income youths. *American Journal of Orthopsychiatry, 79*(1), 19–30.

Buka, S. L., Monuteaux, M., & Earls, F. (2002). The epidemiology of child and adolescent mental disorders. In M. T. Tsuang & M. Tohen (Eds.), *Textbook in psychiatric epidemiology* (2nd ed., pp. 629–655). New York: Wiley-Liss.

Carlson, L. E., Labelle, L. E., Garland, S. N., Hutchins, M. L., Birnie, K., & Didonna, F. (2009). Mindfulness-based interventions in oncology. In F. Didonna (Ed.), *Clinical handbook of mindfulness* (pp. 383–404). New York: Springer Science+Business Media.

Carney, D. R., Cuddy, A. J., & Yap, A. J. (2010). Power posing: Brief nonverbal displays affect neuroendocrine levels and risk tolerance. *Psychological Science, 21*(10), 1363–1368.

Carsley, D., Khoury, B., & Heath, N. L. (2018). Effectiveness of mindfulness interventions for mental health in schools: A comprehensive meta-analysis. *Mindfulness, 9*(3), 693–707.

Cash, S. J., & Bridge, J. A. (2009). Epidemiology of youth suicide and suicidal behavior. *Current Opinion in Pediatrics, 21*, 613–619.

Centers for Disease Control and Prevention. (2015). National suicide statistics. Retrieved from *www.cdc.gov/violenceprevention/suicide/statistics/index.html.*

Chentsova-Dutton, Y. E., Ryder, A. G., & Tsai, J. (2014). Understanding depression across cultural contexts. In I. H. Gotlib & C. L. Hammen (Eds.), *Handbook of depression* (3rd ed., pp. 337–354). New York: Guilford Press.

Chiesa, A., & Serretti, A. (2011). Mindfulness based cognitive therapy for psychiatric disorders: A systematic review and meta-analysis. *Psychiatry Research, 187,* 441–453.

Copeland, W. E., Keeler, G., Angold, A., & Costello, E. J. (2007). Traumatic events and posttraumatic stress in childhood. *Archives of General Psychiatry, 64,* 577–584.

Costello, E. J., Mustillo, S., Angold, A., Erkanli, A., & Keeler, G. (2003). Prevalence and development of psychiatric disorders in childhood and adolescence. *Archives of General Psychiatry, 60,* 837–844.

Crijnen, A. A. M., Achenbach, T. M., & Verhulst, F. C. (1999). Problems reported by parents of children in multiple cultures: The Child Behavior Checklist syndrome constructs. *American Journal of Psychiatry, 156*(4), 569–574.

Cservenka, A., & Brumback, T. (2017, June). The burden of binge and heavy drinking on the brain: Effects on adolescent and young adult neural structure and function. *Frontiers in Psychology, 8,* 1111.

Danielson, M. L., Bitsko, R. H., Ghandour, R. M., Holbrook, J. R., Kogan, M. D., & Blumberg, S. J. (2018). Prevalence of parent-reported ADHD diagnosis and associated treatment among U.S. children and adolescents, 2016. *Journal of Clinical Child and Adolescent Psychology, 47,* 199–212.

Davidson, R. J., & Kasczniak, A. W. (2015). Conceptual and methodological issues in research on mindfulness and meditation. *American Psychologist, 70,* 581–592.

Diamond, A. (2013). Executive functions. *Annual Review of Psychology, 64,* 135–168.

Dickie, E., Brunet, A., Akerib, V., & Armony, J. (2013). Anterior cingulate cortical thickness is a stable predictor of recovery from post-traumatic stress disorder. *Psychological Medicine, 43,* 645–653.

Dimidjian, S., Hollon, S. D., Dobson, K. S., Schmaling, K. B., Kohlenberg, R. J., Addis, M. E., . . . Gollan, J. K. (2006). Randomized trial of behavioral activation, cognitive therapy, and antidepressant medication in the acute treatment of adults with major depression. *Journal of Consulting and Clinical Psychology, 74,* 658–670.

Dougherty, D. M., Marsh, D. M., Moeller, F. G., Chokshi, R. V., & Rosen, V. C. (2000). Effects of moderate and high doses of alcohol on attention, impulsivity, discriminability, and response bias in immediate and delayed memory task performance. *Alcoholism: Clinical and Experimental Research, 24,* 1702–1711.

Droutman, V. (2015). *Effect of mindfulness training on attention, emotion-regulation and risk-taking in adolescence.* Doctoral dissertation, University of Southern California, Los Angeles, CA. Available from ProQuest Dissertation Publishing (Document No. 10014568).

Dube, S. R., Miller, J. W., Brown, D. W., Giles, W. H., Felitti, V. J., Dong, M., & Anda, R. F. (2006). Adverse childhood experiences and the association with ever using alcohol and initiating alcohol use during adolescence. *Journal of Adolescent Health, 38,* e1–e10.

Ehrenreich, J. T., & Gross, A. M. (2002). Biased attentional behavior in childhood anxiety: A review of theory and current empirical investigation. *Clinical Psychology Review, 22,* 991–1008.

Elder, T. E. (2010). The importance of relative standards in ADHD diagnoses: Evidence based on exact birth dates. *Journal of Health Economics, 29,* 641–656.

Emmons, R. A. (2009). Gratitude. In H. T. Reis & S. Sprecher (Eds.), *Encyclopedia of human relationships* (pp. 774–777). Thousand Oaks, CA: SAGE.

Esmailian, N., Tahmasian, K., Dehghani, M., & Mootabi, F. (2013). Effectiveness of mindfulness-based cognitive therapy on depression symptoms in children with divorced parents. *Journal of Clinical Psychology, 3,* 47–57.

Fedewa, A., & Ahn, S. (2011). The effects of physical activity and physical fitness on children's achievement and cognitive outcomes: A meta-analysis. *Research Quarterly for Exercise and Sport, 82,* 521–535.

Felitti, V. J., Anda, R. F., Nordenberg, D., Williamson, D., Spitz, A., Edwards, V., . . . Marks, J. S. (1998). Relationship of childhood abuse and household dysfunction to many of the leading causes of death in adults. *American Journal of Preventive Medicine, 14,* 245–258.

Finkelhor, D., Turner, H. A., Shattuck, A. M., & Hamby, S. L. (2013). Violence, crime, and abuse exposure in a national sample of children and youth: An update. *JAMA Pediatrics, 167,* 614–621.

Flook, L., Goldberg, S. B., Pinger, L., Bonus, K., & Davidson, R. J. (2013). Mindfulness for teachers: A pilot study to assess effects on stress, burnout, and teaching efficacy. *Mind, Brain, and Education, 7*(3), 182–195.

Fox, G. R., Kaplan, J., Damasio, H., & Damasio, A. (2015). Neural correlates of gratitude. *Frontiers in Psychology, 6,* 1491.

Franco, C., Amutio, A., López-González, L., Oriol, X., & Martínez-Taboada, C. (2016). Effect of a mindfulness training program on the impulsivity and aggression levels of adolescents with behavioral problems in the classroom. *Frontiers in Psychology, 7,* 1385.

Germer, C. K., & Neff, K. D. (2013). Self-compassion in clinical practice. *Journal of Clinical Psychology, 69,* 856–867.

Germer, C. K., & Neff, K. D. (2014). Cultivating self-compassion in trauma survivors. In V. M. Follette, J. Briere, D. Rozelle, J. W. Hopper, & D. I. Rome (Eds.), *Mindfulness-oriented interventions for trauma: Integrating contemplative practices* (pp. 43–58). New York: Guilford Press.

Godsey, J. (2013). The role of mindfulness based interventions in the treatment of obesity and eating disorders: An integrative review. *Complementary Therapies in Medicine, 21*(4), 430.

Gold, E., Smith, A., Hopper, I., Herne, D., Tansey, G., & Hulland, C. (2010). Mindfulness-based stress reduction (MBSR) for primary school teachers. *Journal of Child and Family Studies, 19,* 184–189.

Goodman, M. S., Madni, L. A., & Semple, R. J. (2017). Measuring mindfulness in youth: Review of current assessments, challenges, and future directions. *Mindfulness, 8,* 1409–1420.

Goodman, M. S., Madni, L. A., & Semple, R. J. (2019). Measuring mindfulness. In V. G. Carrión & J. Rettger (Eds.), *Applied mindfulness: Approaches in mental health for children and adolescents* (pp. 55–72). Arlington, VA: American Psychiatric Association.

Gotink, R. A., Chu, P., Jan, J. V. B., Benson, H., Fricchione, G. L., & Hunink, M. G. M. (2015). Standardised mindfulness-based interventions in healthcare: An overview of systematic reviews and meta-analyses of RCTs. *PLOS ONE, 10*(4), e0124344.

Goyal, M., Singh, S., Sibinga, E. M. S., Gould, N. F., Rowland-Seymour, A., Sharma, R., . . . Haythornthwaite, J. A. (2014). Meditation programs for psychological stress and well-being: A systematic review and meta-analysis. *Journal of the American Medical Association, 174,* 357–368.

Grasso, D., Greene, C., & Ford, J. D. (2013). Cumulative trauma in childhood. In J. D. Ford & C. A. Courtois (Eds.), *Treating complex traumatic stress disorders in children and adolescents: Scientific foundations and therapeutic models* (pp. 79–99). New York: Guilford Press.

Greenberg, M. T., Weissberg, R. P., O'Brien, M. U., Zins, J. E., Fredericks, L., Resnik, H., & Elias, M. J. (2003). Enhancing school-based prevention and youth development through coordinated social, emotional, and academic learning. *American Psychologist, 58,* 466–474.

Gregg, J. A., Callaghan, G. M., Hayes, S. C., & Glenn-Lawson, J. L. (2007). Improving diabetes self-management through acceptance, mindfulness, and values: A randomized controlled trial. *Journal of Consulting and Clinical Psychology, 75*(2), 336–343.

Grossman, P. (2008). On measuring mindfulness in psychosomatic and psychological research. *Journal of Psychosomatic Research, 64,* 405–408.

Grossman, P. (2010). Mindfulness for psychologists: Paying kind attention to the perceptible. *Mindfulness, 1*(2), 87.

Hanh, T. N. (1991a). *The miracle of mindfulness: An introduction to the practice of meditation* Boston: Beacon Press.

Hanh, T. N. (1991b). *Peace is in every step: The path of mindfulness in everyday life.* New York: Bantam Books.

Hanh, T. N. (2009). *The blooming of a lotus: Guided meditation for achieving the miracle of mindfulness.* Boston: Beacon Press.

Haydicky, J., Shecter, C., Wiener, J., & Ducharme, J. M. (2015). Evaluation of MBCT for adolescents with ADHD and their parents: Impact on individual and family functioning. *Journal of Child and Family Studies, 24*(1), 76–94.

Haydicky, J., Wiener, J., Badali, P., Milligan, K., & Ducharme, J. M. (2012). Evaluation of a mindfulness-based intervention for adolescents with learning disabilities and co-occurring ADHD and anxiety. *Mindfulness, 3,* 151–164.

Hilton, L., Maher, A. R., Colaiaco, B., Apaydin, E., Sorbero, M. E., Booth, M., . . . Hempel, S. (2016). Meditation for posttraumatic stress: Systematic review and meta-analysis. *Psychological Trauma: Theory, Research, Practice, and Policy, 9*(4), 453–460.

Hodges, M., Godbout, N., Briere, J., Lanktree, C. B., Gilbert, A., & Kletzka, N. T. (2013). Cumulative trauma and symptom complexity in children: A path analysis. *Child Abuse and Neglect, 37,* 891–898.

Hofmann, S. G., Sawyer, A. T., Witt, A. A., & Oh, D. (2010). The effect of mindfulness-based therapy on anxiety and depression: A meta-analytic review. *Journal of Consulting and Clinical Psychology, 78,* 169–183.

Holt, M. K., Finkelhor, D., & Kantor, G. K. (2007). Multiple victimization experiences of urban elementary school students: Associations with psychosocial functioning and academic performance. *Child Abuse and Neglect, 31,* 503–515.

Huguet, A., Ruiz, D., Haro, J., & Alda, J. (2017). A pilot study of the efficacy of a mindfulness program for children newly diagnosed with attention-deficit hyperactivity disorder: Impact on core symptoms and executive functions. *International Journal of Psychology and Psychological Therapy, 17,* 305–316.

Hutcherson, C. A., Seppala, E. M., & Gross, J. J. (2008). Loving-kindness meditation increases social connectedness. *Emotion, 8,* 720–724.

Hwang, Y.-S., Bartlett, B., Greben, M., & Hand, K. (2017). A systematic review of mindfulness interventions for in-service teachers: A tool to enhance teacher wellbeing and performance. *Teaching and Teacher Education, 64,* 26–42.

James, W. (1890). *The principles of psychology.* New York: Dover. (Reprinted 1950)

Jastrowski Mano, K. E., Salamon, K. S., Hainsworth, K. R., Anderson Khan, K. J., Ladwig, R. J., Davies, W. H., & Weisman, S. J. (2013). A randomized, controlled pilot study of mindfulness-based stress reduction for pediatric chronic pain. *Alternative Therapies in Health and Medicine, 19*(6), 8.

Jayakody, K., Gunadasa, S., & Hosker, C. (2014). Exercise for anxiety disorders: Systematic review. *British Journal of Sports Medicine, 48,* 187–196.

Jennings, P. A. (2015). Early childhood teachers' well-being, mindfulness, and self-compassion in relation to classroom quality and attitudes towards challenging students. *Mindfulness, 6,* 732–743.

Jennings, P. A., Frank, J. L., Snowberg, K. E., Coccia, M. A., & Greenberg, M. T. (2013). Improving classroom learning environments by Cultivating Awareness and Resilience in Education (CARE): Results of a randomized controlled trial. *School Psychology Quarterly, 28*(4), 374–390.

Johnson, C., Burke, C., Brinkman, S., & Wade, T. (2016). Effectiveness of a school-based mindfulness program for transdiagnostic prevention in young adolescents. *Behaviour Research and Therapy, 81,* 1–11.

Kabat-Zinn, J. (1994). *Wherever you go there you are: Mindfulness meditation for everyday life.* New York: Hyperion.

Kabat-Zinn, J. (Producer). (2014). Guided mindfulness meditation series 2: Mindful mountain [CD]. Retrieved from *www.soundstrue.com/store/guided-mindfulness-meditation-series-2-3407.html?___SID=U.*

Kessler, R. C., Adler, L. A., Berglund, P., Green, J. G., McLaughlin, K. A., Fayyad, J., . . . Zaslavsky, A. M. (2014). The effects of temporally secondary co-morbid mental disorders on the associations of DSM-IV ADHD with adverse outcomes in the U.S. National Comorbidity Survey Replication Adolescent Supplement (NCS-A). *Psychological Medicine, 44,* 1779–1792.

Kessler, R. C., Coccaro, E. F., Fava, M., Jaeger, S., Jin, R., & Walters, E. (2006). The prevalence and correlates of DSM-IV intermittent explosive disorder in the National Comorbidity Survey Replication. *Archives of General Psychiatry, 63,* 669–678.

Leahy, R. L. (2001). *Overcoming resistance in cognitive therapy.* New York: Guilford Press.

Lee, J., Semple, R. J., Rosa, D., & Miller, L. (2008). Mindfulness-based cognitive therapy for children: Results of a pilot study. *Journal of Cognitive Psychotherapy, 22,* 15–28.

Lee, S. S., Humphreys, K. L., Flory, K., Liu, R., & Glass, K. (2011). Prospective association of childhood attention-deficit/hyperactivity disorder (ADHD) and substance use and abuse/dependence: A meta-analytic review. *Clinical Psychology Review, 31,* 328–341.

Liehr, P., & Diaz, N. (2010). A pilot study examining the effect of mindfulness on depression and anxiety for minority children. *Archives of Psychiatric Nursing, 24,* 69–71.

Lutz, J., Herwig, U., Opialla, S., Hittmeyer, A., Jancke, L., Rufer, M., . . . Bruhl, A. B. (2014). Mindfulness and emotion regulation—an fMRI study. *Social Cognitive and Affective Neuroscience, 9*(6), 776–785.

Mahdi, S., Viljoen, M., Massuti, R., Selb, M.,

Almodayfer, O., Karande, S., . . . Bölte, S. (2017). An international qualitative study of ability and disability in ADHD using the WHO-ICF framework. *European Child and Adolescent Psychiatry, 26*, 1219–1231.

Mak, C., Whittingham, K., Cunnington, R., & Boyd, R. (2018). Efficacy of mindfulness-based interventions for attention and executive function in children and adolescents—a systematic review. *Mindfulness, 9*(8), 59–78.

Marlatt, G. A., & Gordon, J. R. (1985). *Relapse prevention: Maintenance strategies in the treatment of addictive behaviors.* New York: Guilford Press.

Matthys, W., & Lochman, J. E. (2017). *Oppositional defiant disorder and conduct disorder in childhood* (2nd ed.). West Sussex, UK: Wiley-Blackwell.

Maynard, B. R., Solis, M., Miller, V., & Brendel, K. E. (2017, March). Mindfulness-based interventions for improving cognition, academic achievement, behavior and socioemotional functioning of primary and secondary students. Retrieved from *https://campbellcollaboration.org/media/k2/attachments/Campbell_systematic_review_-_Mindfulness_and_school_students.pdf*.

McNeil, L. (1986). *Contradictions of control: School knowledge and school structure.* New York: Routledge & Kegan Paul.

Meiklejohn, J., Soloway, G., Isberg, R., Sibinga, E., Grossman, L., Saltzman, A., . . . Pinger, L. (2012). Integrating mindfulness training into K–12 education: Fostering the resilience of teachers and students. *Mindfulness, 3*, 291–307.

Mendelson, T., Greenberg, M. T., Dariotis, J. K., Gould, L. F., Rhoades, B. L., & Leaf, P. J. (2010). Feasibility and preliminary outcomes of a school-based mindfulness intervention for urban youth. *Journal of Abnormal Child Psychology, 38*, 985–994.

Merikangas, K. R., He, J. P., Burstein, M., Swanson, S. A., Avenevoli, S., Cui, L., . . . Swendsen, J. (2010). Lifetime prevalence of mental disorders in U.S. adolescents: Results from the National Comorbidity Survey Replication—Adolescent Supplement (NCS-A). *Journal of the American Academy of Child and Adolescent Psychiatry, 49*, 980–989.

Miller, A. L. (1999). Dialectical behavior therapy: A new treatment approach for suicidal adolescents. *American Journal of Psychotherapy, 53*, 413–417.

Mirsky, A. F. (1996). Disorders of attention: A neuropsychological perspective. In G. R. Lyon & N. A. Krasnegor (Eds.), *Attention, memory, and executive function* (pp. 71–95). Baltimore: Brookes.

Moffitt, T. E., Arseneault, L., Belsky, D., Dickson, N., Hancox, R. J., Harrington, H., . . . Heckman, J. J. (2011). A gradient of childhood self-control predicts health, wealth, and public safety. *Proceedings of the National Academy of Sciences of the USA, 108*(7), 2693–2698.

Muller, J., & Roberts, J. E. (2005). Memory and attention in obsessive–compulsive disorder: A review. *Journal of Anxiety Disorders, 19*(1), 1–28.

Neff, K. D. (2009). The role of self-compassion in development: A healthier way to relate to oneself. *Human Development, 52*, 211–214.

Neff, K. D. (2011). *Self-compassion: The proven power of being kind to yourself.* New York: Morrow.

Neff, K. D., & Germer, C. K. (2013). A pilot study and randomized controlled trial of the mindful self-compassion program. *Journal of Clinical Psychology, 69*, 28–44.

Nickerson, A., Aderka, I. M., Bryant, R. A., & Hofmann, S. G. (2012). The relationship between childhood exposure to trauma and intermittent explosive disorder. *Psychiatry Research, 197*(1–2), 128–134.

Oldenburg, D. (1984, December 31). The humble hum and its good vibrations. *The Washington Post,* p. D5.

Patel, R. S., Patel, P., Shah, K., Kaur, M., Mansuri, Z., & Makani, R. (2018). Is cannabis use associated with the worst inpatient outcomes in attention deficit hyperactivity disorder adolescents? *Cureus, 10*(1), e2033.

Pennebaker, J. W. (1997). *Opening up: The healing power of expressing emotions.* New York: Guilford Press.

Pennebaker, J. W. (2000). Telling stories: The health benefits of narrative. *Literature and Medicine, 19*, 3–18.

Peper, E., Lin, I. M., Harvey, R., & Perez, J. (2017). How posture affects memory recall and mood. *Biofeedback, 45*(2), 36–41.

Peters, J. R., Eisenlohr-Moul, T. A., & Smart, L. M. (2016). Dispositional mindfulness and rejection sensitivity: The critical role of nonjudgment. *Personality and Individual Differences, 93*, 125–129.

Petersen, S. E., & Posner, M. I. (2012). The attention system of the human brain: 20 years after. *Annual Review of Neuroscience, 35*, 73–89.

Petter, M., Chambers, C. T., & Chorney, J. M. (2013). The effects of mindful attention on cold pressor pain in children. *Pain Research and Management, 18*(1), 39–45.

Posner, M. I., & Petersen, S. E. (1990). The attention system of the human brain. *Annual Review of Neuroscience, 13*, 25–42.

Raes, F., Griffith, J. W., Van der Gucht, K., & Williams, J. M. G. (2014). School-based prevention and reduction of depression in adolescents: A cluster-randomized controlled trial of a mindfulness group program. *Mindfulness, 5*, 477–486.

Reising, M. M., Bettis, A. H., Dunbar, J. P., Watson, K. H., Gruhn, M., Hoskinson, K. R., & Compas, B. E. (2018). Stress, coping, executive function, and brain activation in adolescent offspring of depressed and nondepressed mothers. *Child Neuropsychology, 24*(5), 638–656.

Roeser, R. W., Schonert-Reichl, K. A., Jha, A., Cullen, M., Wallace, L., Wilensky, R., . . . Harrison, J. (2013). Mindfulness training and reductions in teacher stress and burnout: Results from two randomized, waitlist-control field trials. *Journal of Educational Psychology, 105*(3), 787–804.

Roeser, R. W., Skinner, E., Beers, J., & Jennings, P. A. (2012). Mindfulness training and teachers' professional development: An emerging area of research and practice. *Child Development Perspectives, 6,* 167–173.

Rogers, C. (1961). *On becoming a person: A therapist's view of psychotherapy.* New York: Houghton Mifflin Harcourt.

Rueda, M. R., Fan, J., McCandliss, B. D., Halparin, J. D., Gruber, D. B., Lercari, L. P., & Posner, M. I. (2004). Development of attentional networks in childhood. *Neuropsychologia, 42*(8), 1029–1040.

Ruffault, A., Bernier, M., Juge, N., & Fournier, J. F. (2016). Mindfulness may moderate the relationship between intrinsic motivation and physical activity: A cross-sectional study. *Mindfulness, 7,* 445–452.

Ruffault, A., Czernichow, S., Hagger, M. S., Ferrand, M., Erichot, N., Carette, C., . . . Flahault, C. (2017). The effects of mindfulness training on weight-loss and health-related behaviours in adults with overweight and obesity: A systematic review and meta-analysis. *Obesity Research and Clinical Practice, 11*(5, Suppl. 1), 90–111.

Rynczak, D. (2012). *Effectiveness of mindfulness in reducing impulsivity in youth with attention-deficit/hyperactivity disorder.* Doctoral dissertation, Chicago School of Professional Psychology, Chicago, IL. Available from ProQuest, UMI Dissertations Publishing (UMI No. 3515271).

Saltzman, A. (2014). *A still quiet place: A mindfulness program for teaching children and adolescents to ease stress and difficult emotions.* Oakland, CA: New Harbinger.

Satlof-Bedrick, E., & Johnson, C. N. (2015). Children's metacognition and mindful awareness of breathing and thinking. *Cognitive Development, 36,* 83–92.

Schonert-Reichl, K. A., & Lawlor, M. S. (2010). The effects of a mindfulness-based education program on pre- and early adolescents' well-being and social and emotional competence. *Mindfulness, 1,* 137–151.

Sedlmeier, P., Eberth, J., Schwarz, M., Zimmermann, D., Haarig, F., Jaeger, S., & Kunze, S. (2012). The psychological effects of meditation: A meta-analysis. *Psychological Bulletin, 138,* 1139–1171.

Segal, Z. V., Williams, J. M. G., & Teasdale, J. D. (2002). *Mindfulness-based cognitive therapy for depression: A new approach to preventing relapse.* New York: Guilford Press.

Segal, Z. V., Williams, J. M. G., & Teasdale, J. D. (2013). *Mindfulness-based cognitive therapy for depression* (2nd ed.). New York: Guilford Press.

Semple, R. J. (2019). Yoga and mindfulness for youth with autism spectrum disorder: Review of the current evidence. *Child and Adolescent Mental Health, 24*(1), 12–18.

Semple, R. J., & Burke, C. A. (2011). Treating children and adolescents with mindfulness. In P. C. Kendall (Ed.), *Child and adolescent therapy: Cognitive-behavioral procedures* (4th ed., pp. 411–426). New York: Guilford Press.

Semple, R. J., & Burke, C. (2019). State of the research: Physical and mental health benefits of mindfulness-based interventions for children and adolescents. *OBM Integrative and Complementary Medicine, 4*(1), 1–31.

Semple, R. J., Droutman, V., & Reid, B. A. (2017). Mindfulness goes to school: Things learned (so far) from research and real-world experiences. *Psychology in the Schools, 54,* 29–52.

Semple, R. J., & Lee, J. (2011). *Mindfulness-based cognitive therapy for anxious children: A manual for treating childhood anxiety.* Oakland, CA: New Harbinger.

Semple, R. J., Lee, J., Rosa, D., & Miller, L. F. (2010). A randomized trial of mindfulness-based cognitive therapy for children: Promoting mindful attention to enhance social–emotional resiliency in children. *Journal of Child and Family Studies, 19,* 218–229.

Semple, R. J., & Madni, L. A. (2014). Treating childhood trauma with mindfulness. In V. M. Follette, J. Briere, D. Rozelle, J. W. Hopper, & D. I. Rome (Eds.), *Mindfulness-oriented interventions for trauma: Integrating contemplative practices* (pp. 284–300). New York: Guilford Press.

Semple, R. J., Reid, E. F., & Miller, L. (2005). Treating anxiety with mindfulness: An open trial of mindfulness training for anxious children. *Journal of Cognitive Psychotherapy, 19,* 379–392.

Siegel, D. J. (2007). *The mindful brain: Reflection and attunement in the cultivation of well-being.* New York: Norton.

Siegel, D. J., & Bryson, T. P. (2012). *The whole-brain child: 12 revolutionary strategies to nurture your child's developing mind.* New York: Bantam Books.

Singh, S., & Singh, S. (2014). Effect of mindfulness therapy on attention deficit among adolescents with symptoms of attention deficit disorder. *Indian Journal of Health and Wellbeing, 5*(10), 1165–1172.

Stahl, B., & Goldstein, E. (2010). *A mindfulness-based stress reduction workbook*. Oakland, CA: New Harbinger.

Ströhle, A. (2009). Physical activity, exercise, depression, and anxiety disorders. *Journal of Neural Transmission, 116,* 777–784.

Tang, Y.-Y., Tang, R., & Posner, M. I. (2016). Mindfulness meditation improves emotion regulation and reduces drug abuse. *Drug and Alcohol Dependence, 163*(S1), S13–S18.

Tang, Y. Y., Yang, L., Leve, L. D., & Harold, G. T. (2012). Improving executive function and its neurobiological mechanisms through a mindfulness-based intervention: Advances within the field of developmental neuroscience. *Child Development Perspectives, 6,* 361–366.

Tarrasch, R. (2018, April). The effects of mindfulness practice on attentional functions among primary school children. *Journal of Child and Family Studies, 27*(8), 2632–2642.

Tarrasch, R., Berman, Z., & Friedmann, N. (2016). Mindful reading: Mindfulness meditation helps keep readers with dyslexia and ADHD on the lexical track. *Frontiers in Psychology, 7,* 578.

Teasdale, J. D. (1999). Metacognition, mindfulness and the modification of mood disorders. *Clinical Psychology and Psychotherapy, 6,* 146–155.

Teasdale, J. D., Moore, R. G., Hayhurst, H., Pope, M., Williams, S., & Segal, Z. V. (2002). Metacognitive awareness and prevention of relapse in depression: Empirical evidence. *Journal of Consulting and Clinical Psychology, 70,* 275–287.

Teper, R., Segal, Z. V., & Inzlicht, M. (2013). Inside the mindful mind: How mindfulness enhances emotion regulation through improvements in executive control. *Current Directions in Psychological Science, 22,* 449–454.

Thoreau, H. D. (1863). Life without principle. *The Atlantic Monthly, 12,* 484–495.

Tomoda, A., Navalta, C. P., Polcari, A., Sadato, N., & Teicher, M. H. (2009). Childhood sexual abuse is associated with reduced gray matter volume in visual cortex of young women. *Biological Psychiatry, 66,* 642–648.

Tomoda, A., Polcari, A., Anderson, C. M., & Teicher, M. H. (2012). Reduced visual cortex gray matter volume and thickness in young adults who witnessed domestic violence during childhood. *PLOS ONE, 7*(12), e52528.

Tsafou, K. E., De Ridder, D. T., van Ee, R., & Lacroix, J. P. (2016). Mindfulness and satisfaction in physical activity: A cross-sectional study in the Dutch population. *Journal of Health Psychology, 21,* 1817–1827.

Tucker, M., & Oei, T. P. S. (2007). Is group more cost effective than individual cognitive behaviour therapy?: The evidence is not solid yet. *Behavioural and Cognitive Psychotherapy, 35,* 77–91.

Tuithof, M., ten Have, M., van den Brink, W., Vollebergh, W., & de Graaf, R. (2012). The role of conduct disorder in the association between ADHD and alcohol use (disorder): Results from the Netherlands Mental Health Survey and Incidence Study–2. *Drug and Alcohol Dependence, 123,* 115–121.

U.S. Department of Health and Human Services. (2017). *Child maltreatment 2015*. Washington, DC: U.S. Department of Health and Human Services, Administration for Children and Families, Administration on Children, Youth and Families, Children's Bureau. Retrieved from *www.acf.hhs.gov/programs/cb/research-data-technology/statistics-research/child-maltreatment*.

van de Weijer-Bergsma, E., Formsma, A. R., Bruin, E. I., & Bögels, S. M. (2012). The effectiveness of mindfulness training on behavioral problems and attentional functioning in adolescents with ADHD. *Journal of Child and Family Studies, 21,* 775–787.

van de Weijer-Bergsma, E., Langenberg, G., Brandsma, R., Oort, F. J., & Bögels, S. M. (2014). The effectiveness of a school-based mindfulness training as a program to prevent stress in elementary school children. *Mindfulness, 5,* 238–248.

Viglas, M., & Perlman, M. (2018). Effects of a mindfulness-based program on young children's self-regulation, prosocial behavior and hyperactivity. *Journal of Child and Family Studies, 27*(4), 1150–1161.

Wells, A. (2008). Metacognitive therapy: Cognition applied to regulating cognition [Special issue]. *Behavioural and Cognitive Psychotherapy, 36,* 651–658.

Willard, C., & Saltzman, A. (Eds.). (2015). *Teaching mindfulness skills to kids and teens*. New York: Guilford Press.

Williams, J. M. G., Teasdale, J. D., Segal, Z. V., & Kabat-Zinn, J. (2007). *The mindful way through depression: Freeing yourself from chronic unhappiness*. New York: Guilford Press.

Yin, X., Zhao, L., Xu, J., Evans, A. C., Fan, L., Ge, H., . . . Liu, S. (2012). Anatomical substrates of the alerting, orienting and executive control components of attention: Focus on the posterior parietal lobe. *PLOS ONE, 7*(11), e50590.

Index

Note. *f* or *t* following a page number indicates a figure or a table.

Absent-minded experiences, 22–23. *See also* Autopilot
Abuse
 attentional problems and, 215
 emotion regulation and impulse control and, 222
 overview, 232
 pathway through, 231–238
 stress disorders and, 232–233
 symptoms and, 232–238, 234*t*
Academic performance, 245–246
Acceptance
 cultivating your own practice in mindfulness and, 13
 of emotions, 123
 Mindful Hearing (activity 38), 104
 Pathway through Depression, 206
 postactivity discussions and, 9–10
 radical acceptance, 118–119
 SEAT (Sensations, Emotions, Actions, and Thoughts) acronym and, 18
Actions, 27. *See also* SEAT (Sensations, Emotions, Actions, and Thoughts) acronym
Activities. *See* Concluding Activities; Introductory and Core Activities; Mindful Awareness Activities; Mindfulness of Emotions; Mindfulness of the Body Activities; Mindfulness of the Breath Activities; Mindfulness of Thoughts; Sensory-Based Mindfulness Activities; *individual activities*
Acute stress disorder (ASD), 233
Adjustment disorder (AD), 233
Administrator buy-in, 12–13
Advanced Deepening Activities. *See also* Mindful Awareness Activities; Mindfulness of Emotions; Mindfulness of Thoughts; Sensory-Based Mindfulness Activities
 attentional problems and, 220
 depression and, 209
 emotion regulation and impulse control and, 230
 stress and anxiety and, 200
 trauma, abuse, and neglect and, 237–238
Adverse childhood experiences (ACEs), 232. *See also* Abuse; Neglect; Trauma

Aggressive disorders, 221–226, 223*t*–225*t*
Alcohol use. *See* Substance use
Anger. *See also* Frustration and Anger, Mindfulness of (Part I) (activity 49); Frustration and Anger, Mindfulness of (Part II) (activity 50); HALT (Are you Hungry, Angry/Anxious, Lonely, or Tired?) acronym
 breathing exercises and, 37
 emotion regulation and impulse control and, 221–222
 envy and, 167
 vocabulary for, 149–150
Antisocial personality disorder (ASPD), 222
Anxiety. *See also* Worry
 activities for, 199–200
 attentional problems and, 214
 breathing exercises and, 37
 closing eyes during a practice and, 26
 A Cup of Mindfulness (activity 3), 24
 at different ages, 197–198
 drawing-based activities and, 93
 HALT (Are you Hungry, Angry/Anxious, Lonely, or Tired?) acronym and, 60–61
 Mindful Body Relaxation (activity 23), 62–64
 Mindful Listening and Speaking (activity 31), 79
 Mindful Silliness (activity 12), 43
 Mindfulness of the Body Activities and, 42
 Mindfulness of Worry and Anxiety (Part I) (activity 45), 130–135, 177
 Mindfulness of Worry and Anxiety (Part II) (activity 46), 135–139, 178–179
 movement activities and, 50–51
 overview, 131
 pathway through, 195–200
 symptoms of, 195–197, 196*t*
 thoughts and rumination and, 56
 vocabulary for, 131, 136
Anxiety disorders, 197
Appreciation of the Group (activity 57), 189–190
 attentional problems and, 220
 emotion regulation and impulse control and, 230
 stress and anxiety and, 200
 trauma, abuse, and neglect and, 238

Art-based activities
 Appreciation of the Group (activity 57), 189–190
 Mindful Seeing (Part I) (activity 34), 91–94, 94*f*
 Mindful Seeing (Part II) (activity 35), 97–98
 What Does Mindfulness Mean to Me Now? (Part II): Drawing (activity 55), 185–187
 What Does Mindfulness Mean to Me? (Part I) (activity 2), 20–22
Attachment disorders, 222, 233
Attentional functioning
 A Cup of Mindfulness (activity 3), 22–24
 Finding Five New Things (activity 25), 66–68
 Mindfulness of the Body Activities and, 42
 overview, 3, 17, 211–218, 213*t*, 216*t*–217*t*
 pathway through, 211–220
 research support for mindfulness and, 241–243, 246
 symptoms of, 212–218, 213*t*, 216*t*–217*t*
 trauma, abuse, and neglect and, 237
Attention-deficit/hyperactivity disorder (ADHD)
 emotion regulation and impulse control and, 222
 overview, 212–213, 213*t*
 research support for mindfulness and, 242–243
 substance use and, 215
Authenticity, 13
Autopilot
 anger and frustration and, 154
 anxiety and worry and, 137
 attending skills and, 67
 cultivating mindfulness with practice and, 22–23
 eating mindfully and, 84–85, 88–90
 Mindfulness of Thoughts (activity 41), 116
 overview, 19, 30
 reactions and, 123
 seeing mindfully and, 91–98, 94*f*
 temporary nature of emotions and, 127–128
 walking activity and, 48

256

Avoidance, 127–128, 195, 197–198, 234*t*
Awareness. *See also* Discomfort,
    Mindfulness of (activity 28); Everyday
    Life, Mindfulness in (activity 24);
    Finding Five New Things (activity
    25); Listening and Speaking, Mindful
    (activity 31); The Mindful STOP
    (activity 30); Mindfulness of the
    Body Activities; Pleasant Events,
    Mindfulness of (activity 26); Present
    moment awareness; Unpleasant
    Events, Mindfulness of (activity 27);
    Urges, Mindfulness of: Urge Surfing
    (activity 29)
  anger and frustration and, 154–155
  body awareness, 42
  eating mindfully and, 88
  emotional awareness, 123
  Here-and-Now Stones (activity 58),
    190–191
  overview, 2, 17
  Pathway through Depression, 206, 208
  SEAT (Sensations, Emotions, Actions,
    and Thoughts) acronym and, 18

Behavioral activation, 206
Behavioral problems. *See also* Social–
    behavioral symptoms
  emotion regulation and impulse control
    and, 225*t*, 226–227
  emotions and, 123
  HALT (Are you Hungry, Angry/Anxious,
    Lonely, or Tired?) acronym and, 60–61
  movement activities and, 51
  stress and anxiety and, 195, 197–198
Belly Breathing (activity 10), 35–36, 37. *See
    also* Breath-based activities
  emotion regulation and impulse control
    and, 229
  stress and anxiety and, 199
  trauma, abuse, and neglect and, 237
Bipolar disorders (BPs), 201. *See also*
    Depression
Bodily needs, 60–61
Body awareness, 42. *See also* Awareness;
    Mindfulness of the Body Activities
Body Relaxation, Mindful (activity 23),
    62–64
  attentional problems and, 220
  depression and, 209–210
  emotion regulation and impulse control
    and, 229
  stress and anxiety and, 200
Body Scan (activity 21), 57–59
  attentional problems and, 220
  depression and, 209, 209–210
  emotion regulation and impulse control
    and, 229–230
  stress and anxiety and, 200
  trauma, abuse, and neglect and, 237
Body sensations. *See also* Body-oriented
    practices; Sensations
  attentional problems and, 219
  Body Scan (activity 21), 57–59
  depression and, 207–208
  embarrassment and, 162
  emotions and, 123
  Mindfulness of Sadness and Loss (Part I)
    (activity 47), 139–143
  Mindfulness of Worry and Anxiety (Part
    I) (activity 45), 130–135
  Mindfulness of Worry and Anxiety (Part
    II) (activity 46), 135–139
  overview, 35–36

  trauma, abuse, and neglect and, 236
  What Does Mindfulness Mean to Me
    Now? (Part III): Journaling (activity
    56), 187–189
Body-oriented practices. *See also* Body
    Relaxation, Mindful (activity 23); Body
    Scan (activity 21); Body sensations;
    Flower Stretch, Mindful (activity 13);
    Lying Down, Mindfulness While
    (activity 18); Matching Movement
    Moments (activity 17); Mindfulness
    of My Feet (activity 20); Mindfulness
    of the Body Activities; Mountain
    Visualization, Mindful (activity 19);
    Movement activities; Movements,
    Mindful (activity 16); Silliness,
    Mindful (activity 12); The Mindful
    HALT (activity 22); Three Minutes
    in My Body (activity 14); Walking,
    Mindful (activity 15)
  depression and, 208
  stress and anxiety and, 199–200
  trauma, abuse, and neglect and, 236, 237
Borderline personality disorder, 222
Brain science, 11, 171
Breath, Mindfulness of (activity 7), 29–32, 40
Breath Counting, Mindful (activity 11), 37–39
  attentional problems and, 219
  emotion regulation and impulse control
    and, 229
  stress and anxiety and, 199
  trauma, abuse, and neglect and, 237
Breath-based activities. *See also* Belly
    Breathing (activity 10); Breath
    Counting, Mindful (activity 11);
    Mindfulness of the Breath Activities;
    Smiling While Waking Up, Mindful
    (activity 9); Stillness activities; Taking
    Three Mindful Breaths (activity 8)
  anger and frustration and, 157
  attentional problems and, 219
  belly breathing, 35–36
  closing eyes during a practice and, 228
  emotion regulation and impulse control
    and, 229
  metacognitive awareness and, 244
  Mindfulness While Lying Down (activity
    18), 53–54
  overview, 3
  Pathway through Depression, 208
  Pathway through Stress and Anxiety, 199
  sadness and, 141, 142
  stress and anxiety and, 198
  trauma, abuse, and neglect and, 237
Butterfly pose, 50
Buy-in
  from administrators and organizations,
    12–13
  introductory practices and, 17
  from kids and teens, 10–12

CALM (Chest, Arms, Legs, Mind)
    Reminder, 63–64
Cannabis use. *See* Substance use
Cat and cow pose, 50
Chattering mind, 56–57. *See also*
    Rumination; Thoughts
Checking in with needs, 60–61
Childhood trauma. *See* Trauma
Choice
  anger and frustration and, 154–155, 156–157
  closing eyes during a practice and, 26, 30
  embarrassment and, 164
  envy and, 168

  frustration and, 152
  listening activities and, 25
  Mindfulness of Worry and Anxiety (Part
    I) (activity 45), 130–135
  overview, 18
  postactivity discussions and, 9–10
  sadness and, 146–148
  What Does Mindfulness Mean to Me
    Now? (Part III): Journaling (activity
    56), 187–189
Classroom environment, 140
Closing eyes during a practice
  anxiety and worry and, 26
  choice and, 26, 30
  trauma, abuse, and neglect and, 235
Cobra pose, 50
Cognitive approach, 198, 244
Cognitive symptoms. *See also* Symptoms
  depression and, 202, 203*t*, 207–208
  emotion regulation and impulse control
    and, 223*t*
  stress and anxiety and, 196*t*, 197
Cognitive triad, 205–206
Comparisons, 165–170
Compassion. *See also* Compassion, Mindful
    (activity 54); Kindness
  cultivating your own practice in
    mindfulness and, 13
  embarrassment and, 159–160, 164
  everyday awareness and, 66
  listening mindfully and, 80
  Mindfulness of Embarrassment (activity
    51), 159–165
  Mindfulness of Envy (activity 52), 165–170
  sadness and, 139, 142–143
  trauma, abuse, and neglect and, 237–238
  vocabulary for, 173–174
Compassion, Mindful (activity 54), 173–175
  attentional problems and, 220
  depression and, 209
  stress and anxiety and, 200
  trauma, abuse, and neglect and, 237–238
Concluding Activities. *See* Maintenance,
    Generalization, and Concluding Activities
Conduct disorder (CD), 215, 221, 222
Confidence, 43–44
Confidentiality, 8–9
Connection, 77–80
Conversations, 77–80
Critical mind, 17, 21
Criticizing others, 21
A Cup of Mindfulness (activity 3), 22–24.
    See also Introductory and Core
    Activities
  attentional problems and, 219
  stress and anxiety and, 199
  trauma, abuse, and neglect and, 236
Curiosity, 9–10, 18

Decision making, 60–61
Deepening activities. *See* Advanced
    Deepening Activities
Depression. *See also* Sadness
  activities for, 42, 69, 79, 207–210
  envy and, 167
  overview, 201
  pathway through, 201–210
  suicide risk management and, 207
  symptoms of, 201–202, 203*t*–205*t*
Describing activities
  Finding Five New Things (activity 25),
    66–68
  Mindful Eating (Part I) (activity 32),
    84–88

Describing activities *(cont.)*
  Mindful Eating (Part II) (activity 33),
    88–90
  Mindful Seeing (Part II) (activity 35),
    94–98
  Mindful Touching (activity 36), 98–102
  Mindfulness of Smells (Part I) (activity
    39), 106–111
  What Does Mindfulness Mean to Me
    Now? (Part III): Journaling (activity
    56), 187–189
Development activities. *See* Intermediate
  Development Activities
Developmental factors
  attentional problems and, 215, 217
  depression and, 202
  emotion regulation and impulse control
    and, 226
  introducing mindfulness to children and
    teens and, 18–19
  pathways to mindfulness and, 193
  research support for mindfulness and,
    244–245
  social–emotional development and, 244–245
  stress and anxiety and, 197–198
  trauma, abuse, and neglect and, 233, 235
Dialectical behavioral therapy for
  adolescents (DBT-A), 227
Diaphragmatic breathing, 37. *See also* Belly
  Breathing (activity 10)
Discomfort, 72–73, 127–128, 159–165, 200
Discomfort, Mindfulness of (activity 28),
  72–73
  attentional problems and, 219
  stress and anxiety and, 200
Discussions, 47–48
Disinhibited social engagement disorder
  (DSEs), 233
Disordered eating. *See* Eating, disordered
Disruptive disorders, 221–226, 223t–225t
Dissociation, 50–51, 215, 234t, 236
Distorted thoughts, 198. *See also* Thoughts
Downward facing dog pose, 49
Drawing-based activities
  Appreciation of the Group (activity 57),
    189–190
  Mindful Seeing (Part I) (activity 34),
    91–94, 94f
  Mindful Seeing (Part II) (activity 35),
    97–98
  Pathway through Stress and Anxiety, 199
  What Does Mindfulness Mean to Me
    Now? (Part II): Drawing (activity 55),
    185–187
  What Does Mindfulness Mean to Me?
    (Part I) (activity 2), 20–22
Drug use. *See* Substance use

Eating, disordered
  depression and, 202
  Mindful Eating (Part I) (activity 32), 87
  Mindfulness of Urges: Urge Surfing
    (activity 29), 75
  Pathway through Depression, 207
  stress and anxiety and, 195
Eating, Mindful (Part I) (activity 32), 84–88
  emotion regulation and impulse control
    and, 229
  stress and anxiety and, 200
Eating, Mindful (Part II) (activity 33), 88–90
  attentional problems and, 219
  depression and, 209
  emotion regulation and impulse control
    and, 229
  stress and anxiety and, 200

Eating practices, 66, 75. *See also* Eating,
  Mindful (Part I) (activity 32); Eating,
  Mindful (Part II) (activity 33)
Embarrassment, Mindfulness of (activity
  51), 159–165
  attentional problems and, 220
  depression and, 209
  stress and anxiety and, 200
Emotion regulation, 221–226, 221–230,
  223t–225t
Emotional awareness, 123. *See also*
  Awareness
Emotional symptoms. *See also* Symptoms
  depression and, 202, 203t, 209
  emotion regulation and impulse control
    and, 224t
  overview, 216t
  stress and anxiety and, 196t, 197
Emotions. *See also* Compassion, Mindful
  (activity 54); Embarrassment,
  Mindfulness of (activity 51); Envy,
  Mindfulness of (activity 52);
  Frustration and Anger, Mindfulness
  of (Part I) (activity 49); Frustration
  and Anger, Mindfulness of (Part II)
  (activity 50); Gratitude, Mindfulness of
  (activity 53); Happiness, Mindfulness
  of (Part I) (activity 43); Happiness,
  Mindfulness of (Part II) (activity 44);
  Mindfulness of Emotions; Sadness
  and Loss, Mindfulness of (Part I)
  (activity 47); Sadness and Loss,
  Mindfulness of (Part II) (activity 48);
  SEAT (Sensations, Emotions, Actions,
  and Thoughts) acronym; Worry
  and Anxiety, Mindfulness of (Part
  I) (activity 45); Worry and Anxiety,
  Mindfulness of (Part II) (activity 46);
  individual emotions
  Body Scan (activity 21), 57–59
  breathing exercises and, 37
  choice and, 18
  emotion regulation and impulse control
    and, 227
  Mindful Body Relaxation (activity 23),
    62–64
  Mindful Hearing (activity 38), 103–106
  Mindfulness of Discomfort (activity 28),
    72–73
  Mindfulness of My Feet (activity 20),
    56–57
  Mindfulness of Smells (Part II) (activity
    40), 111–114
  overview, 27
  Pathway through Depression, 208
  responses to, 154–155
  temporary nature of, 127–128, 169
  transforming feelings, 183
  trauma, abuse, and neglect and, 236
  vocabulary for, 104
  What Does Mindfulness Mean to Me
    Now? (Part III): Journaling (activity
    56), 187–189
Empathy, 139–143, 159–165. *See also*
  Compassion
Envy, Mindfulness of (activity 52), 165–170,
  209
Ethical considerations, 235
Events, 68–71, 82, 83
Everyday awareness. *See also* Awareness;
  Everyday Life, Mindfulness in (activity
  24); Present moment awareness
  Finding Five New Things (activity 25),
    66–68
  Mindful Hearing (activity 38), 106

Mindfulness of Pleasant Events (activity
  26), 68–70, 82
Mindfulness of Unpleasant Events
  (activity 27), 70–71, 83
Everyday Life, Mindfulness in (activity 24),
  65–66
  attentional problems and, 219
  emotion regulation and impulse control
    and, 230
Executive functioning, 211, 216t, 241–243.
  See also Attentional functioning
Exercise, 154
Expectations
  choice and, 18
  cultivating your own practice in
    mindfulness and, 13
  Mindfulness of Pleasant Events (activity
    26), 69
  Mindfulness of Smells (Part II) (activity
    40), 113
  overview, 8
Exploration, 123
Exposure with response prevention,
  197–198
Expression of selves, 13, 139–140, 142–143,
  148–149

Fear, 50–51, 135–139. *See also* Anxiety;
  Worry
Feeling (touching), 98–102
Feelings. *See* Emotions
Finding Five New Things (activity 25),
  67–68, 81
  attentional problems and, 219
  depression and, 209
  emotion regulation and impulse control
    and, 230
  stress and anxiety and, 200
Flower Stretch, Mindful (activity 13), 43–44
  depression and, 209
  stress and anxiety and, 199
  trauma, abuse, and neglect and, 237
Focus
  Finding Five New Things (activity 25),
    66–68
  Pathway through Depression, 206, 208
  Pathway through Stress and Anxiety, 199
  SEAT (Sensations, Emotions, Actions,
    and Thoughts) acronym and, 18
Frustration, 149–150, 167. *See also* Anger;
  Frustration and Anger, Mindfulness
  of (Part I) (activity 49); Frustration
  and Anger, Mindfulness of (Part II)
  (activity 50)
Frustration and Anger, Mindfulness of (Part
  I) (activity 49), 148–154, 182–183
  attentional problems and, 220
  depression and, 209
  stress and anxiety and, 200
  trauma, abuse, and neglect and, 237–238
Frustration and Anger, Mindfulness of (Part
  II) (activity 50), 154–158, 184
  attentional problems and, 220
  depression and, 209
  stress and anxiety and, 200

Generalization. *See* Maintenance,
  Generalization, and Concluding
  Activities
Generalized anxiety disorder (GAD), 197.
  See also Anxiety
Gratitude, 170–173, 189–190
Gratitude, Mindfulness of (activity 53), 170–173
  attentional problems and, 220
  depression and, 209

emotion regulation and impulse control and, 230
stress and anxiety and, 200
Grounding activities, 50–51
Guided imagery exercises, 167–168, 169–170
Guilt, 172–173

HALT (Are you Hungry, Angry/Anxious, Lonely, or Tired?) acronym, 60–61
Handouts
 Finding Five New Things (activity 25), 81
 Mindful Smiling While Waking Up (activity 9), 41
 Mindfulness of Frustration and Anger (Part I) (activity 49), 182–183
 Mindfulness of Frustration and Anger (Part II) (activity 50), 184
 Mindfulness of Happiness (Part I) (activity 43), 176
 Mindfulness of Judgments (activity 42), 122
 Mindfulness of Pleasant Events (activity 26), 82
 Mindfulness of Sadness and Loss (Part I) (activity 47), 180–181
 Mindfulness of the Breath (activity 7), 40
 Mindfulness of Thoughts (activity 41), 121
 Mindfulness of Worry and Anxiety (Part I) (activity 45), 177
 Mindfulness of Worry and Anxiety (Part II) (activity 46), 178–179
Happiness, 70, 125. *See also* Happiness, Mindfulness of (Part I) (activity 43); Happiness, Mindfulness of (Part II) (activity 44)
Happiness, Mindfulness of (Part I) (activity 43), 124–126, 176
 attentional problems and, 220
 depression and, 209
Happiness, Mindfulness of (Part II) (activity 44), 127–130
 attentional problems and, 220
 depression and, 209
Hearing, Mindful (activity 38), 103–106, 230
Here-and-Now Stones (activity 58), 190–191
 attentional problems and, 220
 depression and, 210
 emotion regulation and impulse control and, 230
 stress and anxiety and, 200
 trauma, abuse, and neglect and, 238
Histrionic personality disorder, 222
Hopelessness, 206
Hormones, 43–44
Household dysfunction, 232
Humming, Mindful (activity 37), 102–103
 stress and anxiety and, 199
 trauma, abuse, and neglect and, 237
Hunger, 60–61
Hyperactivity, 212–213, 213t. *See also* Attention-deficit/hyperactivity disorder (ADHD)
Hyperarousal, 236
Hypomania, 201

Imagery. *See* Guided imagery exercises; Visualization activities
Impulse control
 attention-deficit/hyperactivity disorder (ADHD) and, 213t
 HALT (Are you Hungry, Angry/Anxious, Lonely, or Tired?) acronym and, 60–61

Mindfulness of My Feet (activity 20), 56–57
 overview, 221–226, 223t–225t
 pathway through, 221–230
Inattention. *See* Attentional functioning
Intermediate Development Activities. *See also* Mindfulness of the Body Activities; Mindfulness of the Breath Activities; Sensory-Based Mindfulness Activities
 attentional problems and, 219
 depression and, 208–209
 emotion regulation and impulse control and, 229–230
 stress and anxiety and, 200
 trauma, abuse, and neglect and, 237
Intermittent explosive disorder (IED), 221, 222
Introduction to Mindfulness (activity 1), 219
Introductory and Core Activities. *See also* *individual activities*
 attentional problems and, 219
 A Cup of Mindfulness (activity 3), 22–24
 depression and, 208
 Introduction to Mindfulness (activity 1), 17–19
 Listening to Silence (activity 4), 24–25
 overview, 17
 stress and anxiety and, 199–200
 summary of activities, 239–240
 Taking a Mindful Posture (activity 5), 26
 Taking a Mindful SEAT (activity 6), 27–28
 trauma, abuse, and neglect and, 236–237
 What Does Mindfulness Mean to Me? (Part I) (activity 2), 20–22
Intrusive thoughts, 37. *See also* Thoughts
Irritability, 221–222

Jealousy. *See* Envy, Mindfulness of (activity 52)
Judging mind, 17, 20–21, 31–32. *See also* Judgments; Thoughts
Judgments. *See also* Judgments, Mindfulness of (activity 42); Thoughts
 choice and, 18
 eating mindfully and, 88–90
 Mindful Hearing (activity 38), 103–106
 Mindful Seeing (Part II) (activity 35), 94–98
 Mindful Touching (activity 36), 98–102
 Mindfulness of Smells (Part I) (activity 39), 106–111
 Mindfulness of Smells (Part II) (activity 40), 111–114
 Mindfulness of Unpleasant Events (activity 27), 70–71
 SEAT (Sensations, Emotions, Actions, and Thoughts) acronym and, 18
 vocabulary for, 95–96, 99, 104, 112
 What Does Mindfulness Mean to Me Now? (Part III): Journaling (activity 56), 187–189
 worry and, 133–134
Judgments, Mindfulness of (activity 42), 117–120, 122
 attentional problems and, 219, 220
 depression and, 210
 stress and anxiety and, 200
 trauma, abuse, and neglect and, 237

Kindness, 19, 31–32, 66, 160. *See also* Compassion; Empathy; Self-directed kindness

Labeling of objects, 94–98
Learning disabilities (LDs), 214
Legal considerations, 235

LGBTQ children and teens, 201
Listening activities, 134–135, 160–161, 230. *See also* Hearing, Mindful (activity 38); Humming, Mindful (activity 37); Listening and Speaking, Mindful (activity 31); Listening to Silence (activity 4)
Listening and Speaking, Mindful (activity 31), 77–80, 219
Listening to Silence (activity 4), 24–25. *See also* Introductory and Core Activities
 attentional problems and, 220
 depression and, 209
 emotion regulation and impulse control and, 230
 stress and anxiety and, 200
 trauma, abuse, and neglect and, 237
Loss, 139–143, 144–148, 180–181
Lying Down, Mindfulness While (activity 18), 53–54
 attentional problems and, 220
 emotion regulation and impulse control and, 229–230
 stress and anxiety and, 200

Maintenance, Generalization, and Concluding Activities
 Appreciation of the Group (activity 57), 189–190
 attentional problems and, 220
 depression and, 209–210
 emotion regulation and impulse control and, 230
 Here-and-Now Stones (activity 58), 190–191
 overview, 185
 stress and anxiety and, 200
 trauma, abuse, and neglect and, 238
 What Does Mindfulness Mean to Me Now? (Part II): Drawing (activity 55), 185–187
 What Does Mindfulness Mean to Me Now? (Part III): Journaling (activity 56), 187–189
Mania, 201
Marijuana use. *See* Substance use
Matching Movement Moments (activity 17), 51–53
 attentional problems and, 219
 emotion regulation and impulse control and, 230
 trauma, abuse, and neglect and, 237
Medication, 206
Meditations, 54–56
Memories, 111–114
Metacognition, 198, 243–244
Mindful Awareness Activities. *See also* Advanced Deepening Activities
 Finding Five New Things (activity 25), 67–68, 81
 Mindful Listening and Speaking (activity 31), 77–80
 The Mindful STOP (activity 30), 76–77
 Mindfulness in Everyday Life (activity 24), 65–66
 Mindfulness of Discomfort (activity 28), 72–73
 Mindfulness of Pleasant Events (activity 26), 68–70, 82
 Mindfulness of Unpleasant Events (activity 27), 70–71, 83
 Mindfulness of Urges: Urge Surfing (activity 29), 73–76
 overview, 65
Mindful breathing activities. *See* Breath-based activities

The Mindful HALT (activity 22), 60–61
  depression and, 209
  emotion regulation and impulse control
    and, 229
  stress and anxiety and, 200
Mindful movement activities. See
    Movement activities
The Mindful STOP (activity 30), 76–77, 237
Mindfulness. See also individual activities
  cultivating your own practice in, 13
  introducing to children and teens, 18–19
  overview, 2, 3–6, 4t, 17, 20–21, 30
Mindfulness of Emotions. See also
    Advanced Deepening Activities;
    Emotions
  Mindful Compassion (activity 54),
    173–175
  Mindfulness of Embarrassment (activity
    51), 159–165
  Mindfulness of Envy (activity 52),
    165–170
  Mindfulness of Frustration and Anger
    (Part I) (activity 49), 148–154, 182–183
  Mindfulness of Frustration and Anger
    (Part II) (activity 50), 154–158, 184
  Mindfulness of Gratitude (activity 53),
    170–173
  Mindfulness of Happiness (Part I)
    (activity 43), 124–126, 176
  Mindfulness of Happiness (Part II)
    (activity 44), 127–130
  Mindfulness of Sadness and Loss (Part I)
    (activity 47), 139–143, 180–181
  Mindfulness of Sadness and Loss (Part
    II) (activity 48), 144–148
  Mindfulness of Worry and Anxiety (Part
    I) (activity 45), 130–135, 177
  Mindfulness of Worry and Anxiety (Part
    II) (activity 46), 135–139, 178–179
  overview, 123
Mindfulness of My Feet (activity 20), 56–57
  attentional problems and, 219
  emotion regulation and impulse control
    and, 229
  stress and anxiety and, 200
  trauma, abuse, and neglect and, 237
Mindfulness of the Body Activities. See also
    Intermediate Development Activities;
    Movement activities
  Body Scan (activity 21), 57–59
  Matching Movement Moments (activity
    17), 51–53
  Mindful Body Relaxation (activity 23),
    62–64
  Mindful Flower Stretch (activity 13),
    43–44
  The Mindful HALT (activity 22), 60–61
  Mindful Mountain Visualization (activity
    19), 54–56
  Mindful Movements (activity 16), 49–51
  Mindful Silliness (activity 12), 42–43
  Mindful Walking (activity 15), 45–48
  Mindfulness of My Feet (activity 20),
    56–57
  Mindfulness While Lying Down (activity
    18), 53–54
  overview, 42
  Three Minutes in My Body (activity
    14), 44
Mindfulness of the Breath Activities.
    See also Breath-based activities;
    Intermediate Development Activities
  Belly Breathing (activity 10), 35–36
  emotion regulation and impulse control
    and, 229

Mindful Breath Counting (activity 11),
    37–39
Mindful Smiling While Waking Up
    (activity 9), 34–35, 41
Mindfulness of the Breath (activity 7),
    29–32, 40
  overview, 29
  stress and anxiety and, 199
Taking Three Mindful Breaths (activity
    8), 32–33
Mindfulness of Thoughts. See also
    Advanced Deepening Activities;
    Thoughts
  Mindfulness of Judgments (activity 42),
    117–120, 122
  Mindfulness of Thoughts (activity 41),
    115–117, 121
  overview, 115
  trauma, abuse, and neglect and, 237
Mind's eye, 92–93
Mood disorders, 201. See also Depression
Mood regulation, 43–44
Motivation
  attentional problems and, 218
  buy-in from kids and teens and, 10–12
  depression and, 202, 205, 206
  introductory practices and, 17
Mountain Visualization, Mindful (activity
    19), 54–56
  attentional problems and, 220
  depression and, 209
  emotion regulation and impulse control
    and, 229
  stress and anxiety and, 199–200
  trauma, abuse, and neglect and, 237
Movement activities. See also Mindfulness
    of the Body Activities
  to counteract sleepiness, 26
  emotion regulation and impulse control
    and, 229
  Mindful Movements (activity 16), 49–51
  Mindful Silliness (activity 12), 42–43
  overview, 42
  Pathway through Depression, 208–209
  Pathway through Stress and Anxiety,
    199–200
  trauma, abuse, and neglect and, 236–237
Movements, Mindful (activity 16), 49–51
  attentional problems and, 219
  depression and, 209
  emotion regulation and impulse control
    and, 229
  stress and anxiety and, 199
  trauma, abuse, and neglect and, 237
Music, 103–106, 134–135, 154

Narcissistic personality disorder, 222, 226
Needs, 60–61
Negative space drawings, 94, 94f. See also
    Drawing-based activities
Negative thoughts. See also Thoughts
  being kind to yourself and, 31–32
  depression and, 207–208
  Mindfulness of Pleasant Events (activity
    26), 69
  Mindfulness of Unpleasant Events
    (activity 27), 70–71
  Pathway through Depression, 205–206,
    207
Neglect
  attentional problems and, 215
  emotion regulation and impulse control
    and, 222
  overview, 232
  pathway through, 231–238

stress disorders and, 232–233
symptoms and, 232–238, 234t
Neurotransmitters, 43–44

Observing skills
  eating mindfully and, 84–88
  Mindful Eating (Part II) (activity 33),
    88–90
  Mindful Hearing (activity 38), 103–106
  Mindful Touching (activity 36), 98–102
  Mindfulness of Smells (Part I) (activity
    39), 106–111
  overview, 3, 20–21
  seeing mindfully and, 91–98, 94f
  vocabulary for, 91–92, 99, 104, 108
Obsessive–compulsive disorder (OCD),
    197, 214
Open-ended questions, 9–10
Openness, 18, 104
Oppositional defiant disorder (ODD), 221,
    222
Optimism, 207
Organizational factors, 12–13, 217
Overreactivity, 56–59

Pain, 197, 208
Panic, 199
Passive resistance, 12. See also Resistance
Pathway through Attention Problems,
    201–210, 218–220, 239–240. See also
    Attentional functioning
Pathway through Depression, 201–210,
    239–240. See also Depression
Pathway through Problems of Emotion
    Regulation and Impulse Control,
    221–230
Pathway through Stress and Anxiety, 195–
    200, 239–240. See also Anxiety; Stress
Pathway through Trauma, Abuse, and
    Neglect, 231–238, 239–240
Pathways to mindfulness
  attention problems, 211–220
  depression, 201–210
  emotion regulation and impulse control,
    221–230
  overview, 4–6, 193–194
  stress and anxiety, 195–200
  summary of activities, 239–240
  trauma, abuse, and neglect, 231–238
Peer relationships
  Concluding Activities and, 185
  gratitude and, 172–173
  sadness and, 139–140, 142–143
Persistent complex bereavement disorder
    (PCBD), 233
Persistent depressive disorder (PDD), 201.
    See also Depression
Personality disorders, 222, 228
Phobias, 197
Physical activities
  A Cup of Mindfulness (activity 3), 22–24
  Taking a Mindful Posture (activity 5), 26
  Taking a Mindful SEAT (activity 6),
    27–28
Physical sensations. See Body sensations;
    Sensations
Physiological symptoms. See also Symptoms
  depression and, 202, 204t
  overview, 217t
  stress and anxiety and, 196t, 197, 199
  trauma, abuse, and neglect and, 234t, 236
Playfulness, 42–43, 51–53, 199
Pleasant events
  depression and, 208
  eating mindfully and, 88

Mindfulness of Pleasant Events (activity 26), 68–70, 82
temporary nature of emotions and, 127–128
Pleasant Events, Mindfulness of (activity 26), 68–70, 82
depression and, 209
trauma, abuse, and neglect and, 238
Poetry, 93–94
Posttraumatic stress disorder (PTSD), 198, 222, 232–238, 234t
Posture, 26, 27–28
Present moment awareness. *See also* Awareness; Everyday awareness
Finding Five New Things (activity 25), 66–68
Mindfulness in Everyday Life (activity 24), 65–66
Mindfulness of Worry and Anxiety (Part II) (activity 46), 135–139
overview, 19
Program overview, 1–6, 4t, 6–13
Progressive muscle relaxation, 209–210. *See also* Body Relaxation, Mindful (activity 23)
Psychological symptoms, 197

Radical acceptance, 118–119. *See also* Acceptance
Reactive attachment disorder (RAD), 233
Reactivity
Body Scan (activity 21), 57–59
emotions and, 123
Mindfulness of Frustration and Anger (Part I) (activity 49), 148–154
Mindfulness of My Feet (activity 20), 56–57
reactions and, 154–158
trauma, abuse, and neglect and, 236
worry and, 133–134
Reassurance, 163–164, 195
Reexperiencing symptoms, 234t
Refocusing of attention, 18, 66–68. *See also* Focus; Wandering mind
Relationships, 172–173
Relaxation
attentional problems and, 220
Body Scan (activity 21), 57–59
emotion regulation and impulse control and, 229
Mindful Body Relaxation (activity 23), 62–64
stress and anxiety and, 197–198
Research support for mindfulness
buy-in from administrators and organizations and, 12
buy-in from kids and teens and, 11
emotion regulation and impulse control and, 227
executive function and attention and, 241–243
funding for, 241, 242f
metacognitive awareness and, 243–244
mindfulness in schools, 245–246
overview, 5, 241, 246–247
social–emotional development and, 244–245
teachers and, 246
Resiliency, 246
Resistance, 11–12, 227
Responses, 154–158, 155
Risk factors, 207
Risk management, 8–9, 207
Risky behaviors, 202
Role models, 11, 148–149
Rumination, 56–57. *See also* Thoughts

Sadness. *See also* Depression; Sadness and Loss, Mindfulness of (Part I) (activity 47); Sadness and Loss, Mindfulness of (Part II) (activity 48)
choice and, 146–148
envy and, 167
overview, 145–146
vocabulary for, 140, 141–142
Sadness and Loss, Mindfulness of (Part I) (activity 47), 139–143, 180–181
depression and, 209
trauma, abuse, and neglect and, 237–238
Sadness and Loss, Mindfulness of (Part II) (activity 48), 144–148
depression and, 209
trauma, abuse, and neglect and, 237–238
Safety, 8–9, 226, 231
Schools, 245–246
SEAT (Sensations, Emotions, Actions, and Thoughts) acronym
Mindfulness of Frustration and Anger (Part I) (activity 49), 151–152
Mindfulness of Judgments (activity 42), 119–120
overview, 17–18
postactivity discussions and, 10
Taking a Mindful SEAT (activity 6), 27–28
Seeing, Mindful (Part I) (activity 34), 91–94, 94f
attentional problems and, 219
depression and, 209
stress and anxiety and, 200
Seeing, Mindful (Part II) (activity 35), 94–98, 200
Seeing mindfully. *See* Seeing, Mindful (Part I) (activity 34); Seeing, Mindful (Part II) (activity 35); Sensory-Based Mindfulness Activities
Self-awareness, 94–98
Self-compassion, 173–175, 206, 237–238. *See also* Compassion
Self-confidence, 43–44
Self-consciousness, 199, 208
Self-directed kindness, 19, 31–32. *See also* Kindness
Self-efficacy, 43–44
Self-esteem, 172
Self-harm, 195, 202, 235
Sensations. *See also* Mindfulness of the Body Activities; Sensory-Based Mindfulness Activities
belly breathing and, 35–36
Body Scan (activity 21), 57–59
emotions and, 123
Mindful Touching (activity 36), 98–102
Mindfulness of Discomfort (activity 28), 72–73
Mindfulness of Smells (Part II) (activity 40), 111–114
Mindfulness of the Breath (activity 7), 30–31
Mindfulness of Worry and Anxiety (Part II) (activity 46), 135–139
overview, 27
Pathway through Depression, 207, 208
What Does Mindfulness Mean to Me Now? (Part III): Journaling (activity 56), 187–189
Sensory-Based Mindfulness Activities. *See also* Advanced Deepening Activities; Intermediate Development Activities
Mindful Eating (Part I) (activity 32), 84–88
Mindful Eating (Part II) (activity 33), 88–90

Mindful Hearing (activity 38), 103–106
Mindful Humming (activity 37), 102–103
Mindful Seeing (Part I) (activity 34), 91–94, 94f
Mindful Seeing (Part II) (activity 35), 94–98
Mindful Touching (activity 36), 98–102
Mindfulness of Smells (Part I) (activity 39), 106–111
Mindfulness of Smells (Part II) (activity 40), 111–114
overview, 84
Settling skills, 3
Shame, 159–165
"Shoulds," 165–166
Shyness, 79, 199, 208
SIFT (Sensations, Images, Feelings, and Thoughts) acronym, 10, 119–120
Silliness, Mindful (activity 12), 42–43
emotion regulation and impulse control and, 230
stress and anxiety and, 199
trauma, abuse, and neglect and, 236–237
Sleep problems, 197, 199, 207–208
Sleepiness during a practice, 26, 60–61
Smelling mindfully. *See* Sensory-Based Mindfulness Activities; Smells, Mindfulness of (Part I) (activity 39); Smells, Mindfulness of (Part II) (activity 40)
Smells, Mindfulness of (Part I) (activity 39), 106–111
depression and, 209
emotion regulation and impulse control and, 230
stress and anxiety and, 200
Smells, Mindfulness of (Part II) (activity 40), 111–114
depression and, 209
emotion regulation and impulse control and, 230
stress and anxiety and, 200
Smiling practice, 34–35
Smiling While Waking Up, Mindful (activity 9), 34–35, 41, 199–200
Social anxiety, 79
Social norms, 139–140, 142–143
Social–behavioral symptoms. *See also* Behavioral problems; Symptoms
depression and, 202
emotion regulation and impulse control and, 225t
overview, 217t
stress and anxiety and, 195, 197–198
Social–emotional development, 244–245, 246
Somatic symptoms, 208. *See also* Symptoms
Sounds, 102–103, 134–135. *See also* Listening activities
Stillness activities, 53–54, 199–200. *See also* Breath-based activities
STOP (Stop, Take a breath, Observe, and Plan and Proceed) acronym, 76–77
Stress. *See also* Anxiety; Trauma
activities for, 199–200
attentional problems and, 214
at different ages, 197–198
management of, 246
Mindful Body Relaxation (activity 23), 62–64
pathway through, 195–200
stress disorders and, 232–233
symptoms of, 196t
thoughts and rumination and, 56

Substance use
   attentional problems and, 215
   depression and, 202
   emotion regulation and impulse control
      and, 222, 226
   stress and anxiety and, 195
Substance use disorders (SUDs), 222, 226
Suicide risk management, 207. *See also*
      Depression
Symptoms
   of attentional functioning problems,
      212–218, 216*t*–217*t*
   of depression, 201–202, 203*t*–205*t*
   emotion regulation and impulse control
      and, 221–226, 223*t*–225*t*
   of stress and anxiety, 195–198, 196*t*
   suicide risk management and, 207
   trauma, abuse, and neglect and, 232–236,
      234*t*

Tactile sensations, 98–102. *See also*
      Sensations
Taking a Mindful Posture (activity 5),
      26. *See also* Introductory and Core
      Activities
   emotion regulation and impulse control
      and, 229
   stress and anxiety and, 199
   trauma, abuse, and neglect and, 237
Taking a Mindful SEAT (activity 6), 27–28.
      See also Introductory and Core
      Activities
   attentional problems and, 219, 220
   emotion regulation and impulse control
      and, 229
   stress and anxiety and, 199
   trauma, abuse, and neglect and, 237
Taking Three Mindful Breaths (activity 8),
      32–33
   attentional problems and, 219, 220
   emotion regulation and impulse control
      and, 229
   stress and anxiety and, 199
Task-based activities, 22–24
Teachers, 246
Teaching tips
   attentional problems and, 217–218
   depression and, 205–206
   emotion regulation and impulse control
      and, 226–227
   stress and anxiety and, 198
   trauma, abuse, and neglect and, 235
Tension, 62–64
Thinking errors, 198. *See also* Thoughts
Thoughts. *See also* Judgments; Judgments,
      Mindfulness of (activity 42);
      Mindfulness of Thoughts; SEAT
      (Sensations, Emotions, Actions, and
      Thoughts) acronym
   being kind to yourself and, 31–32
   choice and, 18
   counting with the breath and, 37
   depression and, 207–208
   embarrassment and, 159–165
   emotions and, 123
   Mindful Listening and Speaking (activity
      31), 77–80
   The Mindful STOP (activity 30), 76–77
   Mindfulness of Discomfort (activity 28),
      72–73
   Mindfulness of My Feet (activity 20), 56–57
   Mindfulness of Pleasant Events (activity
      26), 69

Mindfulness of Sadness and Loss (Part I)
      (activity 47), 139–143
Mindfulness of Smells (Part I) (activity
      39), 106–111
Mindfulness of Smells (Part II) (activity
      40), 111–114
Mindfulness of Thoughts (activity 41),
      115–117, 121
Mindfulness of Unpleasant Events
      (activity 27), 70–71
Mindfulness of Worry and Anxiety (Part
      I) (activity 45), 130–135
   overview, 28
Pathway through Depression, 205–206, 208
SEAT (Sensations, Emotions, Actions,
      and Thoughts) acronym and, 18
self-criticism and, 21
stress and anxiety and, 198
trauma, abuse, and neglect and, 231
What Does Mindfulness Mean to Me
      Now? (Part III): Journaling (activity
      56), 187–189
Thoughts, Mindfulness of (activity 41),
      115–117, 121, 219
Three mindful breaths exercise, 32–33
Three Minutes in My Body (activity 14), 44
   attentional problems and, 219
   trauma, abuse, and neglect and, 237
Tiredness during a practice, 26, 60–61
Tobacco use. *See* Substance use
Touching, Mindful (activity 36), 98–102
   attentional problems and, 219
   emotion regulation and impulse control
      and, 230
   trauma, abuse, and neglect and, 237
Transition times, 77
Trauma
   attentional problems and, 215
   depression and, 206
   dissociation and, 215
   emotion regulation and impulse control
      and, 222, 227–228
   Mindfulness of the Body Activities and,
      42
   movement activities and, 50–51
   overview, 232
   pathway through, 231–238
   stress and anxiety and, 198
   stress disorders and, 232–233
   symptoms and, 232–238, 234*t*
Tree pose, 50
Triggering moments, 77, 154–155, 158, 184
Trust, 11–12

Unhappiness, 17. *See also* Happiness
Unpleasant events, 70–71, 83, 88, 127–128
Unpleasant Events, Mindfulness of (activity
      27), 70–71, 83, 209
Unworthiness, 172–173
Urges, Mindfulness of: Urge Surfing
      (activity 29), 73–76
   attentional problems and, 220
   emotion regulation and impulse control
      and, 230
   trauma, abuse, and neglect and, 237

Visualization activities
   Mindful Compassion (activity 54),
      174–175
   Mindful Mountain Visualization (activity
      19), 54–56
   Mindful Seeing (Part I) (activity 34),
      91–94, 94*f*

Mindfulness of Embarrassment (activity
      51), 161, 164–165
Mindfulness of Envy (activity 52),
      167–168
Mindfulness of Frustration and Anger
      (Part II) (activity 50), 154–158
Mindfulness of Judgments (activity 42),
      117–120
Mindfulness of Thoughts (activity 41),
      116–117
Mindfulness of Urges: Urge Surfing
      (activity 29), 74–75
Mindfulness of Worry and Anxiety (Part
      I) (activity 45), 132–134

Walking, Mindful (activity 15), 45–48
   depression and, 209
   emotion regulation and impulse control
      and, 229
   stress and anxiety and, 199
   trauma, abuse, and neglect and, 237
Walking exercises, 45–48, 66, 236. *See also*
      Walking, Mindful (activity 15)
Wandering mind, 17, 18, 31. *See also*
      Refocusing of attention
What Does Mindfulness Mean to Me
      Now? (Part II): Drawing (activity 55),
      185–187
   attentional problems and, 220
   depression and, 210
   emotion regulation and impulse control
      and, 230
   stress and anxiety and, 200
What Does Mindfulness Mean to Me Now?
      (Part III): Journaling (activity 56),
      187–189
   attentional problems and, 220
   depression and, 210
   emotion regulation and impulse control
      and, 230
   stress and anxiety and, 200
   trauma, abuse, and neglect and, 238
What Does Mindfulness Mean to Me?
      (Part I) (activity 2), 20–22. *See also*
      Introductory and Core Activities
   attentional problems and, 219
   emotion regulation and impulse control
      and, 229
   stress and anxiety and, 199
Worry, 131, 136. *See also* Anxiety; Worry
      and Anxiety, Mindfulness of (Part
      I) (activity 45); Worry and Anxiety,
      Mindfulness of (Part II) (activity 46)
Worry and Anxiety, Mindfulness of (Part I)
      (activity 45), 130–135, 177
   depression and, 209
   stress and anxiety and, 200
   trauma, abuse, and neglect and, 237–238
Worry and Anxiety, Mindfulness of (Part II)
      (activity 46), 135–139, 178–179
   depression and, 209
   stress and anxiety and, 200
   trauma, abuse, and neglect and,
      237–238

Yoga. *See also* Movements, Mindful
      (activity 16)
   attentional problems and, 219
   depression and, 209
   emotion regulation and impulse control
      and, 229
   stress and anxiety and, 199–200
   trauma, abuse, and neglect and, 236